I0131606

ALL·IN·ONE

HCISPP®
HealthCare Information Security and Privacy Practitioner

EXAM GUIDE

Sean P. Murphy

**Mc
Graw
Hill**

New York   Chicago   San Francisco
Athens   London   Madrid   Mexico City
Milan   New Delhi   Singapore   Sydney   Toronto

McGraw Hill is an independent entity from (ISC)²ᵐ and is not affiliated with (ISC)² in any manner. This study/training guide and/or material is not sponsored by, endorsed by, or affiliated with (ISC)² in any manner. This publication and accompanying media may be used in assisting students to prepare for the HCISPP exam. Neither (ISC)² nor McGraw Hill warrants that use of this publication and accompanying media will ensure passing any exam.

McGraw Hill books are available at special quantity discounts to use as premiums and sales promotions, or for use in corporate training programs. To contact a representative, please visit the Contact Us pages at www.mhprofessional.com.

HCISPP® HealthCare Information Security and Privacy Practitioner All-in-One Exam Guide

Copyright © 2021 by McGraw Hill. All rights reserved. Except as permitted under the Copyright Act of 1976, no part of this publication may be reproduced or distributed in any form or by any means, or stored in a database or retrieval system, without the prior written permission of publisher, with the exception that the program listings may be entered, stored, and executed in a computer system, but they may not be reproduced for publication.

All trademarks or copyrights mentioned herein are the possession of their respective owners and McGraw Hill makes no claim of ownership by the mention of products that contain these marks.

(ISC)²®, HCISPP®, CISSP®, CCSP®, CAP®, ISSAP®, ISSEP®, ISSMP®, SSCP® and CBK® are trademarks or registered trademarks of (ISC)² in the United States and certain other countries. All other trademarks are trademarks of their respective owners.

1 2 3 4 5 6 7 8 9   LCR   24 23 22 21 20

Library of Congress Control Number: 2020941364

ISBN   978-1-260-46006-3
MHID   1-260-46006-1

Sponsoring Editor	**Technical Editor**	**Production Supervisor**
Wendy Rinaldi	Lori Reed-Fourquet	Thomas Somers
Editorial Supervisor	**Copy Editor**	**Composition**
Janet Walden	Lisa Theobald	Cenveo Publisher Services
Project Manager	**Proofreader**	**Illustration**
Revathi Viswanathan,	Richard Camp	Cenveo Publisher Services
Cenveo® Publisher Services	**Indexer**	**Art Director, Cover**
Acquisitions Coordinator	Claire Splan	Jeff Weeks
Emily Walters		

Information has been obtained by McGraw Hill from sources believed to be reliable. However, because of the possibility of human or mechanical error by our sources, McGraw Hill, or others, McGraw Hill does not guarantee the accuracy, adequacy, or completeness of any information and is not responsible for any errors or omissions or the results obtained from the use of such information.

*To my wife, Melissa, my son, Sean II, and daughter, Emily…
this is for you. Over all the years, the laughs, the travels, the
accomplishments, and the sacrifices…this book is not possible
without your love and support. Lord willing and the creek don't rise,
there is much more to come. Just know I do it all for you, because of
you. I love you Dunkenfluegels.*

ABOUT THE AUTHOR

Sean P. Murphy, FACHE, CPHIMS, CISSP-ISSMP, CIPP/IT, HCISPP, is currently a senior vice president at Boeing Employees Credit Union (BECU) and serves as the organization's chief information security officer. Prior to joining BECU, Sean held several senior-level health information privacy and security officer positions in various organizations. He is a healthcare information security expert with nearly 25 years of experience in the field, serving at all levels of healthcare, from community hospital, to international integrated delivery system levels securing government and commercial delivery systems. Sean retired from the US Air Force Medical Service Corps after reaching the rank of Lieutenant Colonel. He has served as CIO and CISO in the military, in civilian healthcare organizations, and now in the financial sector, but his proudest professional accomplishment was his service as a senior mentor to the Afghan National Police Surgeon General's Office in 2008–2009 in support of Operation Enduring Freedom. He has a master's degree in business administration (advanced IT concentration) from the University of South Florida, a master's degree in health services administration from Central Michigan University, and a bachelor's degree in human resource management from the University of Maryland. Sean is an active member of (ISC)² and has thrice earned (ISC)² certification. He was part of the consortium of security industry, healthcare, academic, and government experts that came together to develop the first exam and establish the HCISPP credential. Since then, he has authored and contributed to several information security and healthcare information protection books, including *Healthcare Information Security and Privacy* (McGraw Hill Professional, 2015) and *Official (ISC²) Guide to the CISSP CBK* (2015). He is a past chairman of the HIMSS Privacy and Security Committee and is a fellow and a leader on the US Department of Health and Human Services Healthcare and Public Health Sector Coordinating Council (HPH SCC) Joint Cyber Security Working Group (JCWG).

About the Technical Editor

Lori Reed-Fourquet is a principal at e-Healthsign, LLC, consulting in health informatics. She is the convener for ISO/TC 215/WG 4 on health informatics privacy, security, and safety. She also serves as planning co-chair for IHE Quality, Research, and Public Health committee and is an active member of the IHE Patient Care Coordination committee and the HL7 Patient Administration, HL7 Structured Documents, and HL7 Public Health Work Groups. Lori has been working in medical and health informatics for more than 20 years, serving in numerous leadership capacities and creating successful collaborations, pilots, and deployments involving diverse healthcare communities in competing markets. She was part of the contracting team to the Office of the National Coordinator for Health Information Technology (ONC) security and privacy and standards harmonization initiatives as part of the United States' efforts to advance nationwide interoperable health information technology. She serves as a technical assessor for ANSI-ASQ National Accreditation Board (ANAB), an ONC-approved accreditor for the Permanent Certification Program for Health Information Technology. She has developed health information exchange (HIE) security and privacy policies for multiple HIE initiatives, including those in the United States and Saudi Arabia. She holds a master's degree in computer science from Rensselaer Polytechnic Institute.

CONTENTS AT A GLANCE

CONTENTS

ACKNOWLEDGMENTS

There is an old expression that says when you find a turtle sitting atop a fence post, you can be sure of one thing: the turtle did not get there by himself. That expression has described the positive things that have happened in my life. This book is no different. Although there is one name on the cover, many others have provided direct and indirect material that you will find within. While I cannot mention everyone, there are a few I really have to acknowledge specifically.

Over the past 20 years, numerous people have worked in the medical device security arena, specifically, and healthcare information privacy and security, generally. Most were voices in the wilderness. I know because I commiserated over too many adult beverages with leaders who were the first to identify and describe the requirements to secure medical devices and protect patients. Medical device manufactures were not quick to engineer security controls into their devices. In fairness, purchasers were not asking for security controls, and changes to medical devices after final designs and approvals from the US Food and Drug Administration (FDA) are obtained are infeasible. That was 20 years ago, but we are still having many of the same conversations. The good news is that many more people are having these conversations, the FDA has taken a prominent position on the issues, the US government has identified healthcare information networks as part of the nation's critical infrastructure, and patient safety is connected to medical device security. More purchasers want to ensure that the devices meet security standards.

Having said all that, this book is not possible without the mentorship and example set by Mike Nielsen, a fellow Air Force Medical Service Corps (MSC) retiree. Mike's awareness and passion for medical device security goes back before "it was a thing." Mike was at the forefront of the Department of Defense joint-medical services (Army, Navy, and Air Force) working with the FDA and medical device manufacturers, particularly in the picture archiving and communication system (PACS) and teleradiology world before just about anyone. Anyone. He was advocating for integrating the old Rainbow Series standards into medical devices to test and evaluate them under the FDA's *Purple Book: Lists of Licensed Biological Products*, and then the US Department of Defense (DoD) Information Technology Security Certification and Accreditation Process (DITSCAP) for certification and accreditation. (It makes me feel old to find reference material for the Rainbow Series archived at a web site called "The Wayback Machine." But that is evidence of just how long we have been on notice about security vulnerabilities with Internet-connected medical devices.) Mike's voice can be heard throughout this book, especially in the areas of medical device security and clinical engineering as security professionals.

I can't continue without mentioning my utmost appreciation for, and undying gratitude to, Wendy Rinaldi—my editing consultant, acquisitions editor, and taskmaster throughout the entire process. Acknowledgment is a tiny portion of the debt I owe her for her patience and tenacity. This book would never have happened if she did not continue to give me chance after chance to get the work done. I also need to thank Lisa Theobald, Emily Walters, Lori Reed-Fourquet, and Janet Walden, who did a tremendous job juggling the various revisions and edits to keep the project moving along. There were a lot of moving parts in this effort, and this team was magnificent in keeping all the plates spinning. I also benefitted from their, in many cases extensive, professional editing suggestions and phraseology. If readers find this book easy to consume, it is only because of Lisa, Emily, Lori, and Janet.

I will always provide the following acknowledgment: Everyone who works in healthcare information security owes a debt of gratitude to Mr. Lynn McNulty, especially if you have or aspire to earn HCISPP. I must acknowledge Lynn's vision and support, although now posthumously. I will always remember meeting Lynn in a pub and mapping out the need for healthcare-specific information protection measures of workforce competency. Yes, this was on the back of a napkin—and not figuratively, but literally. He believed in the concept that protecting healthcare information required different competencies than other industries. He was the genesis of the HCISPP at (ISC)² along with Hord Tipton. From their leadership, my work emerges. Lynn believed in the ramblings and passion of this healthcare information security professional when very few others thought there was a need for a differentiation between information security domains. He built the bridge between (ISC)² and the concept of credentialing healthcare information security practitioners outside of the normal information security credentialing process, with the goal of beginning to measure workforce competency in healthcare information security and privacy. Without Lynn, this day would never have come. Without him, however, I will continue on in his spirit of building relationships, growing professionalism, and securing sensitive information in healthcare. We all miss you, Lynn.

INTRODUCTION

If you are reading this introduction, you are probably one of two types of people. The first type is someone who has worked in healthcare for a few years and whose responsibilities are becoming more dependent on information technology—and therefore information security. Perhaps you work in healthcare records management, and your organization is on its first or second evolution of the electronic healthcare record. You have been chosen to provide your records management expertise to the new digital system. Congratulations! You are clearly valued in your organization. And this book will serve you, because it will address, in a practical manner, your concerns about moving from paper-based records to digital, networked systems.

The second type of person is someone who has worked in information technology in healthcare or an industry other than healthcare. Perhaps you are a network operator who previously worked for a local bank or supermarket. Now you have the opportunity to be the firewall administrator for the community hospital. Congratulations to you as well! You are now an important person in the delivery of healthcare. You may not consider yourself a healthcare provider, but you are, and you most certainly directly support those personnel who provide patient care. Within this book, you will learn of the importance to patient care and healthcare business of providing information security and privacy in a healthcare organization. When it comes to healthcare provision, the actions or inactions of information technology practitioners can impact patient safety or clinical quality.

For those of you who do not fit into the two categories I mentioned, do not worry. This material is very much applicable to your pursuit to elevate your competency and your dedication to the profession. Having performed healthcare information security and privacy work for about two decades, I offer this book as a collection of lessons learned as much as anything else. Here, you will find real scenarios, actual issues, and practical solutions. I name no names to protect the innocent. In sum, I grew up in healthcare information security and still maintain a "healthcare first" attitude. When perfectly acceptable information security practices are applied to healthcare without considering the impact on patient care or provider practices, healthcare delivery and the patient often suffer. My goal is to provide constructive, practical guidance for professionals like you to balance the need to protect patient information and deliver quality patient care safely. Of course, an outcome of your study of this material is to obtain certification. This designation demonstrates that you understand that competent healthcare information security and privacy professionals can, in fact, enable better healthcare, improve outcomes, and advance organizational initiatives.

The contents of this book cover the entire exam outline according to the International Information System Security Certification Consortium, or (ISC)^2. Each chapter is aligned with one of the seven domains tested by the HCISPP exam, as listed here, along with the percentage of questions you will see on the exam:

Domain	Exam Questions
1. Healthcare Industry	12%
2. Information Governance in Healthcare	5%
3. Information Technologies in Healthcare	8%
4. Regulatory and Standards Environment	15%
5. Privacy and Security in Healthcare	25%
6. Risk Management and Risk Assessment	20%
7. Third-Party Risk Management	15%

Beyond the relative importance (ISC)[2] assigns to each domain based on the exam construction, you will find practical information in this book. As you work on a daily basis, and depending on your position in your organization, you may find the information presented in some chapters more valuable than information in other chapters. For this reason, I wrote these chapters with a philosophy that each chapter is 100 percent important to an HCISPP in the workplace, even if the exam applies unequal weighting. You can thank me later if the extra material also helps you in your day-to-day practices.

I hope you will enjoy reading this material as much as I have enjoyed constructing it. I welcome your feedback on any and all of the information in this book. In many ways, what you will read is the result of many discussions and commiseration sessions I have had over the years with like-minded colleagues and friends. Those conversations continue, I am glad to say. Add your voice. After you dig into the contents, let me know what you think about this book. The easiest way to reach me is on LinkedIn at https://www.linkedin.com/in/seanmurphy092009.

Why Become an HCISPP

I am passionate about the need for and value of the discussions in this book for two reasons. Some people enter healthcare from other industries, and they must understand the business of healthcare before they are able to provide healthcare information security. Others come from health information management and privacy roles as their responsibilities for protecting information include more use of digital assets and information technologies that require security controls for electronic information.

Certification demonstrates competency. But more importantly, certification through (ISC)[2] demonstrates a commitment to the profession: to sit for the exam, you must meet standards, and to maintain the credential, you must continue to meet standards through continued professional education. HCISPP as a stand-alone certification demonstrates a practitioner's experience and dedication to healthcare information security and privacy. The quality of the HCISPP is backed by (ISC)[2] as the credential-granting organization. The organization maintains accreditation for the quality of HCISPP through the rigid ANSI/ISO/IEC 17024 standard, *Personnel Certification – Documents and Resources*.

I was proud and fortunate to participate in the first iteration of the HCISPP credentialing process. The group that came together to discuss the ideal HCISPP candidate, job task analysis, exam questions, and even the name of the credential were leaders and practitioners with a common goal. The group comprised authorities from the United States and international government and private sectors, along with academic subject matter experts. Our focus was on a credential that specifically differentiates the healthcare information security and privacy professional within the security and privacy vocations. We wanted to provide recognition for professionals who demonstrated high levels of competency within the (ISC)² domains. After more than a year, the group hammered out the first version of HCISPP to a terrific acceptance by the healthcare industry.

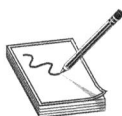

NOTE You may wonder why the credential is titled "HealthCare Information Security and Privacy Practitioner," or HCISPP. It was difficult to find a credential title that did not result in an acronym that was already taken. We also had to avoid acronyms that could possibly endure ridicule, such as Certified Healthcare Information Privacy and Security, whose acronym would be CHIPS. Although abbreviating HealthCare as HC might seem like extra, some who noticed that without the C in HCISPP, we would result in an acronym that might be maligned by a less mature audience. In the end, we chose HCISPP and it has endured—but the process was a lot like naming a child.

Before you sign up to take an exam, make sure you understand and meet the prerequisites. As I said earlier, HCISPP is a stand-alone credential. It is also meant to be a practitioner-level recognition. That does not mean it is easy or a low bar. Before you take the HCISPP exam, (ISC)² requires at least two years of experience, and one of those years must be in healthcare. Every candidate must have worked as an employee, and not as a volunteer, in information security or privacy roles. There is no expectation that a candidate has experience or expertise in all of the domains in the HCISPP Common Body of Knowledge (CBK). However, the prerequisites include that the experience must come from at least one of the domains related to privacy, security, and compliance. There are some caveats, too, as legal experience can satisfy requirements concerning compliance. If you have worked in information management functions, that experience can be substituted for the privacy competencies.

How to Use This Book

When I wrote my first book in 2015, it was among just a handful of books about healthcare information security and privacy available at the time. I had hoped that this would change over time and more books would be available to choose from, but it really has not. If you look at the supplemental references (ISC)² includes on its web site (www.isc2.org), you can exhaust the list pretty quickly. An Internet search on terms such as "healthcare information security and privacy" turns up a few more options. The good news is that this book covers the material you need if your purpose is to achieve certification. The organization of the book matches the published organization of the HCISPP exam domains.

Each chapter covers one domain. However, the book is intended for more use over a longer lifespan:

- This book will help those of you who are experiencing firsthand the integration of healthcare, biomedical engineering, information security, information technology, and privacy.
- It is a terrific desk reference for those of you who already have a few years in a healthcare information security and privacy position.
- The material is valuable as part of a curriculum in healthcare information security and privacy in universities, colleges, and technical education workshops and seminars.

As you read through the book, you may note that there are some biases or rationales for how some material was emphasized beyond what may be testable. In no case does the material detract from your exam preparation, but as an HCISPP you may find these lessons learned useful in how you approach your job.

All Healthcare Is Local (Like Politics)

For the most part, we are guided more by our organizational policies and experiences than by theoretical practices and higher level regulatory pressures. That said, organizational policies and procedures should be based on laws and directives from regulators. To be effective as a healthcare information security and privacy professional, however, you will be guided more by organizational policies and procedures. This is why experience in the healthcare field is so important toward measuring competency.

With that in mind, one of the underlying themes of this book is the role you will play in developing and implementing organizational policies. As you read this book, take the opportunity to think about your own organizational policies and procedures around information protection:

- What policies and procedures are in place?
- What are their stated purposes?
- What regulations do they comply with?
- What are the roles and responsibilities presented?

Following are some of the types of policies you should look for:

- Information security program
- Information risk management
- Incident reporting process
- Information governance (information management council, configuration control board, and so on)
- Notice of privacy practices

By focusing on the organization's policies, the book has a practical application. As you read and study, you may encounter information that does not reflect how your organization does things. There is always room and need for some variation. By comparing and gathering internal sources, you will gain a better appreciation of the general organization and structure of information protection, which should be evident in all healthcare organizations. (If nothing else, you may identify opportunities for improvement!) Again, internal policies and procedures are typically linked to a requirement that is external to the organization, such as the US Health Insurance Portability and Accountability Act (HIPAA) or the Canadian Personal Health Information Protection Act (PHIPA). Therefore, this book recognizes how important internal guidance is in understanding the application of overarching national or international regulatory frameworks and directives.

EXAM TIP You should know that (ISC)² can test only on general policies and procedures as they align with regulations. Do not get confused if you come across a scenario that is "not how your organization" would act or react. Remember to consider the general requirements of policies and procedures as well as applicable regulatory requirements.

Publicly Available Sources Are Prioritized

Each chapter ends with a references section to provide a citation for where certain facts and statements can be verified. Along with the specific citations, you may find it useful to explore the material the citations come from to explore additional topics and content in those sources.

The majority of the references provided in the book are publicly available. In most cases, they are offered here with the intent of suggesting further reading. Not only are they listed to cite a particular point made, but they also point you to a wealth of additional material you may want to access. In this way, the book helps expand your knowledge base. No single book can cover every topic in sufficient detail, but narrowing the universe of information down to a manageable list of sources is possible. At the same time, obscure, hard-to-find, and proprietary sources of information are likely not available to any of us on a day-to-day basis, so these constitute a small and necessary portion of the book's source material. The sources listed are intended to augment the material and be applicable to healthcare. Among the references are the following:

- National Institute of Standards and Technology 800 series, with special emphasis on
  - SP 800-122, *Guide to Protecting the Confidentiality of Personally Identifiable Information (PII)*
  - SP 800-66 Rev. 1, *An Introductory Resource Guide for Implementing the Health Insurance Portability and Accountability Act (HIPAA) Security Rule*
  - SP 800-61 Rev. 2, *Computer Security Incident Handling Guide*
  - SP 800-53 Rev. 4, *Security and Privacy Controls for Federal Information Systems and Organizations* (updated 2015)

- SP 800-39, *Managing Information Security Risk: Organization, Mission, and Information System View*
- SP 800-37 Rev. 2, *Risk Management Framework for Information Systems and Organizations: A System Life Cycle Approach for Security and Privacy*
- International Association of Privacy Professionals (IAPP) Privacy Advisor, accessed at https://iapp.org/news/privacy-advisor

International Coverage

If you work in the United States, you undoubtedly are concerned with HIPAA and its amendments. In this book, you will find ample material to guide you in the relevant areas of HIPAA compliance. However, as the provision of healthcare becomes global and many US healthcare providers expand their markets overseas, international healthcare laws and procedures become relevant to US-based healthcare workers. Add to that the growing market for electronic health records and cloud-based services, to name a few, that are outside the United States, and you can see that, although healthcare is still local in nature, it requires an international perspective as well.

At the same time, the target audience of this book includes all of our international colleagues in healthcare. The fact is we all share the same convergence of

- Paper-based records to digital
- Regulatory pressures to protect sensitive information
- Workforce professions with new information protection responsibilities
- Increased networking and interoperability

Because we share these common concerns, this book is inclusive of an international healthcare information security and privacy professional audience. Some may think there is too much of an international focus. Others will think there is not enough. In the end, the intent is to at least acknowledge the common concerns we all have and the similar framework and approaches we take. A special point of emphasis, this book was written as the European Union Data Protection Directive (DPD) was superseded by the General Data Protection Regulation (GDPR). More importantly, the (ISC)² HCISPP exam includes coverage of EU DPD. There are several areas where the inclusion of EU DPD may seem confusing as we have transitioned to GDPR in practice. However, for purposes of the exam, knowing about EU DPD is necessary.

Emphasis on Risk Management

One of the central responsibilities in the practice of healthcare information security and privacy is managing information risk:

- Knowing the standards-based assessment tools
- Understanding the importance of assessing the organization and third parties

- Comprehending the process of mitigating vulnerabilities
- Communicating findings throughout the organization
- Continually assessing the organization and the risk management program for improvement

These basic concepts are foundational, and a large portion of this text is dedicated to them. This is on purpose, as risk management proficiency is a practical skill that you must have. I am not the first author to point out that no silver bullet exists—there is no perfect process or technology that will prevent all data incidents and breaches. Perfection is not the goal. Compliance is not equal to security either. What is key is your proficient application of risk management to your organization to protect, detect, correct, and recover as quickly as possible, with minimal impact, and at the least cost to the organization.

If you do these things, which are hard, your role as a healthcare information security and privacy professional can be rewarding and vital to improved patient care, enhanced organization-wide quality, and reduced costs over the long run. Not to mention, the work can be a lot fun!

Exam Expectations

It probably goes without saying that the major hurdle to becoming an HCISPP is passing the exam. You can expect a three-hour exam. You can take necessary breaks to use the restroom, but you should try and minimize these as much as possible. You may have plenty of time, but in the proctoring environment, coming and going during the exam is a pain. If there are a lot of exam-takers in the room, you may experience significant delays as the proctor has to provide secure exit and entry during the exam to ensure that candidates do not access material or bring it back into the testing area.

The exam has 125 multiple-choice questions, based on short questions and some longer scenarios. Keep in mind that approximately 25 of the questions are trial or test questions, provided to evaluate their usefulness in future exams. These questions do not count against your score. You probably will not be able to tell which questions are experimental. That said, if you come across a question that seems incomprehensible or you simply do not know the answer, do not agonize. Maybe it is an experimental question. I like to take that approach so I can concentrate better on the questions I do know. The exam is worth 1000 points, and a passing score is 700. Again, stay positive and spend energy on questions about which you feel confident. You will not get every single question right.

A final thought: If you have the experience and you have studied this book well, you are well on your way to demonstrating your professionalism and expertise in protecting health information. You will soon join the vast and growing network of credentialed healthcare information protection professionals worldwide by earning the HCISPP. The credential itself continues to top the lists of desirable certifications in health IT and security. My best wishes for your success.

CHAPTER 1

Healthcare Industry

This chapter covers Domain 1, "Healthcare Industry," of the HCISPP certification. After you read and study this chapter, you should be able to:

- Understand the general organization of the United States healthcare system as well as select international healthcare delivery systems.
- Recognize the roles that make up the healthcare delivery system and how these interact with the information security professional.
- Understand the systems and taxonomies used to provide coding of healthcare information and to facilitate exchange of information in patient care delivery and payment.
- Be aware of the financial components of delivering and sustaining healthcare operations.
- Comprehend privacy and security aspects within health information management.
- Describe the information protection implications of third-party relationships in healthcare organizations.
- Appreciate the relationship between information privacy and security concepts with respect to foundational health data management approaches.
- Identify the standards and formats for data interoperability and exchange in clinical operations.

Over the past few decades, the complexity of a typical healthcare organization has increased. Beginning with the earliest hospitals and clinics, operations included direct patient care, hospitality, food service, janitorial, and engineering, to name a few ancillary functions. While those functions may be provided by third-party suppliers today, they are still imperative to caring for patients. Today, the complexity is increased as organizations form into integrated delivery systems where payers, providers, and other components are organized into one entity. This results in a very diverse workforce.

In many communities, the healthcare systems that reside in the area are primary employers or sources of income. This is important to know from a healthcare information protection perspective because the stakes are high and the organization must remain solvent. A data breach or cybersecurity event can erode trust or cause financial penalties that shift resources from patient care.

An extremely rich mixture of highly educated and talented physicians, nurses, administrators, and medical technicians provide direct and indirect patient care. Adding to the complexity, the numerous environments in which healthcare is delivered bring even more diversity to the categories of caregivers and support personnel that are necessary. Healthcare is delivered in hospitals, clinical offices, specialty diagnostic centers, and even the home. The challenges are equally complex for those of us who are charged with protecting the information privacy and security along with these medical professionals in the multitude of environments. One solution does not fit all scenarios to safeguard individually identifiable health information. This chapter will introduce and provide a brief overview of these categories of healthcare organization staff and their various qualifications.

Along with the complexity of the healthcare organizations, the reliance on third-party relationships has increased. This chapter presents an overview of the role and impact that third-party organizations play in healthcare. From suppliers of services to emerging technologies that augment employed staff and increase capabilities, the healthcare organization has many external relationships. A significant number of these are considered critical to operations. Relationships can be established by contracts, partnerships, or subsidiaries to the organization. It becomes interesting when the third party serves multiple industries, with healthcare being only one of them. Cloud service providers are a great example of a third party that has become integral to healthcare organizations. The growing pains for both sides have provided learning examples.

We will start with an introduction to the types of third-party relationships and related services on which healthcare organizations depend. Later, we will focus on the management processes available to address third-party–supplier risk to the healthcare organization.

Types of Organizations in the Healthcare Sector

From the origins of sanitariums and spas, which were more like warehouses for the sick and dying, our modern healthcare system has evolved rapidly into a very complex, highly technical, and essential component of communities and public health. Healthcare is less about a place than a process today. It can be delivered in hospitals, homes, and via mobile phones. Patients expect access to care in multiple settings and on-demand. Providers' expectations and demands are increasingly decentralized, digital, and instantaneous. Those who work in the healthcare sector understand the current reality of what a healthcare organization can be, compared to what a healthcare organization was only two or three decades ago.

Let's start with an overview of the major participants in the delivery of healthcare, which involves distinct groups: patients, providers, payers, and external stakeholders (such as suppliers, regulators, and the surrounding community). These groups play key roles that distinguish them from others even as the point of care may evolve.

Patients

No discussion about healthcare and healthcare information security and privacy starts without an acknowledgment of the patient. In the simplest terms, the patient is why we do what we do. A patient is a person who seeks assistance with matters of health (physical and mental), improvement of health status, or treatment of illness. The care patients seek can be preventative in nature, interventional, rehabilitative, or in recovery from a previous incident.

People can serve different roles on behalf of a patient. Proxies and advocates often assist the patient in navigating the provider and payer systems. These individuals may be family members, members of volunteer organizations, or commercial business entities. The key point is that these entities act primarily on behalf of the patient because the patient care system is complex, or the individual patient needs assistance to participate in their care. The central transaction in healthcare is the conversation between provider and patient. We protect information to ensure that the interchange is complete, protected, and maintained for all the different, legitimate uses of the information.

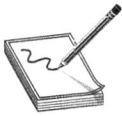

> **NOTE** "Healthcare consumer" is an evolving term that reflects the increasing levels of involvement patients have in their own care. Think of a patient as someone who is currently receiving care. A healthcare consumer can be a current patient. But the term also includes the rest of the population, who are all potential patients who must evaluate the choices they have in using the healthcare delivery system.

A patient can have an inpatient or an outpatient status. An *inpatient* is administratively admitted to the healthcare organization for 24 hours or more. In these cases, a *bed* is traditionally the unit of measure for occupancy rates. For periods of less than 24 hours, the patient is considered in *outpatient* status. Outpatient status is also known as *ambulatory*. In some cases, a patient may be admitted in an *observation* status, which can last up to 48 hours without formal admission as an inpatient. Many patients enter the healthcare system through the emergency department. Typically, the admission status of these patients is determined once they are stabilized. For example, a patient who visits an emergency room is considered an outpatient status if the patient is released within 24 hours.

Outpatient care is provided in numerous types of healthcare settings, including hospitals, medical clinics, associated facilities, and even their own home environments. Increasingly, many surgical and treatment procedures are safe and possible outside of the traditional hospital setting. Advances in technology have reduced the need for inpatient admissions. This evolution has fostered changes in where care can be provided. Today you can find urgent care centers in shopping centers, and patients can undergo some surgical procedures outside a hospital facility. This evolution has been fostered by changes in favorable regulatory guidance and reimbursement rules.

The patient can also be viewed through the lens of the data that constitutes a healthcare facility's identity. This is important, because a protecting a patient's identifiable information is significantly different from information protection and other security and privacy concerns applicable and important in other industries. For example, a patient can be identified by his or her name, date of birth, Social Security number, or home address. These identifiers are similar across other data collection activities of personally identifiable information (PII). However, patients can also have unique information referencing genetic code, billing codes, treatment codes, and images, to name just a few data elements. If PII is disclosed in an unauthorized manner or to an unauthorized viewer, the disclosure violates patient privacy and can also be used to fraudulently receive medical services or alter a medical record. Such disclosure can be a problem in terms of identity theft, financial impact to a patient and a provider organization, and patient safety.

Compounding the issue is that, unlike PII, most protected health information (PHI) is difficult to change (if not impossible) if it has been corrupted or misused in some way. For example, a bank account or even a Social Security number can be replaced, although the unauthorized disclosure of this information is a problem. The disclosure of a patient's medical history, however, is far more difficult to remedy. If the information is spoofed by someone in order to fraudulently receive healthcare services, the actual patient will have difficulty fixing the problem. In some cases, the imposter receives care, and that care is integrated into the victim's medical record. The addition of this information could result in patient safety and care issues (such as blood type mismatches, drug interactions, and so on). If certain diagnoses such as mental health issues or highly sensitive diseases are disclosed, that element of privacy and confidentiality cannot be regained or remedied.

Providers

"Provider" is a broad term that may refer to a single healthcare provider, such as a physician, nurse, or therapist who helps in identifying, preventing, or treating an illness or injury. The term can also describe an organization that employs, contracts, or organizes people who deliver services to patients. Various types of organizations deliver healthcare as providers, such as hospitals, specialized clinics, and even home healthcare agencies. As mobile applications and cloud-based technologies become more advanced, virtual healthcare provider organizations are emerging. In these virtual organizations, caregivers are linked with patients without regard to geographic location. The technology platform *is* the healthcare organization. By 2022, the virtual healthcare market in the United States is anticipated to earn revenues of $3.5 billion.[1]

When multiple types of provider organizations, both inpatient and outpatient services, are organized into a coordinated system of clinics and hospitals, they are called *integrated delivery systems*. These systems can be organized into a single corporate structure, or the systems can provide care, services, or supplies under terms of contracts and other legally binding agreements. The systems are established to increase efficiency and reduce redundancy in providing quality healthcare.

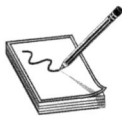

NOTE In most countries and for the majority of uses, the terms "doctor" and "physician" are synonymous. In the context of daily conversation, both describe credentialed healthcare providers. In some countries such as England, there is a distinction between the two: a person is either a doctor or a physician based on level of education, specialty focus, or other advancement through academic examination.

At this point, you know the central transaction in healthcare. The interaction between provider and patient is foundational to the entire system. Understanding the fundamental importance of patient-provider communications can help guide information security professionals. Our role is to look for solutions that improve the communications while maintaining security. At the same time, we must avoid actions that negatively impact the physician-patient interactions.

If you walk into any provider organization, you will notice a wide variety of occupations involved. There are people performing roles ranging from janitorial services to open-heart surgery. There are teams cleaning rooms and others delivering babies. People perform clinical, administrative, or support services to care for patients. The variety of occupations and different levels of education and competency that exist in healthcare differentiates the healthcare industry from many other industries. The US government identifies almost 50 different categories of healthcare practitioners, technologists, and healthcare support occupations.[2] This is in addition to the numerous business and information technology types of professionals that constitute the healthcare organization workforce that must work together efficiently and effectively. From the lowest skilled, entry-level employee to the most senior executive or seasoned physician, the entire organization works in an interconnected way to provide patient care. The following sections cover several of the major categories of healthcare organization occupations you should know about.

Nurses

Nursing is the largest occupational category in any healthcare provider organization. Nursing staff serve a variety of roles and responsibilities, and more than half of US nurses work in provider organizations. In the United States, almost 3.5 million nursing professionals are in the workforce today, accounting for nearly three of every five healthcare professional and technical jobs in the country.[3] Nurses are a professional category of caregiver, with many countries requiring specific education and licensing requirements. Although there are millions of nurses in the workforce, the demand for nursing remains unmet. Presently, there may be as many as 200,000 unfilled nursing jobs in the United States, primarily because of the lack of nursing educators and education resources. In 2018, the American Association of Colleges of Nursing reported that US nursing schools turned away more than 75,000 qualified applicants from baccalaureate and graduate nursing programs because of an insufficient number of faculty, clinical sites, classroom space, and clinical preceptors, as well as budget constraints.[4] General categories of nursing include nurses' aides, licensed practical nurses, registered nurses, and nurse practitioners.

Nurses are essential and influential in the delivery of healthcare. They have impressive levels of education, training, and certification and are indispensable in every aspect of clinical workflow. Beyond direct patient care, nurses are also invaluable when serving in administrative and executive functions of the healthcare business. In the healthcare industry, nurses are prominent in the exam room as well as in the board room. Nursing professionals are highly sought after, and many nurses serve in areas outside of direct patient care. Nurses working in health education roles, in privacy and security areas, and in data analytics are not uncommon.

Nurses' Aides Nurses' aides provide a great deal of patient care in a variety of health-care settings from the physician's office, to the hospital, to long-term care environments. As an occupation that is related to hospital orderlies and attendants, nurses' aides perform services that include moving, repositioning, and lifting patients. They may also provide numerous patient services related to personal care, feeding, bathing, comforting patients, and keeping patients at ease. The education level of most nurses' aides is post-high school (a diploma or certificate). It is not uncommon for healthcare organizations to require at least a competency exam that the nurses' aide also needs to pass.

Registered Nurses and Certified Registered Nurses The care that registered nurses (RNs) provide is more directly involved in coordinating with physicians and other healthcare providers. Whether in an emergency room (ER) or an intensive care unit (ICU), RNs are working at the front lines of patient care. RNs also have a large role in educating patients and the public about health status, post-discharge instructions, and a variety of other concerns related to healthcare. Of course, RNs work in the same environments as all other nurses, but because of their additional education, training, and credentialing, RNs can work independently in some nontraditional healthcare environments such as correctional facilities, schools, and summer camps. Most commonly, RNs receive a bachelor's degree in nursing. It is possible, however, to obtain RN licensure with an associate degree in nursing or a diploma from select nursing programs. All RNs must obtain a license by passing a national RN licensing exam.

An advanced registered nursing career track is the certified registered nurse anesthetist (CRNA). These nurses can provide anesthesia to patients for any surgery or procedure that requires it. Whereas this responsibility was previously reserved for physicians, CRNAs enable small-market and rural hospitals to control costs by reducing staffing expense while maintaining the standard of care. To become a CRNA, the process includes obtaining a bachelor's degree in nursing or an equivalent, often obtaining a master of science degree in nursing (MSN), and being a licensed RN. Additionally, a CRNA must have clinical experience in an acute care setting. They need to demonstrate one year of experience in an area such as the ICU as opposed to long-term care or rehabilitation units. In addition to all this, they also must complete an accredited nurse anesthesia educational program. Finally, they are required to pass a national certification examination.

A second example of an advanced registered nurse specialty is the certified nurse midwife (CNM). This nurse usually has completed a bachelor's degree and an MSN program. The board certification is in the profession of midwifery. CNMs specialize in providing care such as birthing services for women who are not experiencing high-risk pregnancies.

Nurse Practitioners Within the nursing profession, the role of nurse practitioner (NP) has emerged to extend and expand the capabilities of caregivers due to workforce shortages and advances in medicine. RNs may undergo additional training to be able to diagnose medical conditions, order treatment, prescribe drugs, and make referrals much as a physician would. To become an NP, one must first be an RN. Then, after additional, advanced classroom and clinical education, the RN is credentialed as an NP.

The types of practices in which NPs work are almost limitless. They serve in primary care settings such as pediatrics, family practice, and geriatrics and in specialty care areas such as OB/GYN, oncology, dermatology, and pain management.

To become an NP, the RN must obtain an MSN or the doctor of nursing practice (DNP) degree. Then the candidate must pass a national board certification exam. The NP will take the exam based on the specific clinical focus area of their educational program—in other words, if the program concentrated on geriatrics, the certification exam would do the same. Once these hurdles are cleared, the board-certified NP can apply for additional credentials, such as a Drug Enforcement Agency (DEA) registration number to be able to prescribe controlled substances in addition to the medications the NP licensing allows.

> **CAUTION** About a quarter of US nurses are union members. The unionization of the nursing profession is important to healthcare delivery and may impact information privacy and security. For example, implementing a policy that does not allow access to personal e-mail using company computers may result in a union protest, called a grievance. The grievance does not invalidate the appropriateness of the security control, but it does add complexity and delay to the eventual policy implementation.

Licensed Practical/Vocational Nurses A licensed practical nurse (LPN) or a licensed vocational nurse (LVN) works under the supervision of an RN. The choice of occupational title depends on the US state in which the nurse is employed. The duties and qualifications are the same for LPN and LVN. These nurses must complete a year-long (typically) certified educational program. Often these programs are affiliated with a teaching hospital that provides some hands-on experience for the students. After they complete the program, students must pass an additional licensing exam. LPNs and LVNs work in every area of healthcare provision—in hospitals, of course, but they also may provide care in skilled nursing facilities, rehabilitation centers, or even a patient's home. Through home healthcare, the continuum of care extends from the hospital back into the patient's normal living environment, which has a demonstrated positive impact on outcomes.

Physicians

Physicians have been providing healthcare since as far back as time has been recorded. Hippocrates, in around 350 BC, is considered the "father of modern medicine."[5] In contrast, modern nursing began in the nineteenth century—although the services of nursing in patient care have certainly taken place as long as people have been sick and injured.

From the very beginning to today, the central relationship in healthcare has been between the doctor and the patient. A physician's main role is to diagnose and treat injuries and illnesses for their patients. Surgeons, who are a specialized type of physician, treat patients by operating to treat injuries, diseases, and deformities. Almost all physicians obtain a bachelor's degree and then complete four more years in an accredited medical school. There has always been a measure of importance placed on applied performance under the guidance of a current physician. So, after medical school, on-the-job training continues as an intern for a year. Then the student must complete a residency, usually focusing on a specialty or area of increased proficiency, such as cardiology or internal medicine.

TIP Residency is a key difference between the requirements of nurses, including NPs and CRNAs, and physicians. This distinction is changing as more NP residencies are becoming available and recommended, even if they are not required.

Like a nurse, a doctor must obtain a license to practice and hold the credential of doctor of medicine (MD) or doctor of osteopathic medicine (DO). It is also common for MDs and DOs to take additional exams for board certification. There are board certifications (sometimes more than one) for all the various specialties. After training and licensing is completed, physicians are permitted to prescribe medications and order, perform, and interpret diagnostic tests independently. In addition, each physician is also required to be credentialed specifically to practice in a particular hospital or healthcare organization. This is an internal function of the healthcare organization. Organization personnel verify the background and qualifications of the physician and grant the physician privileges to practice medicine within the organization.

As mentioned, a physician can be a general practitioner with responsibilities in family medicine, internal medicine, or other primary care types of areas. Otherwise, based on additional, focused training and experience, physicians and surgeons (called specialists) can concentrate on an individual disease or condition, or on a specific physiologic system. To help illustrate the number and variety of these specialties, Table 1-1 contains some of the most common specialties with a brief description. The specializations listed in Table 1-1 are not comprehensive. There is variation internationally as countries may differ in how they subdivide and recognize specialty practices. The common factor for determining specialization, however, is according to the defined group of patients, diseases, skills, or philosophy on which the physician focuses.

Specialty	Description
Anesthesiologist	During surgery, safely delivers anesthesia to patients and monitors them through the procedure
Cardiologist	Focuses on diseases and conditions of the heart and cardiovascular systems
Dermatologist	Specializes in conditions of the skin and are very important in early detection of skin cancers
Emergency/Trauma	Specializes in treating a variety of acute injury, trauma, emergencies, and so on, 24 hours a day, every day of the year

Table 1-1 List of Specialist Physicians with Descriptions

Specialty	Description
Endocrinologist	Treats issues involving glands such as the thyroid and hormonal issues that impact growth, mood, and metabolism
Epidemiologist	Identifies the spread of new diseases and how a virus mutates, and establishes mitigations and interventions to address threats and potential incidents and active outbreaks
Neurologist	Specializes in disorders of the brain such as Parkinson's disease and Alzheimer's disease
Neurosurgeon	Performs neurological surgery to treat central and peripheral nervous system diseases and the brain
Obstetrician/Gynecologist (OB/GYN)	Handles conditions related to the female reproductive system, including pregnancy and childbirth
Oncologist	Diagnoses and treats cancer patients, with further specialization in one or more specific cancer types or patient categories
Ophthalmologist	Diagnoses and treats eyes and various eye defects and blindness; performs eye surgeries
Orthopedic surgeon	Performs examinations and surgeries on bones, joints, and other bone-related conditions such as arthritis and osteoporosis
Pathologist	Studies samples of cells for abnormalities using DNA, tissue, blood, and so on; also performs autopsies to determine cause of death
Pediatrician	Concentrates on general medical issues pertaining to children (birth to adolescent)
Psychiatrist	Treats mental illnesses and behavioral health issues
Radiologist	Specializes in reading and interpreting X-rays or other imaging technologies to provide diagnoses
Plastic surgeon	Performs corrective and reconstructive surgeries and procedures; may specialize in cosmetic surgery to adjust patients' physical appearance, sometimes called a plastic surgeon
Podiatrist	Concentrates on issues with gait, feet, and ankles, and their impact on overall physical health; important in the care of diabetics with wound issues of the feet and toes
Pulmonologist	Focuses on lung conditions and ventilator support for ICU patients
Surgeon	Practices general surgery to treat trauma, transplant organs, or any number of other surgeries; may choose to concentrate in one or two areas—all specialists may at one time or another perform surgeries
Urologist	Focuses primarily on urinary problems such as urinary tract infections; provides diagnoses and treatments for male reproductive system conditions

Table 1-1 List of Specialist Physicians with Descriptions *(continued)*

CAUTION In some industries, it is acceptable to reward those who refer business to you. However, in the United States, paying for healthcare referrals is a crime. To avoid violating the law and improve patient care, physicians can align into organized physician services. The results are independent healthcare delivery organizations that provide comprehensive services without geographic borders. These groups are affiliated through contracts and agreements to serve large, defined patient populations. Examples of the physician-led groups include independent physician associations, medical foundations, medical service organizations, and physician hospital organizations.

National Provider Identifier (NPI) Standard

The US Health Insurance Portability and Accountability Act (HIPAA) establishes an identification standard for providers called the National Provider Identifier (NPI). The NPI is a unique identification number for healthcare organizations subject to HIPAA for administrative and financial transactions. It is permanently assigned to the provider regardless of location or job changes. The NPI is a 10-position, intelligence-free numeric identifier (a 10-digit number). This means that the numbers do not carry other information about healthcare providers, such as the state in which they live or their medical specialty. Providers cannot use other types of identifiers even if the use predates HIPAA. The NPI must be shared by providers with other providers, health plans, clearinghouses, and any entity that may need it for billing purposes. The purpose of the NPI is to improve the efficiency and effectiveness of electronic transmission of healthcare information.

Physician Assistants

The physician assistant (PA) is another provider role that has evolved separately by broadening the nursing role. Collectively, the NP, CRNA, and PA are often called "physician extenders" because they have absorbed traditional roles and responsibilities reserved for physicians to help increase the availability of advanced care. Physician extenders have also proven invaluable by often improving quality (certainly not lessening it), reducing costs, and increasing access. The PA is recognized as another general category of healthcare professional or staff who also has a license to practice medicine under the guidance of a physician. This recognition is not universal across international health systems. Primarily a US healthcare physician extender, the PA may not be recognized in other countries.

Most often, a candidate for PA already has a bachelor's degree, but some programs confer one as part of completing the PA curriculum. In any case, PA programs typically require approximately two to three years of schoolwork with clinical rotations in all areas of PA practice, such as internal medicine, family practice, emergency medicine, and so on. In some cases, a graduating PA decides to specialize in a specific clinical area and obtains additional training and experience. This process is similar to physicians gaining experience through specialty rotations but involves a much shorter length of time. PAs provide the same patient care functions as a physician, but they must work under the direction and oversight of a physician. One difference is in performing surgery: a PA can aid a physician-surgeon but cannot conduct the surgery independently. As with all nurses and physicians, there is a licensing requirement for PAs.

Medical Technicians

When you hear someone referred to as a medical technician, it is similarly overarching, like doctor or nurse. There are numerous subcategories of medical technicians that fully describe the expertise and technical aptitude of any particular area. First, the general category of medical technician describes the kind of work done in clinical laboratories performing tests and exams. A medical technician has practical knowledge and ability in a particular clinical area. They also must be able to understand medical data produced by their specific equipment and how it relates to the patient. They are the first line of interpreters of results. While they do not make diagnoses, they can certainly reduce error and rework when they recognize inaccuracies in data, such as in a blood bank or microbiology laboratory. Another type of medical technician operates medical devices in support of performing procedures in the specific clinical practice. This would include diagnostic imaging, cardiac catheterization, and hemodialysis. The reports and findings of tests and examinations made by all of these different types of medical technicians are used by physicians to diagnose and treat patients. It is important to note that even with sophisticated testing technologies and highly skilled medical technicians, the actual interpretations and diagnoses remain the role of the physician.

Biomedical Technicians and Clinical Engineers   Biomedical technicians and clinical engineers are the personnel who maintain (and operate) medical devices. One of the key differences between these types of medical technicians and the technicians discussed in the preceding section is that biomedical technicians and clinical engineers typically do not require extensive training on human anatomy, physiology, and clinical technique. With respect to education, clinical engineers have an educational requirement that exceeds that for a biomedical technician, including a four-year degree at least. A biomedical technician, much like other medical technicians, may have a two-year degree or a certificate of training from a healthcare vocational training program. In any case, both clinical engineers and biomedical technicians work in conjunction with other medical technicians to operate and maintain all of the various medical devices and technologies safely in the healthcare organization.

EXAM TIP   You probably will not be tested in depth on occupations in the healthcare setting. This material is provided because understanding roles and responsibilities is vital to the HCISPP. For example, as medical device security is one of the most pressing issues related to healthcare information security and privacy, understanding the role of biomedical technicians and clinical engineering is as predictive of your success as mastering only what might be testable.

Other Provider Types with Specific Access

Based on how they provide clinical services to the patient, several other healthcare providers and support personnel handle protected health information. All the following providers require varying levels of licensure and certification requirements as well. Some jurisdictions internationally still require physicians to serve in these roles.

- **Emergency medical technicians** EMTs require special training to provide first response to emergency situations and handle traumatic injuries and medical care at accident scenes and other locations.

- **Social workers** This profession concentrates on patients' quality of life and subjective wellbeing and administer to individuals, groups, and communities. Areas of practice include research, counseling, crisis intervention, and teaching.

- **Psychologists** A medical professional, they provide patient care with respect to behavior and mental processes and counselling services, and they may conduct research within academic settings.

- **Psychiatrists** An MD that focuses on examining and treating disorders of the mind or mental health. They can prescribe medication. Their evaluation of the patient consists of a consideration of symptoms and complaints to determine if the origin is physical illness or injury, mental disorders, or a combination.

- **Pharmacists** These professionals are responsible for dispensing medications and ensuring their proper and safe use. They are an integral part of the healthcare team in that they often provide meaningful education and counseling for patients who are receiving medication. A doctor of pharmacy (PharmD) degree from an accredited pharmacy program is required. This is followed by successfully passing licensure exams.

Administration

No healthcare organization could succeed without another significant part of the healthcare workforce—the administration. There are many examples of providers who perform administrative roles in the organization, such as chief medical officer physicians or department managers who started their careers as medical technologists. However, many administrative positions are held by people not trained as providers but with education and experience focused on clerical, managerial, and executive competencies.

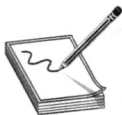

NOTE Healthcare administrators include professionals with academic training and certifications in information technology, information security, and data science, as examples. They may have little training or experience in healthcare, but they still play important roles in patient care and safety. These members of administration can be chief information officers, chief information security officers, chief data officers, or any of the people that serve on their teams.

Administration describes all the various people that administratively support the provision of healthcare. At every level of the healthcare organization, from the chief executive officer to the ward clerk, administrative individuals provide appropriate levels of management and leadership. At the most senior level, administration refers to the management of internal and external forces to achieve specific goals. One of the key responsibilities for senior administrators is to recruit and retain quality physicians, to ensure appropriate staffing levels, and to manage performance. Below this level, the administration strives to achieve their objectives and allocate resources appropriately. Much like all the other healthcare professions, administrators can have a general focus across many areas, such as a chief operating officer or a physician's office manager. On the other hand, many administrators specialize in a given area, such as information technology or finance.

In terms of education and training, the path to administrative positions mirrors that of other healthcare professions and categories. For more senior-level positions, at least a bachelor's degree is needed. In many cases, especially in a specialty area such as information technology or finance, a graduate degree is often preferred. It is also preferred that administrators in these positions have previous experience working in healthcare organizations. For other administrative positions, a combination of a high school diploma and on-the-job training is required. Board certification is available to administrators of all types, from general administrators, to information technology, to finance. The certification of administration personnel provides a common framework for peer-to-peer relationships with healthcare provider colleagues.

Environmental Services

Without janitorial or housekeeping services, a healthcare organization could not open its doors. The regulatory and patient safety issues that healthcare organizations face make environmental concerns very important, especially because these types of services, including maintenance, alterations, and construction, happen in areas where patients are or will be.

Environmental service personnel also provide laundry operations and linen distribution. Coupled with housekeeping services, these personnel integrate in the overall management of beds within the organization. How quickly a room or a bed can be made ready after a patient is discharged can mean significant added revenue, but if this is done incorrectly, patient safety, satisfaction, and outcomes can suffer because rooms are transitioned quickly, but they lack cleanliness, for example. Infection control plays a large role and can be a huge revenue drain on healthcare organizations considering the number of hospital-acquired infections and readmissions that can result from a lack of proper cleanliness.

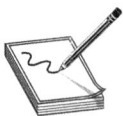

NOTE With respect to credentialing and certifying cybersecurity professionals in the United States, the National Initiative for Cybersecurity Education (NICE) has been established to, among other things, advocate for and recommend a framework for educating the future cybersecurity workforce. This framework will draw from the credentialing and certification processes already established and recognized in healthcare and other industries, albeit not just in information technology. For more information, see https://niccs.us-cert.gov/footer/about-nice.

Healthcare Clearinghouse

A medical claims clearinghouse is a third-party system that interprets or "scrubs" claim data between US provider systems and private insurance payers. According to the US Department of Health and Human Services, a healthcare clearinghouse is a "public or private entity, including a billing service, repricing company, or community health information system, which processes non-standard data or transactions received from one entity into standard transactions or data elements, or vice versa."[6] The electronic claims submission clearinghouse intermediates between provider financial charges and insurers' denial or acceptance of the claims for payment. Providers can submit bills directly to health insurers, but many choose to deal with clearinghouses in the middle to increase efficiency. Healthcare clearinghouses are subject to HIPAA and have an important role in addressing information privacy and security during electronic data interchanges.

Healthcare Organizational Behavior

Now that we have discussed the healthcare players and their roles, let's briefly look at how they interact (and why that matters to us). In short, you will want to acknowledge the power and politics in healthcare organizations. As noted in the specific professions, these roles have long histories, and their relationships and interactions have been influenced by political factors as well as clinical practices. Before the mid-twentieth century, the predominant healthcare roles were doctors and nurses. The relationship between the two professions is so intense that a Wisconsin physician, Leonard Stein, famously coined the term "Doctor-Nurse Game" in 1967 to help explain and understand the relationship. The major (and not complimentary) objectives of the game demonstrate the underlying communication problems between doctors, nurses, and, by extension, all allied health professions.[7] Some debate that the game has ended as nursing professions have advanced in status and power within healthcare organizations, but others are not ready to declare that victory.[8]

The evolution of the healthcare workforce has led to complex organizational behavior dynamics. The need for a variety of allied healthcare professions, such as specialized medical technicians and myriad administrative personnel, came from the reliance on and success of clinical and information technology. Healthcare organizations must now more than ever work together.

The connection between organizational behavior and understanding information protection in healthcare is about knowing your customer. The healthcare organization is unlike any other customer or end user a security professional will serve. The interaction of nurses, physicians, administration, and medical technicians consists of multiple perspectives and priorities. Healthcare security professionals must take it all into account with respect to protecting information. You cannot apply information privacy and security in healthcare exactly as it is applied in other critical infrastructure organizations, such as telecommunications or industrial control system industries. To understand why is to master the power and politics at play.

We've established that healthcare starts with the patient, and the central relationship in healthcare is the doctor–patient relationship. Anything that interferes with that relationship must be clinically reasonable (and legally defensible). A successful healthcare information security and privacy practitioner must account for this. For instance, installing the latest vulnerability update for an operating system considered a critical fix is a top priority in most organizations with information systems. The edict to stop work and push out the patch remotely from information technology servers may well be the industry best practice. But in healthcare, that edict may interfere with patient care and can cause patient safety issues. Remember that medical devices are increasingly networked and will require the same vulnerability updates. Imagine what would happen if an automatic push across the organization caused a cardiac catheterization lab system to reboot in the middle of a patient procedure; patient safety could be at risk. (This is one oversimplified example.)

Safely implementing health information technology and security is already identified as a potential issue in healthcare-adverse events (those related to patient safety).[9] The key concept is that a healthcare organization chart, a seniority list, or a corner office will not always illustrate the power within the healthcare organization. When developing and implementing an information protection strategy, you must consider and include input from physicians (who may or may not be employees of the organization), nurses, and anyone else who is providing direct patient care.

Health Insurance

Whether healthcare is funded by a public source, such as the government, or reimbursed by private entities, such as health insurers, someone has to pay the bill for services rendered. Both in the United States and internationally, it is uncommon for an individual to "self-pay," so most payers are commonly described as third parties. In sum, a *payer* is almost always someone other than the patient who finances or reimburses the cost of healthcare.

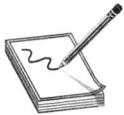

> **NOTE** Some people with health insurance choose to self-pay (also called "pay cash") for certain healthcare services to increase confidentiality of the treatment record. The intention is to shield select information from a health payer, for example. For more information, see "Modifications to the HIPAA Privacy, Security, Enforcement, and Breach Notification Rules Under the Health Information Technology for Economic and Clinical Health Act and the Genetic Information Nondiscrimination Act; Other Modifications to the HIPAA Rules," at https://www.govinfo.gov/content/pkg/FR-2013-01-25/pdf/2013-01073.pdf. Or consult additional information on expanded privacy and security provisions.

Healthcare Across the Globe

Healthcare delivery has patients, providers, and payers in every model in countries around the world. To highlight this, we present several major healthcare systems. Our starting point is the US healthcare system. You will observe a contrast with the US private and public payers with the rest of the global healthcare delivery systems. As a security professional, you are not expected to have a deep understanding of international healthcare systems; a high-level understanding of major components is enough. You may begin to put privacy and security issues into context based on knowing who pays for healthcare and how providers are regulated. There is intentionally no evaluation of one delivery system over another in this book; each has its own merits and opportunities for improvement.

United States

The US healthcare system consists of both private payers and public insurers. What sets the United States apart from the rest of the world is the extent to which healthcare costs are met by private payers, or health insurance companies. Health insurance is a way for individuals to be protected against large medical expenses by joining a larger population where the risk of medical expenses is estimated for the entire group. The insurance company charges a monthly premium applicable to the entire target population. In this way, the costs of medical care are spread out across the group. Under the heading of "private payer," several considerations are described in the following sections.

Indemnity Insurance

This model for insurance payment is based on fee-for-service. A patient receives healthcare services, pays for it at the point of care, and then submits a claim to the insurance company for reimbursement. In this scenario, the patient has the maximum freedom of choice in physicians and other services. Of course, this scenario also results in the highest cost. Indemnity plans usually have an out-of-pocket maximum. Once the beneficiary reaches their annual limit for medical expenses, the insurer pays the entire bill. There is no patient payment for services unless the provider charges more than the usual and customary fee. The patient will be responsible for charges above that amount.

Employer-Based Insurance

The reliance on health insurance in the United States is a relatively recent development. The growth can be directly traced to employers offering coverage as an employment benefit, in addition to salary and other enticements. This may be related to federal government's regulatory pressures to freeze wages during World War II. Employer-based healthcare became increasingly common as a result. Employer-based coverage comes in two types: fully insured plans and self-funded plans. Each version has legal and tax incentives for both employers and employees. The US Census Bureau reported that, in 2015, about 67 percent of the population was covered by private health insurance, and about 56 percent of that group was covered by employer-based health insurance.[10] Figure 1-1 depicts the narrative in the next few paragraphs of US healthcare expenditures by payer type: self-pay, private insurance, Medicare and Medicaid, and other (third-party payers such as non-custodial parental support, state workers compensation, court settlements from a liability insurer, and so on).

Fully Insured Health Plans   In this type of fee-for-service plan, the employer purchases government-licensed insurance that is regulated at the state level depending on the states in which the insurer operates. The federal government has jurisdiction as well. The insurance company collects premiums and bears the financial risk if what the company pays out goes beyond the collected premiums.

Figure 1-1
Distribution of US healthcare expenditures in 2018, by payer (Source: Office of the Actuary in the Centers for Medicare and Medicaid Services)

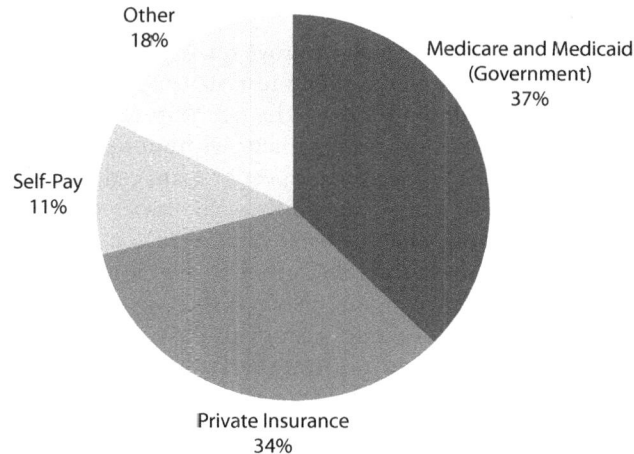

Other
18%

Medicare and Medicaid
(Government)
37%

Self-Pay
11%

Private Insurance
34%

There are three primary types of government-licensed health insurance organizations:

- **Commercial health insurers**   In some cases, these companies, called indemnity insurers, may be owned by stockholders or policyholders (as a mutual insurance company). Aetna is an example of a stock company version of a commercial health insurer.

- **Blue Cross and Blue Shield plans (BCBS)**   About 90 million people are covered by a BCBS plan. Traditionally, they were not-for-profit plans, and many still are today. Some BCBS have organized to be more like commercial, for-profit entities under special state laws by state hospital (Blue Cross) and state medical (Blue Shield) associations. Most plans offer managed care plans, such as health maintenance organization (HMO) and preferred provider organization (PPO) plans, as well as traditional insurance plans.

- **Health maintenance organizations**   HMOs cover approximately 70 million people today. HMOs usually are licensed under special state laws that recognize that HMOs tightly integrate health insurance with the provision of healthcare. HMOs are both provider and payer. Examples include Kaiser Permanente and Harvard Pilgrim.

Self-Funded Employee Health Benefit Plans   In these plans, the employer has the responsibility of paying directly for healthcare services. Funds are reserved to pay claims, and the employer contracts with one or more third parties to administer the insurance benefits. With a self-funded plan, the employer bears most of the financial risk. The employer can contract with an entity called a third-party administrator that specializes in this business. The other options are to contract with health insurers or HMOs to manage the benefits for the employer.

Managed Care

As a mechanism to control cost, improve quality, and increase access, managed care has evolved from an unproven concept almost 50 years ago to a major component of healthcare delivery and resourcing today. The key feature of managed care is in the integration of healthcare provision and payment within one organization. Virtually all private health coverage now involves some aspect of managed care. The managed care organization develops financial incentives to drive patient behavior and provider treatment decisions. At the same time, the managed care organizations rely on objective data analysis to develop treatment protocols that are shared to improve provider practices. Although also intended to control costs and increase efficiency, managed care organizations rely on controlling access to limit waste. Part of this process is a requirement for patients and referring providers to obtain prior authorizations for certain services. Some argue the gatekeeping function of referral management and prior authorizations can be an intrusion into the patient–provider relationship.

The following are the four main types of managed-care options:

- **Health maintenance organization**   Patients are enrolled by paying the HMO a monthly or annual fee. They are then eligible to receive care from providers that have aligned with the HMO. The patient typically has a low or no deductible, but instead a small copayment for each service.

- **Preferred provider organization**   This is a fee-for-service health plan with several providers that have aligned with the PPO. If the patient chooses a participating provider, the cost of medical care is discounted to the enrollee. If not, the health plan pays a lower amount for the provider's service and the patient pays the rest. The patient may incur higher deductibles and coinsurance payments with a PPO. The result is more choice for the patient, yet at a higher cost.

- **Point-of-service (POS)**   This type of plan combines the most attractive elements of both HMOs and PPOs. In exchange for a deductible and higher coinsurance payment on a one-time basis, an HMO enrollee can choose to use a service that is outside the HMO plan. This is in contrast to a strict HMO policy of not reimbursing care received out of network (under the HMO-only model).

- **High-deductible health plan with savings option (HDHP/SO)**   This type of plan usually takes the form of a health savings account (HSA). For a relatively low premium, an enrollee gets catastrophic insurance coverage. For all healthcare received up to catastrophic care, the enrollee must pay a high deductible. To offset this, enrollees are able to save wages before tax in a special type of account to be used to pay any deductibles.

The government is the primary payer in most developed countries and is integral to the overall provision of healthcare. In contrast to other countries, government spending for healthcare in the United States is designed to address populations not served by private insurance. These government-sponsored plans are also typically structured in a managed-care design:

- **Medicaid**   Each US state allocates the money it receives from the federal government to provide medical assistance primarily to the elderly, poor, and disabled. For the most part, recipients are pregnant women, children and babies, people with disabilities, and, in some cases, the elderly poor.

- **Medicare**   Medicare provides insurance coverage for individuals age 65 and older or those who are younger than 65 but have long-term disabilities. It is funded and administered by the federal government. There is no qualification related to income level, only age or disability status.

- **Department of Defense Military Health System (MHS)**   The federal government provides funding for health benefits for active-duty service members and retired service members, as well as their dependents, through the MHS. This network has aspects of direct care (military hospitals) but also purchases healthcare from the commercial sector through a managed-care network called TRICARE.

- **Veterans Health Administration (VHA)**   Veterans of US military service are eligible for care through the federal VHA program, which operates a network of hospitals and treatment centers that provide care specifically to this population.

- **Indian Health Service (IHS)**   Eligible Native Americans may receive care through the IHS within IHS facilities. They may also receive care at non-IHS facilities with payment provided by the federal government.

Depending on what services are covered and the level of reimbursement, many Americans pay premiums for more than one health insurance plan. Often plans overlap. For this reason, healthcare financing in the United States is a complex assortment of programs that can be integrated. A significant concern with the financing system is that it leaves still millions of Americans with too little or no health insurance coverage.

To address the uninsured and underinsured in America, the Patient Protection and Affordable Care Act (PPACA) was enacted in 2010. The law is often abbreviated to the Affordable Care Act (ACA) or nicknamed "Obamacare." The ACA was the most significant reform of US healthcare since Medicare and Medicaid were started in 1965.[11] The exact numbers are hard to obtain, but sources indicate that more than 20 million people have benefitted from the regulatory reform, about half of the estimated population without insurance or enough coverage. The ACA continues to be a hotly debated political topic, even though it was passed into law. Several unsuccessful attempts were made to challenge the act in US courts. Another source of concern is that some studies showed that premiums paid by individuals increased dramatically post-implementation. Figure 1-2 offers a state-by-state view of the changes in how much an individual must pay annually. The sweeping nature of the ACA will continue to drive ongoing changes in the structure and financial operation of healthcare organizations in the United States.

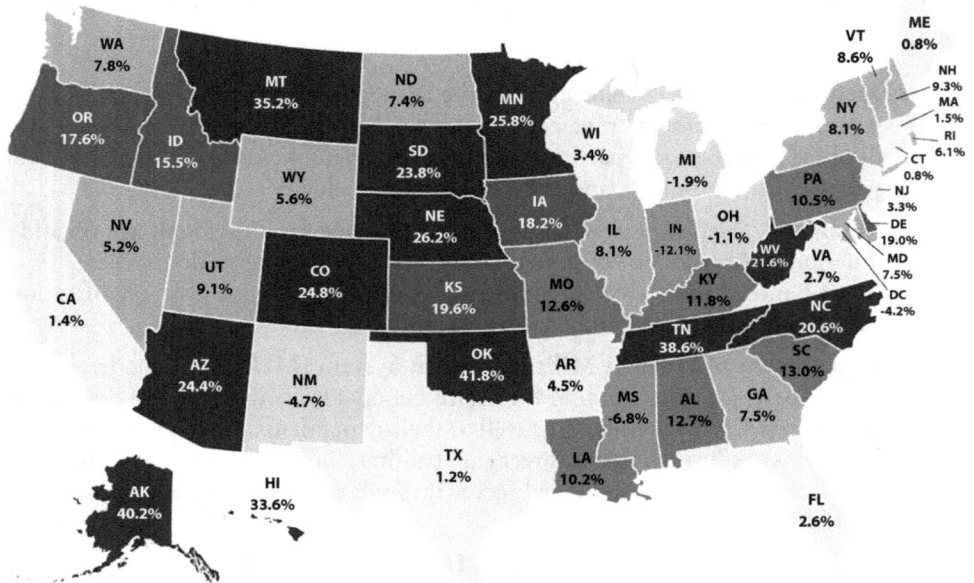

Figure 1-2   Premium growth after ACA (2015–2016) (Source: *Business Insider*)[12]

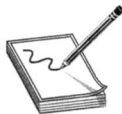

NOTE   Two key provisions of ACA are that insurers must accept all applicants regardless of pre-existing conditions, and an individual mandate requires that everyone purchase a qualified health plan with a minimum of defined "essential health benefits." In January 2019, the individual mandate provision was repealed by Congress. The remainder of ACA components are still in effect.

Internationally, a single-payer system financed by government (public) funds is most common. However, private insurance or self-pay options do exist for some countries. Depending on the country or healthcare system, providers may be able to choose to accept both private and public funds. In some systems, the two types of financing sources operate separately. A select few of those systems are presented in the following sections. Common among these, the government (with few exceptions) collects all healthcare fees and pays all healthcare costs. In short, providers in these countries bill one entity (not the patient) for their services. It is important to understand the financing systems for healthcare delivery on an international level compared as a percentage of each country's gross domestic product (GDP). Figure 1-3 is authored by the Organisation for Economic Cooperation and Development (OECD) and demonstrates overall spending by government and private sources on healthcare.

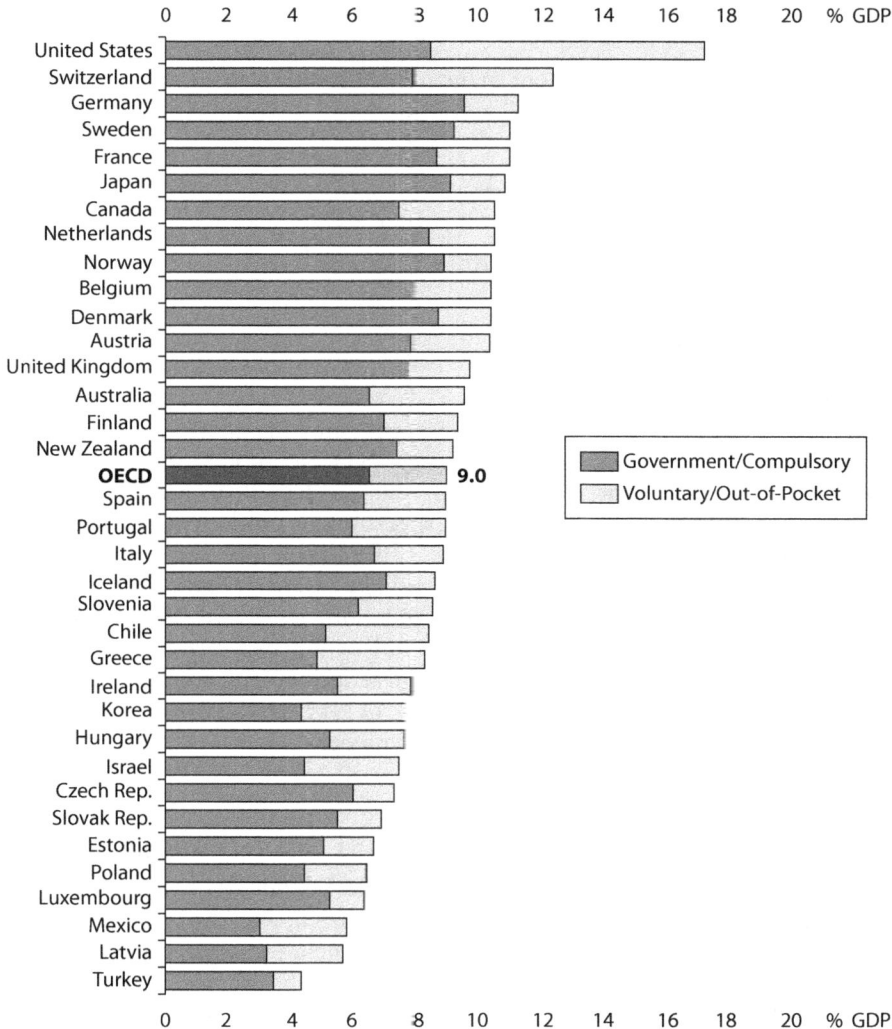

Figure 1-3 Health spending in OECD countries, 2016 (Source: *Health at a Glance 2017, OECD Indicators*)

Canada

Canada's healthcare system is an example of a single-payer system in which the government offers universal coverage. The system is funded through taxes collected. The physicians delivering the care, however, are not government employees and provide services under a fee-for-service model. Canada has a publicly funded Medicare system, with most services provided by the private sector. In this single-payer system, basic services are provided by private doctors (since 2002 private doctors have been allowed to incorporate), who submit claims to the government (payer) for services rendered. The entire fee is paid by the government at the same rate. Each province may opt out of the program, though none currently does.

To be compliant with government mandates, all health plans in Canada must be

- Available to all residents of Canada
- Comprehensive in coverage
- Accessible without financial and other barriers
- Portable within the country and while traveling
- Publicly administered

United Kingdom

The UK's National Health Service (NHS) is a government agency that is organized and resourced to provide universal health coverage. NHS is publicly funded via taxes and is founded on the belief that all citizens have an entitlement to healthcare. Healthcare services include basic services, primary care, specialty care, and inpatient care, along with radiology and laboratory services. That said, private insurance also exists because some types of services are not covered by NHS—usually elective conditions. Approximately seven million people, or 12 percent of the population, are covered by private plans.

In terms of out-of-pocket costs, there are only a few cost-sharing arrangements for publicly covered services. Patients may pay a prescription drug copayment per prescription, while all drugs prescribed for inpatient care in NHS hospitals are free to the patient. NHS dentistry services are also subject to copayments.

European Union

The European Union (EU) does not have any administrative or authoritative role in healthcare. Although each health system is run at an individual member-nation level, the systems are primarily publicly funded through taxation. For the most part, healthcare in the EU is considered universal healthcare. This includes larger systems in Germany, France, Italy, and Spain. There is private funding for healthcare, which is a personal contribution toward meeting anything not funded by taxpayer contribution. This can be totally private funds paid either out-of-pocket or by personal- or employer-funded insurance. Membership in the EU enables citizens to carry a European health insurance card and provides reciprocal emergency healthcare funding for citizens who are visiting other member nations. In fact, this benefit extends to several other European nations that are not currently in the European Union.

EXAM TIP Throughout this text, the European Union (EU) Data Protection Act (DPA) is referenced. This is because at the time of exam publication, the EU DPA was the prevailing regulation and is testable according to the current HCISPP Exam Outline. As of May 25, 2018, the EU replaced the EU DPA and now enforces the General Data Protection Regulation (GDPR). Where applicable, a practical, albeit high-level, comparison of the two regulations is included within this text.

Japan

There is measurably more government control of healthcare in Japan, which also has a universal health coverage model. At a national level, in this model, the pricing of services is set by the government, which also subsidizes local governments, third-party payers, and providers for the cost of providing healthcare (which does not actually equal what the government sets as a fee). The government does this to help these entities implement national-level policies. Japan has 47 prefectures (regions) and 1742 municipalities that operate the nation's healthcare system. However, all of these local healthcare entities adhere to detailed regulations set and enforced at a national level. Although funding is provided by the government, there are gaps in coverage; for instance, some hospitalization costs are not fully covered. Therefore, supplementary private health insurance is held by most of the adult population.

Stakeholders

The healthcare information protection practitioner may require an understanding of the broad impacts of negative events, such as a cybersecurity attack, that can affect entities beyond the healthcare organization. These entities, or *stakeholders,* have an interest in or an impact on the healthcare organization, and they are also affected by events that occur within the healthcare organization. Stakeholders can be many and diverse, from individuals to entire corporations.

Healthcare organizations are critical to the infrastructure of communities. In many communities, the local healthcare organization is probably one of the central institutions in the area and is likely a major employer as well. It is also likely that it is one of the most prevalent buyers and users of services, supplies, and products that are either directly related to patient care or indirectly related to supporting patient care operations.

Local government is also considered a stakeholder, because it has a direct impact on operations in the healthcare organization and is also responsive to things that happen with the facility. In other words, for example, a hospital that shuts down a service such as the emergency room and institutes an alternative care strategy may impact local public administration and policy.

Coding and Classification Systems and Standards

Coding is the transformation of clinical workflow from any type of description in narrative or words into numerical data sets, or codes, that are used for documenting disease descriptions, injuries, symptoms, and conditions. Think of coding in healthcare as a form of translation, from language to numbers. There are many reasons this translation has to be done. One of the most important reasons is the amount of information that is found in healthcare information stores like medical records and billing reports. Using codes to standardize and organize helps providers describe the care they deliver. The translation also assists reimbursement and data surveillance activities by creating and using a taxonomy that contains common meaning.

Related to the use of codes, classification systems facilitate the terminology and taxonomy to be further organized for ease of use. Some of the leading examples of classification systems, such as DRGS and ICD-10, are described in this section. Because the terminology of diagnosis and treatment is so complex, classification systems bridge the gaps in understanding what clinical information means.

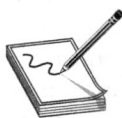

> **NOTE** Healthcare information in narrative form is categorized as *unstructured*. When translated into codes and classification systems, that data is categorized as *structured*. Security tools exist for both forms of data, but structured data tends to be less complicated to identify and safeguard.

The compilation of codes and classification systems culminates in various standards for the common formats and definitions for important data. With all of the complexity between healthcare information technologies, interoperability and systems integration depend on sharing information and collaboration. Standards for the data include rules and procedures that organizations must adopt to share the information appropriately and efficiently. HIPAA is an example of a large set of standards meant to secure and control information exchanges of PHI.

Diagnosis-Related Group (DRG)

A DRG is a classification system used for quality of care and reimbursement matters. It is the basis of the US healthcare system reimbursement under Medicare plans. Patients are classified using DRGs, which helps to identify and organize the types of patients and conditions a healthcare organization treats into cohorts of common diagnoses, also known as a *case mix*. The DRG classification system can standardize the costs incurred by a provider, which influences billing and reimbursements. The following components are used to determine case mix as defined by the US Centers for Medicare and Medicaid Services (CMS):

- **Severity of illness**   A measure of the mortality or incapacity for a patient with a specific disease.

- **Prognosis**   A prediction of the likely outcome of a diagnosis. Included in the prognosis is any probability for changes in severity, positive or negative. Prognosis also consists of an estimate of the patient's quality of life and estimated chances for survival.

- **Treatment difficulty**   Consideration for the complexity or inability for a provider to accurately provide prognosis when examining a patient. The case mix considers the problems that result in treatment including the need to care for the patient very closely until more certainty is obtained.

- **Need for intervention**   The possible outcomes if no intervention to the illness happens.

- **Resource intensity**   Based on a specific illness, the amount of diagnostic, therapeutic, and bed services that are needed to properly treat the patient.

DRGs are designed to replace reimbursement based on fee-for-service billing with the Prospective Payment System (PPS), which uses DRGs and predetermined reimbursement rates for hospitals for services and treatment of specific conditions and to help determine prospective payment rates. There are more than 500 DRG classifications—for example, hernia procedures for a patient age 0 to 17 and fracture of femurs are two examples of DRG classifications. Within a DRG, services and processes should be similar and standard across any group of patients with a particular condition. Adjustments are made for the hospital's case mix, as mentioned earlier, which is a way to account for differences in consumption of resources. Provider organizations are expected to adjust practice patterns to reduce variations that have minimal, if any, demonstrated clinical value. The provider assumes risk for any additional costs that exceed the DRG rate.

Because of concerns with PPSs, other arrangements have been formulated. For example, because of claims that hospitals were discharging patients too early because of DRG guidelines, financing mechanisms known as *bundled payments* emerged. In this model, payers and providers share risk at a more episodic level or per clinical case, tailoring the reimbursements to a specific patient care experience. Another example of a compromise between fee-for-service and lump-sum DRG reimbursements is Accountable Care Organizations (ACOs). In the ACO model, a willing coalition of physicians, healthcare organizations, and other provider groups agree to work together to deliver high-quality care and share financial risk for a common group of patients. ACOs were endorsed by the ACA, and CMS administers the reimbursement program. The ACO is a fee-for-service model, but the use of quality indicators and cost-savings approaches are rewarded with financial incentives such as bonuses for providers.

International Classification of Diseases (ICD)

The International Statistical Classification of Diseases and Related Health Problems, commonly abbreviated to ICD, is the foremost and most widely known hierarchal medical classification system. It is managed under the purview of the World Health Organization (WHO) to categorize diseases so that morbidity and mortality rates can be tracked and reported. The use of ICD codes—14,000 in total—is significant in the digitization of healthcare records and electronic record systems.

For example, code 382.9 is used for "unspecified otitis media," a disorder characterized by inflammation, swelling, and redness in the middle ear. Instead of having to provide all that verbiage, medical billers can communicate the details of the diagnosis for the purposes of payment with a simple number up to six digits long that is internationally understood. Beyond facilitating the reimbursement of healthcare services, standardized codes make data analysis possible by providers and payers alike. ICD classifications of diagnoses and procedures are also suited for output reporting to regulators and for data analysis functions, where data aggregation is advantageous. The resource use and quality of healthcare can be improved by using ICD codes and data analytics to reduce unnecessary tests and services, and health status outcomes can be obtained and compared.

CMS mandated ICD-10 (tenth revision) adoption in the United States as of October 2015. However, because of concerns about the amount of codes, complexity, and cost of implementation, the United States uses a modified version of ICD-10. Published as "ICD-10 Clinical Modification" (ICD-10-CM) and a procedural classification called "ICD-10 Procedure Coding System" (ICD-10-PCS), these variations were developed by the National Center for Health Statistics (NCHS). In 2019, WHO approved ICD-11, which will go into effect in January 2022.

Systematized Nomenclature of Medicine Clinical Terms (SNOMED CT)

Another type of coding standard prevalent in healthcare is SNOMED CT. This is a repository of healthcare terms that is multilingual so it can be used worldwide. It facilitates a capability called semantic interoperability, which is important to the connection of SNOMED CT content to ICD-10, along with other coding standards. The repository contains over 311,000 discrete elements that are used to support accurate coding, retrieval, and analysis to comprehensively support clinical practices.

SNOMED CT is designed for the electronic exchange of clinical health information and is a required standard in the US Healthcare Information Technology Standards Panel and the Office of the National Coordinator for Health Information Technology (ONC) for certification of health information technology (health IT). A key use of SNOMED CT is to create interoperability between electronic health records (EHRs). In contrast to ICD, SNOMED CT is specifically used to describe extensive clinical terminology that is meant more as machine language to construct the EHR. ICD codes are useful for outputs such as medical billing and reporting in public health surveillance. SNOMED CT is a detailed terminology framework of concepts, descriptions, and relationships that works better for developing inputs into healthcare systems, which resemble data flow diagrams or flowcharts. Efforts are underway to integrate SNOMED CT and ICD, possibly when the ICD-11 standard is published.

EXAM TIP You will want to be clear on when coding systems are used: SNOMED CT (during patient care) and ICD (after patient care). SNOMED CT is human language and ICD is numbers and letters.

Additional Coding Systems

Several other coding systems and standards have complementary or specific uses in healthcare. The following sections provide an introductory view of several that serve an administrative and clinical purpose for classification of payment, treatment, and healthcare operations. These may also be imperative for the continued digitization of healthcare information.

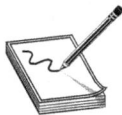

NOTE To increase interoperability of disparate coding systems, the US National Library of Medicine (NLM) has developed the Unified Medical Language System (UMLS) component Metathesaurus, a biomedical thesaurus that attempts to map data and language across standards such as SNOMED CT and ICD. (Such data mapping does not imply that the terms involved are synonymous, however.) The NLM identifies relationships between about 150 source vocabularies to improve the accuracy of current medical practices and electronic data exchange among disparate information sources and databases.

Logical Observation Identifiers Names and Codes (LOINC)

LOINC is a widely accepted coding system specially formulated for identifying laboratory and clinical observations. To be able to exchange observations and measurements electronically across multiple independent lab systems, LOINC uses a universal code system with a maximum field size of seven characters. This results in more than 71,000 LOINC values, which enable data transfer among providers, clinical laboratories, and public health authorities.

Ambulatory Patient Group (APG)

This classification system is used in outpatient services reimbursement. Hospitals may use it for emergency room care that does not become an inpatient admission. Otherwise, the system is used in settings such as same-day surgery clinics and primary care offices. It classifies patients into more than 300 outpatient services. The purpose of the APG system is to outline the resources required to provide necessary care. It is analogous to DRG, which classifies inpatient services

Ambulatory Payment Classification (APC)

APC is mainly a US coding system that is used for Medicare reimbursement. It is applicable only to hospitals and is used as an outpatient prospective payment system. As the DRG system is used to bill inpatient services, when an emergency room or hospital-based service does not lead to a patient admission, outpatients services are billed to Medicare using the APC system. The APC system accounts for every resource used in the outpatient visit. The standard is being considered for wider use in US states under Medicaid reimbursement as well as some private third-party insurers.

Resource Utilization Groups (RUG)

These are commonly used in US long-term care or skilled nursing facilities reimbursed by Medicare and Medicaid. The RUG system consists of categories that reflect levels of resource needs to facilitate risk adjustment and complexity of care factors specific to long-term care. The primary use is for insurance billing purposes. There are 44 classifications that describe variables affecting care, such as patient status and the care needed by activity levels, underlying illnesses, the complexity of the care, and patient cognitive status.

Current Procedural Terminology (CPT)

The CPT system is used by all US healthcare payers and providers to document and report medical, surgical, radiology, laboratory, anesthesiology, and evaluation and management (E/M) services. The CPT is a five-character code that supports reimbursement by listing services provided. The initial version was published by the American Medical Association (AMA) in 1966, and the codes are updated every year. The rules for assigning CPT codes are complex, and there can be variation in how much a provider is reimbursed based on the accuracy and completeness of CPT coding. There are three categories of CPT codes:

- **Category I**   Numeric codes that start at 00100 and end at 99499 and describe a healthcare service and procedure.

- **Category II** Alphanumeric codes that assist with measuring clinical performance if used. They are not mandatory.
- **Category III** Provisional codes used to track emerging technology, procedures, and services.

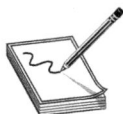

NOTE CMS and the AMA provide for two-character modifiers that can be added to CPT codes to report distinctive situations and to clarify the description of the procedure.

National Drug Code (NDC)

As required by the US Federal Food, Drug, and Cosmetic Act (FD&C Act), drug products are assigned a unique code—an NDC—that is ten or eleven digits in three distinct segments. The codes and corresponding drug identifications are listed in a repository called the NDC Directory, which is maintained by the Food and Drug Administration (FDA). The information in the NDC Directory is updated every day and is used worldwide to identify specific products and sizes by manufacturer. Not every drug has a corresponding NDC; only those that are submitted to the directory and marketed for human use.

CAUTION The FDA makes it clear that just because a drug is found in the NDC Directory it does not mean the FDA has evaluated the data or certified the drug.

Healthcare Common Procedure Coding System (HCPCS)

The Healthcare Common Procedure Coding System (HCPCS) is used much like the ICD system to accomplish medical coding. HCPCS (nicknamed "hick picks") is an outpatient system used to ensure that hospital procedures and physician services are reported and processed in an orderly and consistent manner. (The ICD system is used in some outpatient scenarios, but all inpatient coding.) There are two levels of HCPCS codes. Level 1 codes are, in essence, CPT codes which, as explained earlier, describe products and services healthcare providers deliver. Level 2 codes are used for additional procedures and materials that are not included in Level 1 codes. Examples of items included in Level 2 codes are medical equipment, medical devices, or medical transport.

Revenue Cycle

An understanding of the financial components of healthcare delivery may help you better understand and build security cost–benefit analyses in your organization. The revenue cycle in healthcare includes billing, payment, and reimbursement. Without attention to resource allocation and fair compensation for healthcare services, these services would not happen—at least they would not happen to the extent that the healthcare system of today would have state-of-the-art technology, highly trained professionals, and well-apportioned facilities available.

Claims Processing and Third-Party Payers

If a third party is the payer for healthcare services, claims processing comes into play. For example, in a simplified patient-provider transaction, the provider may charge $100 for a service, and the patient may pay a $25 copay. The remainder of the bill, $75, is sent to the third-party payer as a claim against the insurance or government reimbursement.

The claims process actually begins prior to the patient's appointment. Preapproval is often required, in which the third-party payer must authorize the doctor visit, all or a portion of the services, and any of the recommended follow-up care. Without preapproval, third-party payers can reduce the amount of reimbursement owed, or they may even deny the claim. The patient would then become fully responsible for paying the bill in its entirety.

With preapproval, the normal process for claims would include the physician sending the bill (after copay) to the third-party claims-processing center. Although providers can submit claims manually on paper forms, they more commonly file the claims electronically. Estimates show that electronic claims are three times less expensive than submitting via paper. However, securing the electronic transaction is a concern for healthcare information privacy and security. The claims-processing center compares the patient information and any relevant documentation of the services provided to the explanation of benefits (the policy terms and conditions). Once the third party determines all preapproved services were delivered and covered in the policy, it will submit payment for the remaining balance to the physician.

Payment Models

In the healthcare revenue cycle, claims processing leads to payment or reimbursement for services. The models for these payments have distinct features. In the dominant model, fee-for-service, providers are paid for each service rendered to a patient. This model is used in managed-care plans or when a government payer is involved. Without reiterating how those models work, variations of the fee-for-service model exist and should be understood by healthcare employees. These are discussed in the following sections.

Bundled Payment

Bundled payment is a more predetermined payment model than fee-for-service. In this model, a healthcare provider is compensated based on expected costs for each acute-care episode, not necessarily the actual costs. The parameters of the event, however, are determined by clinical judgment. The episode must have a clear beginning and end, require defined services, and have established clinical guidelines that allow for best practices. Conditions such as cataract surgery, services for end-stage renal disease, and coronary artery bypass grafting (CABG) to improve blood flow to the heart are bundle payment candidates. Bundled payments are central to any healthcare reform debate (in the United States) because of their ability to help reduce healthcare costs, and they are championed by physicians and administrators alike.

Capitation

An even more predetermined compensation model, capitation is a payment arrangement of a set amount for each person covered by the third-party payer. Providers agree in advance to accept a capitated amount, which is a fixed and predetermined payment amount for each person, based on a specified time period in which that person seeks care. A common way to describe this is "per member, per month" system for the provisions of capitation and coverage to which a healthcare provider agrees. To be clear, capitation does not relate to a specific episode of care or event, like fee-for-service and bundled payments. The average expected amount of care for each member that the payer disburses is calculated, and the payer enlists providers that agree to accept this payment. Providers accept a level of risk that they will be able to provide adequate care at some funding amount less than the capitated amount to therefore make a profit. If the amount of care exceeds the capitated amount, the provider takes the loss for excess spending—even if the care was clinically necessary.

The US Evolving Payment Model

Even with alternatives to fee-for-service, additional models of payment (sometimes discussed as part of healthcare reform in the United States) are worth mentioning. The patient-centered medical home (PCMH) and the accountable-care organization (ACO) models are presented here.

In the PCMH model, patient treatment is coordinated by a primary-care manager who makes sure the patient receives appropriate levels of care. This can mean that clinically necessary referrals to specialists or diagnostic tests are vetted by the primary-care manager. As they are approved, these treatments, tests, and referrals are explained to the patient to reduce confusion and help increase the likelihood of patient compliance. Confusion and lack of patient compliance are issues that increase waste and redundancy.

PCMH has a goal of building a relationship for the benefit of the patient that includes physicians, selected family members, and the patient. There is a high degree of integration of information technology and health information exchange (requiring privacy and security considerations). All of these attempt to provide the right care at the right time at the best value from both the perspective of the patient and the provider (healthcare organization).

Physicians, hospitals, and other relevant health service professionals are testing a model that joins them together contractually to provide a broad set of healthcare services. This is an ACO, which is formally organized and applicable currently to Medicare patients only. Even though the ACO may not consist of organizations within the same corporate structure, the intent is to deliver seamless, coordinated care. In fact, as the name states, within the framework of the ACO contract, this organization is accountable to providing such care.

The payment model in healthcare must change from fee-for-service to something more efficient and effective. Churning out services for chronic diseases without regard to improving outcomes can no longer be reimbursed. An ACO (and the PCMH) model strives to improve quality and reduce hospital admissions (and readmissions) and emergency-room visits. In return, costs are contained, and the participating providers can share in the savings.

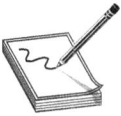

NOTE A common term used to describe the payment models that are being developed is the "value-based payment modifier" (VBPM) model. In the United States, many payment approaches are underway or under development that involve federal and state governments. Other programs are designed by payers of healthcare in the private sector. Generally, the models pay physicians, hospitals, medical groups, and other healthcare providers based on measures including quality, efficiency, cost, and positive patient experience.

Medical Billing

An important component of the healthcare revenue cycle, medical billing is how healthcare providers initiate the process for payment. A claim is generated based on the services and products provided and a medical billing professional sends the payment request to payers, typically a healthcare insurance company, the government, or the individual. Providers may employ a couple different strategies in submitting their bills (or claims for payment). Depending on the size of the provider organization, larger practices tend to submit bills electronically to the payer. In smaller practices, it is more common for the forms to be completed on paper. Because the analog data must be converted to digital before submission, an entity called a clearinghouse receives these paper forms from multiple small practices, converts them to digital files, and submits them to the various payers.

A clearinghouse is not a healthcare provider; it is an entity that works in the middle of the transaction between a healthcare provider and whomever is providing payment or reimbursement. The clearinghouse function is not limited to changing paper-based information to digital. It also serves to improve handling claims and revenue collection of the provider by simplifying the process. For a small practice, having most, if not all, bills rejected because the data fields do not conform to the payers' proprietary format can cause significant financial distress, maybe even bankruptcy. Clearinghouses can serve a significant role in increasing efficiency and reducing errors.

Assuming the data elements are all present and in the correct formatting, another hurdle that providers must overcome in the billing process is medical necessity. Payers review bills to make sure the patient was covered and the services were a medical necessity. The guidelines for medical necessity are established by different state agencies and even by each payer, but all should be located in the federal Medicare statute, which outlines what is reasonable and necessary. In the event a service is deemed not a medical necessity, the claim is denied or rejected, and the provider is notified, usually in the form of explanation of benefits (EOB) or electronic remittance advice (ERA), which also explains why the claim was returned unpaid.

It is clear that in the United States, medical billing is a complex process with almost countless payers and oft-changing regulations. Many argue that this results in measurable additional administrative waste generated in the healthcare system. The administrative burden is necessary, however, and securing these transactions starts with understanding the importance of the interconnections.

Transaction Standards

From the various coding standards such as ICD-10 and CPT, we must be aware that the communication of the codes between provider and payer aligns to transaction standards. As we alluded to in the previous section, rejection of claims happens pretty regularly. Common reasons for rejection are incorrect codes and sometimes non-standard code use. Assuming proper use of transaction standards, you will want to be familiar with how to secure their transfer for continuous and reliable business and clinical operations.

HIPAA Transaction and Code Sets (TCS)

Healthcare information protection professionals are likely aware of the sections of the Health Insurance Portability and Accountability Act (HIPAA) that cover privacy and security standards, just two of the four standards or rules that make up HIPAA. The other sections cover identifiers and transactions and code sets.

The electronic transfer of healthcare information generates information security concerns, so you must have an awareness of this area. The Identifier Rule in HIPAA mandates that uniform identifiers be used for health insurance plans, providers, employers, and patients to facilitate electronic transfer of information. HIPAA TCS are associated rules that also standardize the electronic exchange of healthcare information. The exchanges are computer-to-computer and need no human involvement. The underlying processes are based on electronic data interchange (EDI) standards. The application of this standardizes what types of codes healthcare practitioners use when communicating with payers. For example, HIPAA TCS sets CPT as the standard for procedure codes and ICD as the standard for diagnoses. There are competing code frameworks, but HIPAA TCS forces adoption of one over another. With the Identifier Rule, HIPAA TCS is intended to produce efficiency and cost reduction as part of a concept called "administrative simplification."

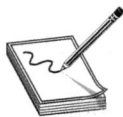

NOTE To improve the efficiency and effectiveness of the healthcare system, Administrative Simplification is a significant mandate that impacts security requirements as the provisions direct standards for TCS and unique identifiers. All the Administrative Simplification Rules are located at US 45 CFR Parts 160, 162, and 164.[13]

ASC X12N Claim Protocol

The American National Standards Institute (ANSI) Accredited Standards Committee (ASC) X12 developed this protocol for HIPAA transactions as part of a larger body of work for all electronic transactions. Many industries including healthcare use X12-based standards as well as adopting X12 XML schemas as they emerge. There are over 315 X12-based standards. X12N—note the N—is the nomenclature used for healthcare claims. As part of administrative simplification, electronic transaction standards mandated or proposed under HIPAA are also compliant with X12 standards. One way to think of the ANSI format is as a form that consists of the HIPAA TCS standards that is then transmitted. The following list is a sample of X12N electronic transaction formats that are part of HIPAA TCS standards:

- Health Care Claims or Equivalent Encounter Information (X12N 837)
- Eligibility for a Health Plan (X12N 270/271)
- Referral Certification and Authorization (X12N 278 or NCPDP for retail pharmacy)
- Health Care Claim Status (X12N 276/277)
- Enrollment and Disenrollment in a Health Plan (X12N 834)
- Health Care Payment and Remittance Advice (X12N 835)
- Health Plan Premium Payments (X12N 820)
- Coordination of Benefits (X12N 837 or NCPDP for retail pharmacy)

ANSI chartered the ASC to oversee the evolution of the X12 standard. ASC X12 version 5010 is the current protocol.

National Uniform Billing Committee (NUBC)

In 1975, the AHA chartered the NUBC because they recognized the need for providers and payers to have and use a common billing form with standardized data. The NUBC was started with the responsibility to create and manage the streamlined billing components. The first uniform bill (UB) was published in 1982 as UB-82, which was updated a decade later by UB-92 after an eight-year hold on any changes during initial adoption. This was the standard for paper-based medical billing until 2004, when UB-04 was available. This version of the standard medical claims form was digitized to support electronic transmission. The current version has 81 separate fields known as form locators (FLs). Each FL has a specific purpose, but some FLs are currently not used.

Reimbursement

Reimbursement is the final step of the revenue cycle. As claims are processed and bills are submitted (and resubmitted), the desired outcome from the provider's perspective is to receive reimbursement for the cost of the healthcare. In a word, reimbursement is repayment for expenses incurred. It is uncommon for reimbursement to equal expenses, however. Healthcare providers and payers continually work together to set rates of reimbursement and adjust them against a standard loosely defined as charges that are "usual, customary, and reasonable." That standard is increasingly squeezed to lower reimbursement rates, which constrains providers that may have capital investments that rely on the margin between cost and repayment. But the counterargument (from payers) is that consistently squeezing reimbursement rates encourages providers to be more efficient and productive.

Workflow Management

Workflow management in the healthcare setting describes the various clinical and business processes providers use. These processes are complex and dynamic. To reduce cost and improve quality, there are efforts to streamline, automate, and reengineer workflow processes with which you should become familiar. Many have information security implications, because with electronic information and EHRs, sensitive data moves through the information system. Often healthcare organizations interoperate, merge, or otherwise create a larger scale of operations. In these cases, workflow management may have information protection challenges in connecting legacy systems, for example. Organizational management of workflow leads to greater efficiency, better access to quality healthcare, and improved patient safety across care settings.

Clinical Workflow

Clinical workflow includes the various processes and patterns of actions clinicians use to deliver healthcare. With regard to electronic information and EHRs, clinical workflow describes how the data moves through the information system, by whom, to whom, when, and how often. Proper management of the workflow assists with compliance and achievement of practice objectives for quality and efficiency. Using health information systems to automate various clinical workflows can have a positive impact on clinical outcomes, minimize medical errors, and reduce costs over time compared to manual processing.

Examples of clinical workflow components include actions taken to register a patient, document patient information gathered during an appointment, develop a treatment plan, prescribe any follow-up tests and medications, provide patient education material, schedule future visits, and process bills or claims, among others. Many processes and subprocesses are involved as a patient moves through the physical organization. The need for electronic data related to these actions must also operate in a synchronized, parallel fashion through the information systems.

Figure 1-4 depicts the general idea of clinical workflow. The figure is intended to illustrate the integrated process involving clinicians, administrative personnel, and technicians, and the example used is not comprehensive. Because there are more interactions and participants in the typical clinical workflow, a single diagram probably cannot depict the entirety of the typical clinical workflow.

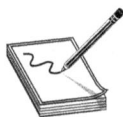

NOTE Workflow management is often accomplished using a workflow management system (WMS). A WMS enables interaction between software, information technologies, telecommunications, and human resources and is key to reducing manual processes and supporting business process reengineering. The healthcare delivery system has benefited from electronic signatures, a significant component made possible by WMS.

Business Process Reengineering (BPR)

Business process reengineering is the review and transformation of central business processes to improve performance measures such as throughput, quality, and efficiency. These improvements typically come from automation of manual processes or the implementation of a new technology. The change is characterized as dramatic, with outcomes that are significant versus incremental. An example is the use of radio-frequency

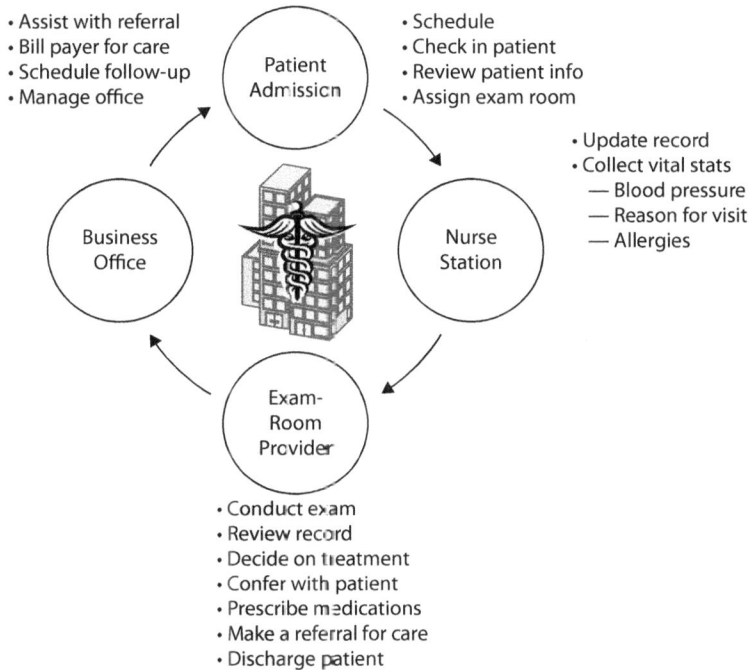

Figure 1-4 Clinical workflow

identification (RFID) logistics systems to track patients, supplies, and equipment via a networked information system.

Some major activities of BPR:

- Focus centrally on customer requirements
- Enable the core process improvements, typically with information technology
- Create business teams with multidepartment representation responsible for an entire process
- Challenge status quo within the organization
- Make the process improvements an enterprise-wide effort

BPR has a continuous cycle that an organization can use to address improvement opportunities. That lifecycle is depicted in Figure 1-5. Notice the lack of a distinct start and stop timeline—BPR should be part of a broader, continuous improvement program in the complex and dynamic healthcare organizational environment.

CAUTION A related concept, business process improvement (BPI) is similar to BPR in use today, except that changes to achieve efficiency and effectiveness do not require complete overhaul of the process in question.

Figure 1-5
BPR lifecycle

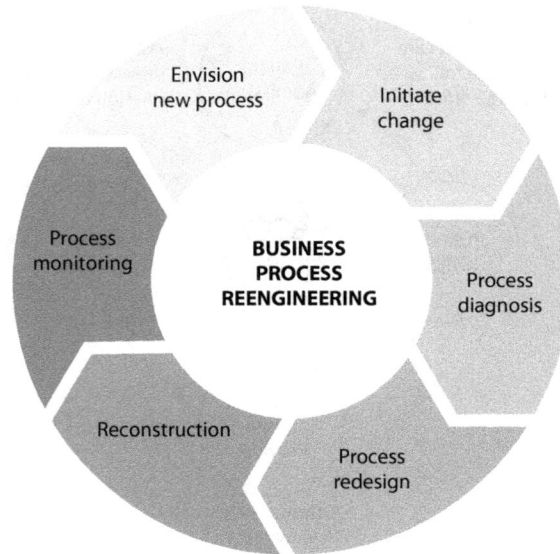

Value Stream Mapping (VSM)

As a business process improvement concept, value stream mapping is rooted in lean-management techniques made popular by Toyota decades ago. VSM is a way to gain improvement by assessing current processes and making changes to arrive at a desired state at a designated time. The focus that leads to improvement involves eliminating waste as much as possible. Although the concept emerged from the manufacturing industry, it has been used in the healthcare environment. The seven categories of waste listed here certainly pertain to healthcare organizations, indicating that value streaming can be relevant and effective in healthcare:

- **Faster-than-necessary pace**   This refers to overproduction, when too much of a good or service is created. The impact is a damaged production flow, quality, and productivity. At the end of the process, storage is required and lead time wastes result.

- **Waiting**   This is the time wasted while goods are not being transported or worked on.

- **Conveyance**   This refers to the transport process by which goods are moved around; specifically important are any instances of double-handling and excessive movement.

- **Processing**   This refers to an overly complex solution for a simple procedure and includes unsafe production. The impact of this category of waste is poor layout and communication and unnecessary motion.

- **Excess stock**   Surplus levels of unnecessary inventory results in greater lead times, increased difficulty identifying problems, and significant storage costs.

- **Unnecessary motion**   Ergonomic waste is to be avoided and requires employees to use excess energy such as picking up objects, bending, or stretching.
- **Correction of mistakes**   Avoid any cost associated with defects or the resources required to correct them.

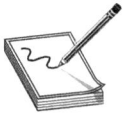

NOTE   You should notice the themes that emerge in this discussion. In terms of proper information protection, value stream mapping would align with building in security controls during any relevant process rather than attempting to bolt them on (repair defects) after the fact.

Regulatory Environment

Healthcare is a highly regulated industry. The US healthcare industry's influential regulators include the US Department of Health and Human Services (HHS), the Centers for Medicare and Medicaid Services (CMS), the Food and Drug Administration (FDA), and the Centers for Disease Control and Prevention (CDC), to name a few. These are just a sample of the government entities with authority to regulate healthcare organizations. These regulators have a principal responsibility over enforcing the law as well as clarifying the guidance they implement. Each plays an important and distinct role as the laws they enact have a specific purpose and scope, although there are examples of overlap.

Federal regulators work in tandem with state level legislatures and local lawmakers such as health departments and state insurance commissioners. In many cases, state governments have enacted legislation that has surpassed or satisfied gaps in federal regulations for healthcare. An example is the state of Massachusetts that mandated health insurance coverage for all its citizens in 2006, before the federal ACA. The Massachusetts law has been amended in several ways since then to make it consistent with the ACA, and for other reasons.

The regulatory environment is not limited to government agencies enforcing laws. Healthcare is impacted by other types of regulatory actors as well, including agencies that assess or audit the payers and providers against standards and acceptable practices. Some standards are mandatory, and others are voluntary, such as standards created by the Joint Commission, formerly the Joint Commission on Accreditation of Healthcare Organizations (JCAHO). However, even voluntary standards often can have the same impact as legal requirements. In the case of the Joint Commission, healthcare organizations have determined that absent JC accreditation (meeting the JC standards) may have a detrimental effect on government reimbursement, payer network inclusion, or patient perceptions.

Another example of external forces that impact healthcare from a regulatory aspect is litigation. From time to time, a legal case will be brought against healthcare organizations. Consider anti-trust cases, for example. Imagine that an independent physician organization brings suit against a large integrated health system that yields influence on those physicians to refer exclusively to the health system or risk some form of penalty later.

Figure 1-6 shows some examples of regulatory pressures that impact healthcare. From a healthcare information protection perspective, you will be most concerned with laws such as HIPAA, and, if you are working in or with member states of the European Union

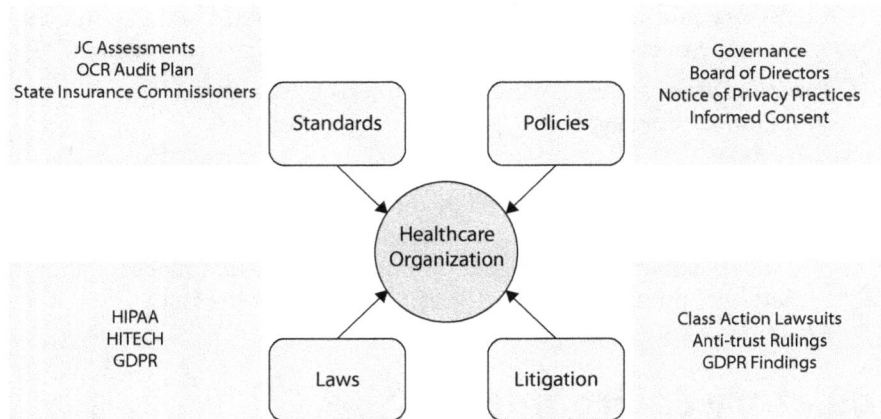

Figure 1-6   Some of the regulatory forces that influence healthcare organizations

(EU), the General Data Protection Regulation (GDPR). Additionally, you will spend the most time learning and adhering to state, local, and organizational regulatory guidance in the form of laws as well as policies and procedures. We will cover this topic in greater depth in Chapter 4. For now, it is enough to have a foundational view that healthcare delivery is accomplished only by simultaneously providing quality patient care, meeting business objectives, and complying with myriad regulatory impacts.

EXAM TIP   For the exam, you should know that the ACA, aka Obamacare, has increased the pace of mergers and acquisitions of healthcare organizations. It is relevant to the information protection professional because these organizational changes involve risk assessment and management of interconnections of legacy systems and other third-party relationships, particularly integration of EHRs.

Patient Rights

Another aspect of the regulatory environment is the protection of patients from various types of harm—for our purposes, harm from unauthorized access to information, loss of sensitive data, and lack of data availability. In fact, some types of cybersecurity issues can result in adverse patient care events. Regulatory oversight helps to provide assurance for patients and the communities in which providers deliver care.

Patient rights are expectations patients should have and obligations providers must respect. They can be written into laws such as the HIPAA Privacy and Security Rules. Patient rights can be specific to an organization and codified in organizational policy. Typically, a patient would receive a copy of relevant patient rights, or they are made available on the provider's web sites.

Following are some examples of patient rights that are applicable to information protection concerns:

- You must get a written explanation of how the provider may use, store, and share the information.

- You must be provided access to your records, obtain copies, and request changes.

- The provider must allow you to limit use or disclosure of your information outside of regular healthcare treatment, payment, and operations.

- The provider must notify you in the event of any information security breaches that are reportable under HIPAA breach notification law.

Patient Care and Safety

Yet another reason why the healthcare industry is regulated so extensively is because of the importance of quality patient care and the need for patient safety. Healthcare information security can be related to these concerns in that data breaches, denial of service (DoS) attacks, and ransomware attacks are just a few of the potential threats to healthcare information security that could negatively impact the quality of patient care and endanger the patient. The potential for harm has been recognized by US regulators. For example, to warn against manipulation of clinical systems and clinical data or even manipulation to patient data, the FDA and the US Department of Homeland Security's Industrial Control Systems Cyber Emergency Response Team (ICS-CERT) issued an alert in 2015, based on a vulnerability where an infusion system could permit an attacker to remotely control a device and alter therapy administration.

The Cybersecurity Information Sharing Act (CISA) was published in an attempt to address the growing threats from cyberattackers in the United States by improving the opportunities for government and private organizations to exchange cybersecurity-related information. This information sharing between government agencies and providers has several benefits specific to healthcare, one of which is reducing the likelihood that a vulnerability in a clinical system or medical device can be exploited. Regulators have begun to enable an environment where risk data can be shared. A notable group working on increased public–private partnerships in healthcare information security is the Health Care Industry Cybersecurity (HCIC) Task Force. The task force members represent a wide variety of government and private sector organizations within the healthcare and public health sector. Participation comes from healthcare providers and payers as well as stakeholders such as privacy advocates and academic researchers. Some of the key participant groups are medical device manufacturers and industry groups related to medical device security. The task force recognizes the connection between healthcare information security and the impact on patient care. It highlighted the following six imperatives in its report to Congress,[14] along with recommendations for best courses of action for public–private partnerships to make improvements:

- Define and streamline leadership, governance, and expectations for healthcare industry cybersecurity

- Increase the security and resilience of medical devices and health IT

- Develop the healthcare workforce capacity necessary to prioritize and ensure cybersecurity awareness and technical capabilities
- Increase healthcare industry readiness through improved cybersecurity awareness and education
- Identify mechanisms to protect R&D efforts and intellectual property from attacks or exposure
- Improve information sharing of industry threats, risks, and mitigations

Public Health Reporting

Sometimes, healthcare organizations collect information from patients that is legitimately needed by public health officials. These are third parties that are not vendors but are most likely government agencies. In the United States, the HIPAA Privacy Rule makes provisions for healthcare organizations to legally disclose protected health information to public health and safety agencies for the benefit of public health. Provisions regarding public health reporting in the United States can be complex and vary among jurisdictions. Generally, public health requires disclosure to identify threats to the health and safety of the total community and individuals. Along with reporting of births or deaths, the Department of HHS in the United States allows public health reporting that consists of the following:[15]

- Child abuse or neglect
- Quality, safety, or effectiveness of a product or activity regulated by the FDA
- Persons at risk of contracting or spreading a disease
- Immunizations, disease registrations (such as cancer), and substance abuse
- Workplace medical surveillance when healthcare is provided at the request of the employer or as a member of the employer's workforce

Similar provisions for public health reporting exist in the EU as well, according to the GDPR, which allows public health reporting for data controllers "pursuant to legal obligation of the controller under GDPR Article 6(1)(c)" and (when) "processing necessary for reasons of public interest in the area of public health . . . such as ensuring high standards of quality and safety of healthcare and of medicinal products" under GDPR Article 9(2)(i)."[16] Allowances for public health reporting is an almost universal exception to the information protection guidelines.

Even though healthcare organizations are generally permitted (and often required) to disclose patient information for public health reporting purposes, there are still things to consider before disclosure. The information provided should be limited to only what is required. In the United States, HIPAA provides guidance for minimum necessary uses and disclosures of and requests for PHI—that is, healthcare organizations must take reasonable precautions to disclose the minimum amount of PHI necessary to accomplish the public health purpose.

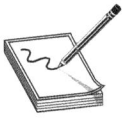

NOTE Public health agencies are not organizations directly subject to HIPAA. However, some activities are subject to the same privacy and security rules. In fact, healthcare organizations are cautious to disclose patient information under the exceptions allowed for in HIPAA. In many cases, they apply equal safeguards as an abundance of caution.

Clinical Research

Clinical research is the investigation of wellbeing and disease in individuals. It is the way we figure out how to prevent, diagnose, and treat illness. Clinical research depicts a wide range of components of examination and study. Basically, it includes human study participants and applies basic research done in labs into new medicines and data to improve patient care. Clinical trials are used for research in the study of disease transmission, physiology and pathophysiology, health services, education, outcomes, and mental health. The safety and effectiveness of treatments and healthcare interventions is known today because of appropriate clinical research. Randomized controlled trials are the basis for "evidence-based medicine." Appropriate clinical research is defined by standards and measures that are collectively known as Good Clinical Research Practice (GCP).

EXAM TIP Remember that a clinical trial is not the same thing as medical care. In a clinical trial, a defined protocol for intervention is followed for all participants. The intervention is not altered for an individual patient's response. Medical care is treatment specific to one patient.

Good Clinical Research Practice (GCP)

To conduct research involving human subjects, the principles of GCP must be followed. There is generally accepted concurrence that GCP is critical to the ethical conduct of clinical research. Human subject protection (HSP) is a core component of GCP. The FDA publishes regulations and procedural guidance on the conduct of clinical trials. In the United States, the FDA has overseen regulatory matters in GCP and has contributed to the international adoption of GCP and HSP principles.

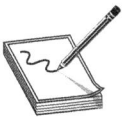

NOTE Through GCP, the public can be more confident that the rights of research participants are respected and their safety is assured. The requirements for GCP are intended to also preserve the integrity of clinical research data.

From an information protection perspective, clinical research differs from public health reporting in terms of use and disclosure of the PHI. Prior consent from participants is not always feasible or possible. In those cases, researchers in the United States can use an internal institutional review board (IRB) or a privacy board to obtain a waiver to any required patient consent. This is a very significant concept that can enable researchers to comply with the HIPAA Privacy Rule and other HSP guidance when researchers need permission. Increased disclosure of patient information is authorized for purposes of clinical research under HIPAA. When the information is used for clinical research, controls that would be required under HIPAA may be absent. You should be aware of the impact of clinical research on any data use scenario. A good IRB or privacy board will use documented protocols and controls to safeguard the protected health information as well as the privacy of research participants. Those would incorporate assurances that the use or disclosure of the patient information adds only a minimum of risk to privacy for the individual. An IRB or privacy board provides oversight in these cases and requires researchers to have the following:

- Alternative controls planned or in place to safeguard protected health information
- Suitable records disposal and destruction plans for patient information when it's no longer needed
- Written statements to prohibit reuse or disclosure of patient information unless permitted by law or the IRB or privacy board
- Sound reasons for why the research is not possible without a waiver to permit access to and use of the patient information

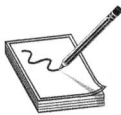

NOTE   The IRB or privacy board will also require a plan for any information that must be kept after the current research to support future research or legal requirements.

An IRB operates under the principles of the Belmont Report, which was written by the National Commission for the Protection of Human Subjects of Biomedical and Behavioral Research as an outcome of the National Research Act of 1974. The Commission was established to examine what fundamental underlying ethical principles should be present in this type of research. The Belmont Report attempts to summarize the findings by the Commission as it disclosed the behaviors the researchers exhibited.

EXAM TIP   You should understand that the Belmont Report is another example of the regulatory environment in the United States and is likewise focused on patient protections. In the Belmont Report, patient protections in clinical research comprise three core principles: respect for persons, beneficence, and justice. This is very similar to how regulators enact guidance for data confidentiality, integrity, and availability in HIPAA. Information protections are present in both and central to regulators' objective for patient safety.

Some clinical research is supplied to a healthcare organization through a third party called a contract research organization (CRO). A CRO provides support to healthcare organizations conducting very specialized types of biopharmaceutical development, pre-clinical research, clinical trials management, and drug safety. For the most part, these advanced research types are done by leading pharmaceutical, biotechnology, and medical device industry companies. The CROs also support academic medical centers, the government, and international organizations. The ability to partner with CROs enables the development and evaluation of all the various trials of safety and efficacy, but not have to have internal staff from the healthcare organization dedicated to the research. For medical devices, the CRO gathers clinical data to support an FDA regulatory premarket submission, drive product adoption, support product reimbursement, or monitor post-market product use. It brings expertise and streamlined processes at a much more cost-effective level than what would be experienced by the healthcare organization if it had to do the same processes itself.

De-identification of Patient Information

Removing any individually identifiable information from the data set helps us be reasonably certain no one can identify someone else based on the remaining information. There are two ways to do this: First is expert determination, in which a person trained in de-identification through complex processes concludes that the algorithms used and the resulting data are sufficiently anonymized and the risk of identification minimal. The second way is simply to remove completely these same categories of identifiable data, which, under the HIPAA Privacy Rule, is called the safe harbor method.

EXAM TIP For the exam, keep in mind that an expert is not defined by current regulations. Relevant experience in statistical, mathematical, or other scientific domains can earn someone expert status. It is an assessment based on the expert's past performance and applicable training in health information de-identification methodologies.

The following list provides the standard categories and sources of data that may be individually identifiable information according to the National Institute of Standards and Technology (NIST) Special Publication (SP) 800-122.

- Name, such as full name, maiden name, mother's maiden name, or alias
- Personal identification number, such as Social Security number (SSN), passport number, driver's license number, taxpayer identification number, patient identification number, and financial account or credit card number
- Address information, such as street address or e-mail address
- Asset information, such as Internet Protocol (IP) or media access control address, or other host-specific persistent static identifier that consistently links to a particular person or small, well-defined group of people
- Telephone numbers, including mobile, business, and personal numbers
- Personal characteristics, including photographic image (especially of face or other distinguishing characteristic), X-rays, fingerprints, or other biometric image or template data (such as retina scan, voice signature, or facial geometry)
- Information identifying personally owned property, such as vehicle registration number or title number and related information

- Information about an individual that is linked or linkable to one of the above (such as date of birth, place of birth, race, religion, weight, activities, geographical indicators, employment information, medical information, education information, and financial information)

Additional health informatics standards in this area also call out risks related to rare data and small sample sizes. For example, ISO 25237, *Health Informatics – Pseudonymization,* contains principles and requirements for privacy protection using pseudonymization services (which replace PII fields with artificial IDs, or pseudonyms) for the protection of personal health information (see the "International Organization for Standardization (ISO) 25237:2017" sidebar). Organizations that perform pseudonymization or rely on organizations that perform such services may find this guidance very helpful. There are several clauses that are central to the ISO 25237 standard. These relate to de-identification components, such as streamlining down to one concept and method for pseudonymization. Other clauses outline the particular policy framework for pseudonymization with minimal requirements for re-identification. As a healthcare information privacy and security professional, you might be most interested in the clause that addresses the risk assessment processes for how effective pseudonymization is and how likely re-identification might be.

International Organization for Standardization (ISO) 25237:2017

ISO 25237:2017 is an example of an international standards document applicable to organizations that want to undertake de-identification or pseudonymization processes or to organizations that make a claim of trustworthiness for operations engaged in pseudonymization services. The guidance contains principles and requirements for privacy protection using pseudonymization services for the protection of personal health information.

Here are some relevant highlights from ISO 25237:2017:

- Defines one basic concept for pseudonymization
- Defines one basic methodology for pseudonymization services, including organizational and technical aspects
- Specifies a policy framework and minimal requirements for controlled re-identification
- Gives an overview of different use cases for pseudonymization that can be both reversible and irreversible
- Guides risk assessment for re-identification
- Provides an example of a system that uses de-identification
- Provides informative requirements for interoperability with regard to pseudonymization services
- Specifies a policy framework and minimal requirements for trustworthy practices for the operations of a pseudonymization service

Another source of guidance on de-identification is the Integrating the Healthcare Enterprise (IHE) "De-Identification Handbook." This material provides an integrated view of the design, approaches, and risks of de-identification as a goal. The end result is proper removal of PHI through various methods such as removing data elements and pseudonymization. The guide also covers re-identification. The general process must be customized and should be adapted to specific situations. There is no universal de-identification profile that fits every organization and situation for data needs. Specifically, this means that each reviewer must create a profile specific to the information being processed, applicable laws and regulations, organizational policies, the operational environment, and more. The design and operation of any de-identification profile or system must be validated and monitored. Validation should occur early in the design phase, again when the system is going live, and during operational use. The characteristics of many data sets change over time, and monitoring production de-identification systems helps ensure that they remain effective over time. It is also important to remember data that is appropriately de-identified for one purpose (such as a clinical trial) may not be correctly de-identified for a new use of the data (such as using the same data set for a public health database).

EXAM TIP When anonymizing data, results that are considered "outliers" can be so unique that they can actually be used to identify an individual. Here's an example: Consider a sample size of a small twelfth-grade class at the local high school (150 students). Anonymize any of the 18 individual identifiers as found in NIST SP 800-122, Section 2.2, that are present in the data set. Then you may be left with data elements such as height, weight, eye color, hair color, and immunizations received. Most likely, those individuals with red hair and blue eyes would be unique enough to be identifiable with just those aggregate (albeit anonymized) data elements. These elements would still require confidentiality protection.

Clinical researchers are afforded some flexibility in the ability to share information legally without gaining prior or additional patient consent. Some of the provisions researchers may apply to use or disclose protected health information without authorization by the research participant are listed here:

- **Limited data sets** Some of the patient information can be excluded, and what remains is the minimum number and types of identifiers needed, if any. You would usually have a data use agreement (DUA) in place for use of a limited data set that would also determine who needs to know the information and for what purposes.

- **Accounting of disclosures** Researchers must keep and be able to provide a record of all information disclosed, by whom, and to whom outside of the research organization (such as another research organization doing similar trials) during the life of the research.

- **Data use agreements** Before the use or disclosure of a limited data set to an external person or organization, the HIPAA Privacy Rule requires the use of a DUA, which outlines several provisions to protect the data because the limited data set is still PHI. The DUA must do the following:

  - Outline for what purpose the data is permitted to be used.

  - Identify authorized recipients and users of the data.

  - Limit additional, unintended uses once the information is disclosed. Exceptions for law enforcement reasons and specifically granted within the DUA are allowed.

  - Extend the obligation to protect the sensitive information from unauthorized disclosure to the authorized recipient. The recipients must extend the same requirement for any further authorized disclosures.

  - The recipient must report unauthorized disclosures to the source that provided the data.

  - If data is de-identified, the recipient should be prohibited from making attempts to re-identify individuals.

  - If the data is breached, the recipient must make reasonable efforts required by law to remedy the event.

EXAM TIP In countries outside of the United States, other types of data may be considered uniquely identifying or protected, such as trade union membership.

Healthcare Records Management

The proper management of healthcare records is an application of the overall information management lifecycle that applies to paper-based records and digital records alike. Healthcare information can be collected and stored on all types of media, such as paper, photography film, optical disks, microfilm, magnetic tapes, CD-ROMs, DVDs, hard disk drives, solid-state drives, floppy disks, or USB flash drives. Records can be retrieved from physical storage in records rooms and warehouses. More commonly today in the digital environment, electronic information is found in application-specific databases, diagnostic biomedical devices, master patient indexes, patient medical records, and health information files. All information has a lifecycle with various phases in which information exists, and healthcare records are no exception.

All phases of healthcare records management require information protection. You need to understand some very important concepts related to the collection, use, storage, and disposal of medical information. The special protections and sensitivity of the healthcare information require certain provisions that may not be present in other information protection policies and procedures outside of healthcare organizations. Mishandling healthcare records can lead to patient safety issues as well as financial penalties or litigation.

A good healthcare records management process enables the organization to protect transactional and historical evidence across the entire continuum of treatment, payment, and operations. An effective records management system can improve provider practices, enhance quality of care, and save resources over time. Following are some specific reasons for a solid healthcare records management system:

- Maintains needed information for as long as the information is useful
- Satisfies requirements for retrieval for forensics and legal discovery
- Lowers costs of management of records over the lifecycle, including destruction
- Ensure business resiliency by providing access to archives that are reliable
- Improves reliability of data backups when information is retrieved
- Collects and maintains ownership and accountability of records

There are many reasons healthcare organizations collect data and maintain records. Obtaining information for records is not normally a problem. Overcollection, however, is usually the concern. Medical record information comes from a variety of sources and is used internally and externally. For example, records resulting from a recording of physician notes and orders are sources, and these same records may be used for data exchange for referrals to other providers or for reimbursement from insurers. Records may be used to report to public health or for collaboration in outside research.

EXAM TIP   Recognize the patient's right to access their own health records and to determine how that information is used. This is an international concern and is contained in the US HIPAA Privacy Rule and GDPR. Also, organizations are required to be able to provide an accounting of disclosures (HIPAA) and records of processing activities (GDPR), as examples.

Record Retention

The lifecycle of records management begins when information is created and ends when the information is no longer needed and properly destroyed. In the time period between, during health records retention, various issues may arise. Health records retention is concerned with how long an organization must maintain a record and for what reasons. The challenge is that there is a scarcity of regulatory guidelines for how long medical records must be maintained in every case. Generally, organizations develop their policy using a patchwork of statutes, regulations, case law, and state medical board position statements. In Table 1-2, an example from the American Health Information Management Association (AHIMA) Retention and Destruction of Health Information brief is provided to depict the types of guidance that exist in the United States for healthcare records custodians.

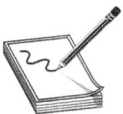

NOTE   In some cases, as shown in Table 1-2, professional industry associations or internal organizational requirements may exceed regulatory or legal requirements.

Federal Requirement	Example of a State Requirement (OK)	Accreditation Requirement	AHIMA Recommendation
Hospitals: Five years. Conditions of Participation 42 CFR 482.24(b)(1).	Healthcare facilities must retain medical records for a minimum of five years beyond the date the patient was last seen or a minimum of three years beyond the date of the patient's death. Oklahoma Dept. of Health Reg. Ch. 13, Section 13.13A.	Joint Commission RC.01.05.01: The hospital retains its medical records. The retention time of the original or legally reproduced medical record is determined by its use and hospital policy, in accordance with law and regulation.	Patient health and medical records (adults): 10 years after the most recent encounter.

Table 1-2 AHIMA Recommendations for the Retention and Destruction of Health Information

As healthcare records have evolved from paper-based to digital, you might think the problems are becoming easier to manage, but this is not always the case. Digital data storage is, of course, relatively inexpensive and accessible compared to having to maintain large rooms filled with paper records. However, there is still a legacy of increasingly inactive paper charts that organizations must address. Managing protection and facilitating the infrequent access to paper is cumbersome and expensive. The second part of the challenge is related to the shift to digital records. Because paper records consume physical space, records retention policies and procedures were created as an imperative to make the best use of physical space. With digital storage, the space required is minimal, and too often, records retention is not established or adapted to these record sets.

EXAM TIP Don't make the mistake to simply transfer paper-based retention rules to electronic data. There may be benefits, such as data analysis, to having different retention standards. Digital healthcare records retention requirements should be based primarily on medical considerations and continuity of care, unless specific regulatory or legal requirements extend the maximum time period.

Once an organization establishes a records retention policy, it needs to communicate the policy to patients along with information about how the patient can access their own information. At a minimum, record retention policies must do the following:

- Help the organization meet all the different requirements for uses of the records. Of course patient care is the primary requirement, but there are legal and research needs that can extend reasons for maintaining the records. For example, records involved in any open investigation, audit, or litigation must not be destroyed until the litigation case has been closed.

- Specify the types of information and the timeframes for keeping the records.
- Differentiate any variances based on the forms of storage, such as paper or electronic media.
- Present destruction options and standard operating procedures that include secure disposal methods.

Destruction of Patient Health Information

A retention schedule will end in a process for safely and securely destroying healthcare records. The destruction process must adhere to legal requirements and organizational policies. This is not a decision or a process that a healthcare information security professional is going to make individually. An information governance guidance is created by clinical and business leaders in the organization who consider the clinical, legal, and operations reasons to maintain records. This guidance must be in place and followed. When a record is no longer needed, it must still be protected until it is destroyed; records are often lost or accessed illegally at this point in the lifecycle because custodians relax controls.

Record retention and destruction processes have ambiguous and conflicting standards to follow. Some regulations and jurisdictions require the organization to create an abstract of the destroyed patient information prior to destruction, notify patients when destroying patient information, or specify the method of destruction used to render the information unreadable. In Chapter 5, you will learn about the technical and operational components of different health records destruction such as purging, degaussing, and data overwriting. Organizations should reassess their methods of destruction annually based on current technology, accepted practices, and availability of timely and cost-effective destruction services.

EXAM TIP Organizations must ensure that paper and electronic records are destroyed with a method that provides for no possibility of reconstruction of information.

An important document that organizations must maintain is the permanent record of the destruction of the health records. Organizations should ensure that they can provide the following for evidence of secure destruction:

- Date of destruction
- Method of destruction
- Description of the disposed records
- Inclusive dates
- A statement that the records were destroyed in the normal course of business
- The signatures of the individuals supervising and witnessing the destruction

EXAM TIP For the exam, remember that under HIPAA, third parties who destroy the healthcare records on behalf of the healthcare organization must adhere to the same secure handling and destruction policies and procedures as the healthcare organization, including providing and maintaining documentation of secure destruction.

Access Control

Access control refers to the safeguards used to limit access to system resources after a user's account credentials and identity have been authenticated and access to the system granted. Three major access control models are used to prevent unauthorized access to healthcare records:

- **Mandatory access control (MAC)** Typically used in military organizations, user access is defined by computer policy, is strictly enforced, and is relatively constant. The owner of the asset is not able to make changes unless the policy is reconfigured. Access control lists store the access properties associated with each computing asset (data, files, record, system, and so on).

- **Discretionary access control (DAC)** The least restrictive control grants the asset owner total control of settings on demand. Users can be granted rights to change access permissions and have control over healthcare records and other medical data. This can pose security risks and threats if used improperly.

- **Role-based access control (RBAC)** This approach is more realistic and is aligned with most risk-based organizational models. User access is limited based on predetermined definitions of what access a person in a job or function should need.

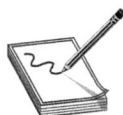

NOTE Rule-based access control is easily confused with role-based access control because it shares an acronym and a similar English pronunciation. Role-based is more common in terms of healthcare records management. However, as EHRs are systems of networked computer systems, you may contend with establishing and managing a secure access model for the EHR that uses rule-based access control to allow or block connections, transactions, and transfers. This access control could be in the form of blocked source IP addresses, allowing certain protocols over one port, or prohibiting e-mail services from the EHR to external recipients.

Authentication, Authorization, and Accounting (AAA)

Three individual access control terms—authentication, authorization, and accounting— are the components of a structure that regulates access to information by administering policies and monitoring use. The objective is to ensure authorized users have legitimate access. These combined processes are a necessity for secure computer and network use.

Authentication is the process of determining that the user who requests access is who they claim to be. This is typically accomplished by requiring a unique set of credentials to gain access, such as a unique username and valid password. If the credentials match what is stored in the identity management database (sometimes called the AAA server), the user is granted access to the network. If the credentials do not match, access to the resource is denied.

Authentication provides the framework for the next component, user *authorization* for performing certain tasks. Once authenticated, the user needs authorization, or a level of permission, to accomplish various actions based on policies. Authorization is the process of enforcing these policies. Each authenticated user may be authorized for different types of access or activities.

To measure resources a user consumes during access, the AAA concludes with *accounting*. A component of auditing in general, accounting documents and reports the consumption of resourcing time and session activity that assists in management of access control.

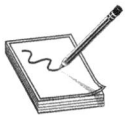

NOTE Remote Authentication Dial-In User Service (RADIUS) is a protocol for authentication and remote access for off-network users and authorizes their access to a system. RADIUS is an example of how network access servers interface with the AAA server to conduct access control for external parties.

The reality is that in many hospitals, if not many healthcare organizations, finely tuned access control is almost impossible. It is nonetheless important, and compliance with access control standards is directed by regulation. You should be aware of the factors that make access control difficult. With an EHR, guarding against unauthorized access to PHI is complex. Patient care is dynamic, personalized, and often involves many hospital employees in many roles. Determining *who needs access* is tough. Access is not predictable or certain for any individual provider, and configuring an EHR to support frequent changes is infeasible. When patient care is provided in an emergency setting, who has access to EHRs is even more difficult to predict with any certainty. As a result, most organizations allow more access than is required; once an employee is authenticated to the EHR, they can access any patient's medical record. This is not an effective implementation of access control.

The other problem is *how much PHI is accessed*. The frequency of access to PHI in an EHR can be several million events per week in a typical provider organization. With so many accesses by too many users with too much access, you can imagine that log management and audit is almost impossible. Trying to find unauthorized access is a daunting task.

Using role-based authority and authorization controls without a firm understanding of healthcare workflow can cause problems. Because many roles in the organization change frequently, the access and privilege process must be flexible. For example, a physician may be a pediatrician, so he or she will have access and privileges to view and edit children's medical records yet be prohibited from accessing adult records in the ICU.

However, if the physician is accessing the system while participating in a medical records peer review process, he or she may be granted temporary, expanded access.

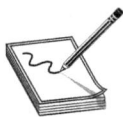

> **NOTE** At minimum, protocols must ensure that patient records, in electronic or paper form, are readily available and producible when legitimate use is required, and that reasonable steps have been taken to ensure that they are protected from theft, loss, and unauthorized use or disclosure, including copying, modification, or disposal.[17]

Least Privilege

The general security objective of least privilege involves granting users the minimum access rights that they need to perform their official duties. In healthcare, that means healthcare records are treated as confidential, access is denied by default, and access must be explicitly granted. How a healthcare organization maintains healthcare records using least privilege will be written as policy, and that policy will state who has access.

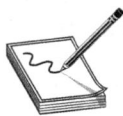

> **NOTE** The phrase "need to know" is sometimes used to describe least privilege.

Separation of Duties

No single user should have the permissions or authorization in the healthcare record system to complete high-risk tasks independently. A good access control system is configured to ensure that no individual has total control of security configurations. Separation of duties prevents against many instances of insider threats and employee mistakes that can lead to compromise of healthcare records. The adherence to separation of duties also mitigates a situation where multiple users with least privilege access join together to increase access to information, which would be unauthorized on an individual basis.

> **EXAM TIP** A review of system activity logs is a necessary security control to audit for execution of privileged functions. EHRs are no exception. Be aware of the need to use those systems' audit logs to detect inappropriate or illegal behavior.

Third-Party Relationships

A discussed earlier, the first party in healthcare is the patient. A physician, a provider group, or another healthcare organization is the second party. Another very important component in the healthcare industry are third parties that supply or operate on behalf of the healthcare organization. These entities comprise any of the external organizations that supply or support the first and second parties in the clinical and business activities involved in healthcare. For those third parties that also handle PHI as part of their business relationships, special privacy and security concerns exist.

Vendors

A vendor is a person or an entity that sells, supplies, or provides a service or product. Most healthcare organizations rely on many vendors. It is impractical, if not impossible, for a healthcare organization to employ or own all the various services and suppliers it needs to operate. For example, a healthcare organization may obtain contracted services for housekeeping and maintenance rather than try to operate those services with employed staff of the organization.

The reliance on these external relationships introduces privacy and security considerations, because the vendors and suppliers will be under the same regulatory obligations that affect the healthcare organization. The healthcare organization will maintain the responsibility to ensure that the external entities comply with these regulations.

Increased emphasis on information protection has moved healthcare organizations and industry oversight authority (including government) to establish cohesive vendor management or credentialing solutions. For instance, in Canada and relative to PHIPA (Personal Health Information Protection Act), there are privacy and confidentiality concerns with sharing of information between healthcare providers and third-party vendors. Canada has established a nationwide vendor credentialing system that enables healthcare providers a level of assurance that third-party vendors understand PHIPA and will comply.

In many cases, a vendor may have many different customers that are not healthcare organizations. Their service or product may or may not be healthcare related. For instance, a vendor can be an office furniture company and may sell all of the interior design and furnishings for a hospital waiting room, administrative offices, and conference rooms. At the same time, a medical supply company that provides durable medical equipment, surgical supplies, and hospital quality beds is also a vendor. The office furniture company undoubtedly sells furniture to a variety of business types, while the medical supply company probably does not have any customers outside of healthcare organizations and practices. For either of these vendor types, the healthcare organization, if large in size and purchasing power, will be a significant customer.

A vendor will employ members of the community based on the vendor's successful relationship with the hospital. For example, the nonprofit Henry Ford Health System in the Detroit metro area specifically emphasizes diversity and minority- and women-owned business in its supply chain database, which consists of more than 300 active vendors in this category.[18] The company's large purchasing power works to support not only the employment rate in the community, but the minority-owned business goals. You can see how the vendor (and the community) depends on the business of healthcare.

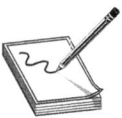

NOTE Although many healthcare organizations try to purchase locally or work with vendors in the community, this is not always possible. National and international companies often provide better pricing and support. A local vendor may still be preferable because of several risk factors of using nonlocal firms, however. National and international firms may be affected by regulations that differ from those supported by the organization. The choice of using an international company may introduce additional data use issues related to trans-border jurisdiction.

Because the relationship between vendors and the healthcare organization is so important and probably very competitive, healthcare organizations establish written policies to govern these relationships. Some of the major components of these policies include the following:

- Definition of the relationship
- Limits to gifts or gratuities
- Establishment and authority for oversight
- On-premises access rules
- Fundraising guidelines

Other special considerations are vendor-specific. For instance, vendors that work with academic medical centers have provisions for publishing by employees, seminar attendance and funding, and honorariums for speaking engagements. All of these provisions are meant to establish and maintain the integrity of the relationships. Unfair advantage of one vendor over another in many communities can mean the difference between a vendor business's success or failure.

Business Partners

A business partner is a particular subcategory of vendor in healthcare organizations. Although business partners provide a product or service for the healthcare organization, the relationship between the healthcare organization and this vendor is not a transactional type. Business partners are characterized as having a longer or recurring relationship with the healthcare organization, commonly described in a contract or formal, written obligation. These relationships are particularly of interest when the business partner handles PHI for the healthcare organization. In the United States, a business partner is sometimes called a business associate. These vendors are subject to, like the healthcare organization, industry-specific privacy laws, such as HIPAA. Therefore, it is crucial for the healthcare organization, as well as any business associates, to understand how they must comply with the relevant regulations, even if the vendor does not serve only the healthcare industry.

Consider a data center provider, for example. The provider may serve the healthcare organization by maintaining all of the data storage, providing applications, and performing backup procedures offsite. The provider may also do this for the local public school system, a retail department store, and other non-healthcare clients. In any case, this vendor must maintain its data center according to the appropriate healthcare regulations, such as HIPAA. This would include signing a special contract, such as a business associate agreement (BAA), that specifically outlines the data center provider's responsibilities and any provisions for noncompliance. You can imagine how complex this can be for a vendor.

Several requirements, with respect to the content of the BAA, follow:[19]

- The business associate must have appropriate safeguards to prevent use or disclosure of information other than as provided for by its contract.
- The business associate must report to the covered entity any use or disclosure of the information not provided for by its contract of which it becomes aware.

- The business associate must ensure that any agents or subcontractors agree to the same restrictions and conditions that apply to the business associate with respect to the individually identifiable health information being processed.

- The business associate must also make available protected health information for patient access and amendment, must make any amendment provided to it from the covered entity, and must provide an accounting of disclosures.

- The business associate must make its internal practices, books, and records relating to the use and disclosure of protected health information available to HHS for purposes of determining the covered entity's compliance.

- At termination of the contract, the business associate must return or destroy all protected health information. The contract must also authorize termination of the contract if the business associate is in material violation.

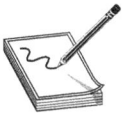

> **NOTE** You'll find an example of the terms and conditions that make up a standard BAA at https://www.hhs.gov/hipaa/for-professionals/covered-entities/sample-business-associate-agreement-provisions/index.html. US healthcare organizations can use that template or modify it with any local specifications as long as the regulatory provisions are met.

The following list provides some examples of business associates. Whether or not they are business associates depends, again, on whether the contract involves the use, disclosure, transmission, or maintenance of PHI.

- Electronic health records and clinical software application vendors who plan, install, and support their products

- Any information technology vendor that provides cloud services to include data storage, application services, security, and hardware management

- Utilization review and management companies that analyze referral patterns and outcomes data to help shape the best and most efficient treatment options

- Physician office answering services that interact with patients and providers on behalf of the healthcare organization

- Data conversion, de-identification, and data analysis service providers

- Medical billing and coding specialists that are not part of the healthcare organization as employees, which can be work-from-home, decentralized businesses

- Academic healthcare researchers, under some circumstances where HIPAA applies

- Third-party medical transcription companies that convert the provider's verbal dictation to a written or digital format

- Health information exchanges (HIEs), e-prescribing gateways, and other health information organizations that standardize transactions and make interchange of information easier

- Companies that destroy documents and computer drives, delete electronic equipment memory, and shred paper records as needed

- Patient safety or accreditation organizations that require access to records for investigations
- Third-party administrators and pharmacy benefit managers that are similar to utilization review firms

Without question, healthcare organizations that are not subject to HIPAA (in other words, international organizations) have third parties that serve as business partners/ associates in relationships that are structured similarly to how they are structured in the United States. International business partner relationships tend to be a little more strategic in nature than a relationship with a vendor that supplies goods and products to the healthcare organization. International business partners extend or supplement healthcare services, and this integrated nature of the partnership is evident in organizations that support both US and Canadian firms (for example). They will attest to complying with US HIPAA (as a business associate) as well as complying with requirements under PIPEDA, Canada's Personal Information Protection and Electronic Documents Act.

EXAM TIP Recognize the legal obligations of third parties in healthcare. Under the HIPAA Omnibus Rule, as of September 23, 2013, business associates and their subcontractors (who are also considered business associates) are directly liable under the law, just like US healthcare organizations (covered entities). This relationship of business associates extends as far as there is PHI being handled "downstream" from the business associates to the third parties they may work with on behalf of the covered entity. Understand that the legal obligation is in effect regardless of whether the covered entity has a compliant BAA in place. Absence of a signed BAA does not excuse any of the downstream business associates if there is a data breach.

Regulators

The role of loc al and national governments is a prime example of a third party with a tremendous impact on healthcare organizations, and it's not reserved for US healthcare. Although the US government, principally through Medicare and Medicaid, is the primary payer, it also heavily regulates the industry. As the governments of most other developed nations fund healthcare completely, government oversight there is more pervasive. In the United Kingdom, for instance, the National Health Service oversees healthcare through the Department of Health, the General Medical Council, and the Nursing and Midwifery Council. Figure 1-7 provides a snapshot of various government agencies' oversight relative to healthcare.

State and Local Government

Most likely, your interaction with the government as a third party will be at the individual state or community level. As the saying goes, politics and healthcare are local, so many of the decisions and events that happen at a national level may not have as much of a direct impact on how you do your job as the local government decisions do. For instance, as

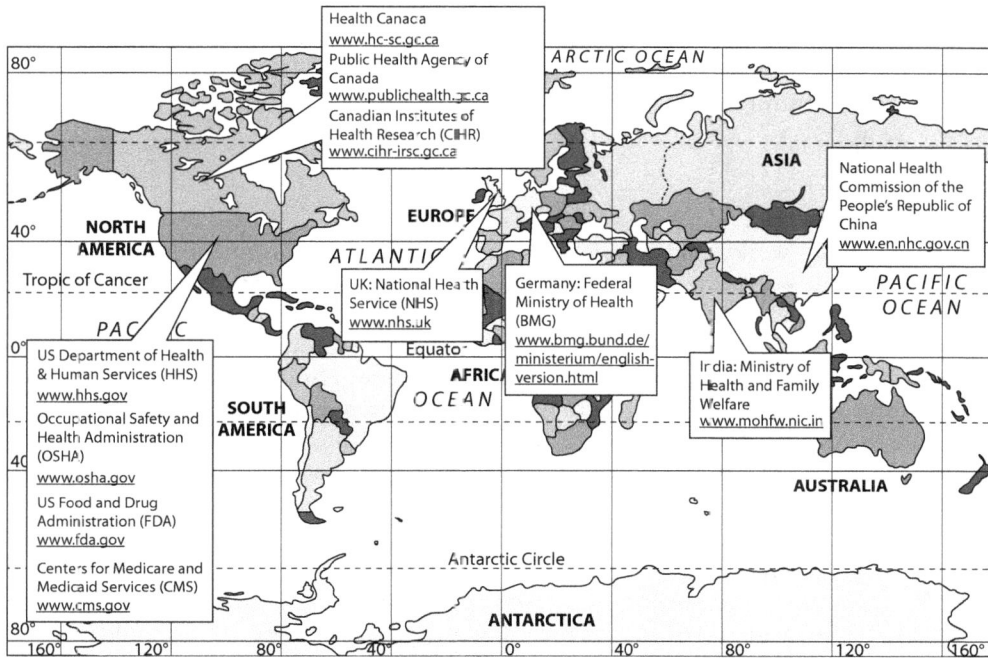

Figure 1-7 Selected government oversight agencies relative to healthcare

a regulatory mechanism, state governments must approve of the building of new facilities or the offering of new services under a provision called "certificate of need." In the United States, as of 2019, 37 states still require the measure, at least in part, to control capital expenditures and, theoretically, control healthcare costs.[20] Their success is arguable, but for a healthcare organization interested in opening a cardio-thoracic surgery ward to increase revenue, for example, not obtaining a certificate of need can be a huge setback. To build the facilities or deliver the service without local government approval can result in fines and penalties, or can at least render the services not reimbursable.

Local governments can also influence healthcare organizations in very positive ways. One way is by partnering on things, such as a community health needs assessment. Such partnerships help both the local government health agencies and the healthcare organization determine a strategic plan for delivering healthcare to the various populations in the community. Local government can allocate where public resources should be expended. The healthcare organization can plan for prevention, intervention, and rehabilitation services targeted to what the community needs. The possible categories are almost infinite, but may include the following:

- At-risk teens initiative
- Community asthma prevention program

- Homeless health initiative
- Injury prevention program
- Poison control center
- Wellness fairs

Law Enforcement

Because you are working in information protection, law enforcement is another direct impact of local government. Although every privacy and security law has a provision for law enforcement access to patient information, it is not unfettered access. Your role may be to provide law enforcement personnel with the information they require based on organizational policies, laws, and their need to know. For instance, disclosure of protected information usually must be in response to written requests from law enforcement officials. It may be difficult to refuse a police officer standing at your desk asking for access to a record of a patient who came through the ER last night, but you may have to do just that.

EXAM TIP One of the most important things you can do as a health information security and privacy practitioner is to know regulatory guidance and your organization's data sharing policies, both of which should be in alignment. Especially in a law enforcement scenario, patient information disclosure can be confusing. If a law enforcement official asks for disclosure of patient information that seems outside of regulator mandates and your organization's policy, you must know to prohibit the disclosure and seek guidance from authorized officials in the organization.

Tort Law and Malpractice

In the United States, the government plays another role as a third party. This role is through the judiciary process and it is a very direct role in healthcare through tort law and malpractice. These are complex concepts that deserve much more attention than can be devoted to them in this text. However, an introduction to the terms and how they add to the highly regulated healthcare industry will help you understand more about how third parties impact healthcare provision. To start, tort law comprises civil (versus criminal) acts that provide patients a remedy against wrongful acts committed against them. We find tort actions in the healthcare industry due to the following:

- Negligence
- Intentional torts
- Infliction of mental distress

For the information privacy and security practitioner, intentional tort is something to note because it covers failure to properly secure information. Although a data breach may be caused by negligence and certainly may cause infliction of mental distress, tort law applies sometimes when failure to ensure confidentiality of patient information is related to intentional acts.

This leads us to malpractice, which is a special kind of tort law that is familiar to healthcare professionals. A malpractice lawsuit is based upon alleged negligence or carelessness by a healthcare provider. The charges can be civil or criminal depending on the nature of the offense. Under the law, *malpractice* is conduct that is considered wrong or unethical based on a standard of professionalism specific to the occupational responsibilities. The conduct is also considered intentional or negligent. Typically, the issue is not information security and does not involve a healthcare information security and privacy practitioner. However, malpractice can be applicable to cybersecurity issues. Cyberattacks and data breaches are sometimes considered impactful to direct patient care and safety. This impact is in addition to the traditional identity theft, data loss, and financial crimes caused by cybersecurity incidents. When a cyberattack results in a patient safety incident, it may be reasonable to consider negligence as a contributing factor in allowing the cyberattack to occur.

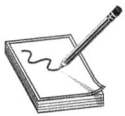

> **NOTE** Providers can purchase insurance against malpractice claims and costs. Such policies may not include coverage of malpractice claims related to a cybersecurity event, however. Providers may choose to purchase additional cybersecurity insurance policies for coverage. Cybersecurity insurance will be covered in greater detail in Chapter 6.

Nongovernment Regulators

When it is said that "healthcare is one of the most highly regulated industries," this means more than just official government oversight. There are several significant examples of nongovernment regulatory third parties that shape healthcare organizations around the world. The focus on improving the safety and efficacy of patient care is one of the primary components that all accreditation organizations have in common. Through peer review and education, accreditation has proven effective in shaping healthcare organizations through third-party relationships.

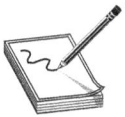

> **NOTE** In this context, *accreditation* describes a voluntary process with findings that are not legally binding for the healthcare organization. This would be in contrast to what a government agency or regulator would conduct—such as an audit or formal inspection with findings that must be mitigated or remedied, for which noncompliance would result in fines and penalties.

Joint Commission The Joint Commission (formerly the Joint Commission on Accreditation of Healthcare Organizations and, previous to that, the Joint Commission on Accreditation of Hospitals) is an independent, not-for-profit organization located in the United States. During the last 25 years, the Joint Commission has begun to develop an international presence as well. For about 100 years, it has accredited and certified healthcare organizations against standards of practice. It currently provides this service for more than 20,000 healthcare organizations and programs in the United States. You may note that the Joint Commission International operates in Spain, particularly, and across Europe. It is, in fact, an extension of the US Joint Commission. Joint Commission accreditation is considered mandatory to demonstrate a healthcare organization's commitment to quality and compliance with performance standards. In fact, in the United States, some reimbursement conditions depend on the organization having a current Joint Commission certification.

Accreditation Association for Ambulatory Health Care   Recognizing the shift from inpatient services to outpatient or ambulatory care settings, another US nongovernment third party began looking at quality and safety issues in physician groups, outpatient clinics, and any other ambulatory patient care centers. The Accreditation Association for Ambulatory Health Care (AAAHC) develops standards with regard to patient safety, quality, value, and measurement of performance. Because its focus is in ambulatory healthcare, its surveys can be particularly efficient and meaningful, with better-equipped, peer-based accreditation processes.

Accreditation Canada   In Canada, a similar organization, Accreditation Canada (formerly known as Canadian Council on Health Services Accreditation, or CCHSA) accredits more than 1000 client organizations ranging from regional health authorities, to hospitals and community-based programs and services. Like the Joint Commission and the AAAHC, the surveyors and auditors are not government employees, and the do not take direction from the government. Both the Joint Commission and Accreditation Canada use experienced professionals to conduct surveys and audits, including physicians, nurses, health executives and administrators, and medical technicians from the allied health professions.

European Union Regulators

The value of accreditation of healthcare organizations is debated in the European Union. Because healthcare is fully funded by the government, third-party accreditation of peers is not uniformly valued or respected. Many believe such efforts should be focused on mandatory compliance verified through government inspection and auditing. Nonetheless, third-party organizations performing accreditation have grown rapidly during the last 30 years in Europe.

To begin to look objectively at the issues, the World Health Organization (WHO) conducted one of the first international studies in 2000. This and subsequent studies have focused more on evidence of accreditation's impact on healthcare organizations' patient care, safety, and quality improvement efforts. Currently, there are eighteen national organizations active in Europe. The trend is in more programs and more participating healthcare organizations and more surveys of healthcare organizations.

Other Third-Party Relationships

In addition to the impacts from external relationships with vendors, business partners, and regulators, other emerging relationships impact the healthcare delivery system. One relationship you should understand is the growing collaboration among (sometimes competing) healthcare delivery systems and security and privacy information sharing groups.

Information Sharing and Analysis Centers

Information Sharing and Analysis Centers (ISACs) are trusted entities that help organizations in the United States protect their organizations and personnel from cyber and physical security threats. The concept of ISACs were specified in Presidential Decision Directive-63 (PDD-63), signed May 22, 1998. The Directive also introduced and endorsed the need for ISACs to partner with government.

Services provided by the typically nonprofit ISACs include collection, analysis, and sharing of actionable threat information. Figure 1-8 shows some of the sources of intelligence that ISACs provide. In the figure, notice the sources of threat intelligence, which include open source and proprietary source intelligence. These sources can contribute to a threat intelligence platform hosted by the sources themselves or by another organization collecting and analyzing the information sent using Structured Threat Information Expression (STIX) and Trusted Automated Exchange of Intelligence Information (TAXII)

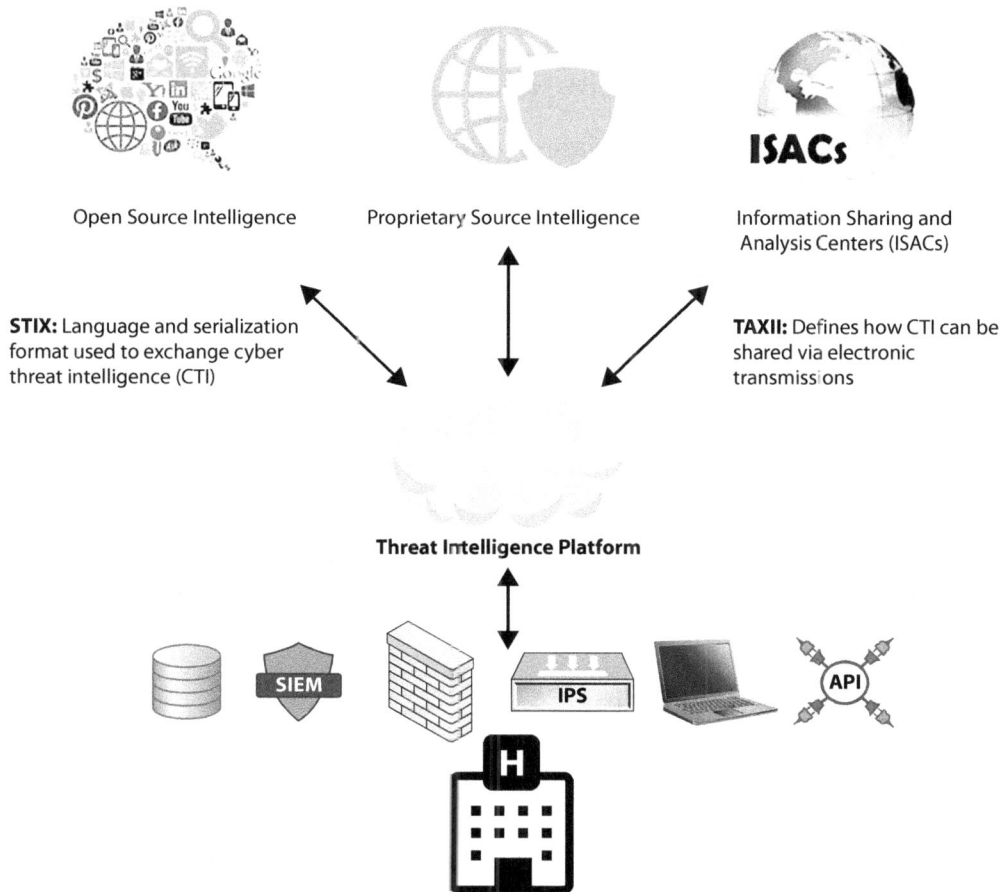

Figure 1-8   Sample threat intelligence service from ISAC

language standards. The threat intelligence platform provides updates to the security tools used by healthcare organizations, many of which are effective for detection, response, and recovery.

A single healthcare organization by itself probably could not provide enough resources to gather and analyze the vast amounts of threat intelligence that an ISAC can provide. In some cases, the ISACs establish the threat levels for their sectors based on the threat warning and incident reporting capabilities they offer.

ISACs are in the business to facilitate information, not sell it. To maintain situational awareness across the various critical infrastructure sectors, ISACs collaborate and share threat and mitigation information with one another and other partners through the National Council of ISACs.

Healthcare Information Sharing and Analysis Center (H-ISAC) The healthcare sector has a devoted ISAC in the H-ISAC, a trusted community of critical infrastructure owners and operators within the health and public health sector. The H-ISAC offers threat intelligence, reporting capabilities, and information sharing, but it devotes extra emphasis to threats and adversary actions that target healthcare and public health. The H-ISAC also expands the surveillance capabilities for the healthcare sector by its integration and collaboration with the entire National Council of ISACs.

Medical Device Innovation, Safety, and Security Consortium (MDISS)

MDISS is a nonprofit public health and patient safety organization focused on medical device cybersecurity. The group takes a collaborative approach, where a threat faced by one organization or medical device is understood to be a threat faced by all. Therefore, the group was established to foster more communication and sharing of practices that will benefit the entire healthcare delivery system. MDISS aims to improve the safety and security of medical devices by assisting their membership with guidance on technology solutions as well as policy and procedures. The organization embraces government–private sector partnerships to leverage industry expertise in device vulnerabilities and government counsel in regulatory requirements. The intention of the group is to be focused on patient safety, approaching medical device security from an epidemiological model, which means looking at the problems from an incident, spread, and control perspective like a disease. This lens is familiar to healthcare public health interventions and is thought to help improve medical device security. This group works together with other collaborative groups such as the H-ISAC, the Healthcare Information and Management Systems Society (HIMSS), and the FDA.

Administering Third Parties

With all of these external forces and third-party relationships shaping the healthcare organization, administering them is a fundamental element in reducing information risk (of unauthorized disclosure). You know that the BAA, which is unique to the United States, is one formal (written) tool that helps reduce information risk. You also need to know about other agreements and documents that are used in the United States and internationally. All are prenegotiated and defined common understandings necessary to protect the confidentiality, integrity, or availability of patient information. A few of note are the service level agreement, the data sharing agreement, and the legal contract.

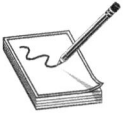

> **NOTE** Formal agreements between healthcare providers and third parties can cover many different types of products and services other than protecting information. For instance, a healthcare organization can have agreements with transportation companies to provide support for moving furniture, equipment, and even patients. There are agreements in place to cover temporary staffing levels from employment agencies. For purposes of our text, we are limiting the content of these types of written agreements to information protection.

Service Level Agreements

The service level agreement (SLA) is a document that outlines the support or products to be provided by the third-party organization and any processes against which the healthcare organization can measure success. Consider network uptime, for example. If the third party agrees to keep the network connected and operating for a particular frequency, that becomes the expectation of the healthcare organization. The measurement can be the frequency—such as 99.999 percent of a full 24-hour day, seven days a week. If the network does not perform to that standard, the healthcare organization may suffer consequences. SLAs also contain remediation steps when things go wrong, including steps for complaint escalation, financial penalties, severance of the agreement, and so on.

Data Sharing Agreements

A data sharing agreement (or data use agreement) is a similarly used document that describes access to and expectations for a third party's use of an organization's patient information. These documents are similar in function to and may be used with a BAA in the United States. It will clearly indicate and limit the specific data elements exchanged, the period of time the data sharing will occur, the systems the third party will access, how the entity will use the data, and provisions for the eventual disposal of the information. These agreements can cover additional parameters, but the main element of the agreement is to protect the healthcare organization by spelling out exactly how the information will or will not be disclosed. This is important because, ultimately, the healthcare organization is responsible for safeguarding the information. In a data sharing agreement, it is imperative to ensure that there is a bona fide and legal "need to know" for the third party.

Chain of Trust Agreements

These agreements are not unique to healthcare. In the United States, this function can be satisfied within the BAA. A chain of trust agreement provides an administrative control via a contract between sender and receiver healthcare organizations for secure information exchange. It establishes the technical controls for information exchange and obliges each party to adhere to them. In this way, both parties agree to ensure the confidentiality and integrity of PHI. If the information exchange involves multiple parties, multiple chain of trust agreements are required.

> **CAUTION** Chain of custody and chain of trust are related concepts. Chain of custody differs in that the documentation is a sufficient legal piece of evidence after the information exchange, such as information disposal, rather than a prospective legal obligation as a chain of trust would be.

Legal Contracts

Finally, the most official and binding of third-party administrative tools is the legal contract. In many ways, the SLA and the data sharing agreement can evolve into a formal contract. Generally speaking, there are four main elements of a contract:

- It must be between two or more parties.
- All parties must be competent to consent.
- The agreement must be something of value.
- The agreement must be lawful.

Where formal contracts differ from an SLA and a data sharing agreement is in the complexity and content. SLAs and data sharing agreements tend to be specifically focused on a service or product, with terms and conditions related to measurements and quality or specific acts and tasks. However, all of these documents are used to set clear expectations, avoid costly legal actions, and provide safe handling of patient information. The formal contract would include more detail about responsibilities, resources, assumptions, and limits of liabilities over the life of the contract. Often the SLA and data sharing agreement serves as an attachment to a formal, long-term contract with a third party (which may provide multiple services).

Understand Foundational Health Data Management

Like any industry that relies on information, healthcare organizations must adhere to proper data management principles. To do this, they should organize their data management around concepts that are considered best practices. Information consisting of data can comprise many different forms in every part of the healthcare organization, including written instructions, treatment plans, images, audio files, video clips, paper documents, and digital files. Successful organizations work to transform the information into a strategic asset, organizing and leveraging it into a resource as valuable as any clinical technology or financial asset it has.

The foundation of a strong healthcare data management program includes four major areas:

- **Data profiling**   This discovery process leads into the data quality process by determining where data quality rules and requirements should focus. Steps in this activity include gathering frequency and basic statistic reports, relationships in tables, phrase and element analysis, and business rules discovery.

- **Data quality**   The objective of this process is to standardize, validate, and verify the data. Adequate checks and oversight must be in place to ensure that data is relevant, accurate, timely, and accessible, to name a few data quality characteristics. The specific techniques of parsing, transformation, verification, and validation help to enable normalization of the data for data integration.

- **Data integration**   Multiple sources of data are combined to obtain an organizational data repository or collection of source data. This effort involves removing duplicate data and consolidating sources using powerful locating and matching technology.

- **Data augmentation**   Once the data reaches this step, the process concludes with enhancing and enriching the data with new data or missing elements. For example, adding demographic, geographic, or credit information can be useful. In this stage, data management algorithms and methods are used for clinical and business data analytics.

In addition to the foundational concepts, your program will need to have policies and procedures that accomplish the following:

- **Governance**   Leadership must be applied to strategically align processes and technology, with a uniform view across the organization. Because data governance is not just an IT issue, a data governance committee must include senior-level executives and specialists from other business and clinical areas (along with IT representatives), who provide vision and authority to the data governance function.

- **Stewardship**   Ownership and accountability are important in managing data. Data is a valuable asset, and all personnel who have and use data must understand their individual roles in ensuring prioritization of data, maintaining trust in data, and reporting and tracking data issues to resolution.

- **Architecture**   Related to the location of data and how it flows through the organization, inventory and documentation make up the first step. Then the organization must identify the stakeholders and the relevant information lifecycle. Additionally, data architecture involves defining the organization's metadata, or its data about data. An element of metadata could be "patient record" and could include multiple elements such as date of birth, appointment date, prescriptions, and so on. Because this information may be used by multiple departments or even across different organizations, having metadata called *patient record number* that is uniformly defined can streamline the myriad processes that rely on these associated data elements.

- **Standards**   With all the business processes and clinical workflows that operate within healthcare, the effort to establish and maintain data with common understanding and meaning is important (and one of the reasons the coding of medical practices with ICD-10, for example, is so essential). Data standards are founded using a combination of regulations, customs, and user acceptance.

- **Security**   Assuring confidentiality, integrity, and availability of data, both in paper form and digital, is a central concern of any data management program. Within healthcare, a lack of protection of data from unauthorized (accidental or intentional) modification, destruction, or disclosure can be a violation of law, a matter of risk to patient safety, or both.

Managing Information Flow and Lifecycle in Healthcare Environments

An *information flow* in healthcare is a pathway that any identifiable piece of information, or of information type that is pertinent in the healthcare domain, follows from sender to recipient and from input to output. Types of information can range from entire databases, to images and sound recordings, to elementary variables related to a patient care event. During the information flow, information is examined, created, updated, and deleted as needed. As illustrated in Figure 1-9, information moves across the continuum of care from patient to provider and then to nonprovider entities in the care path. Healthcare

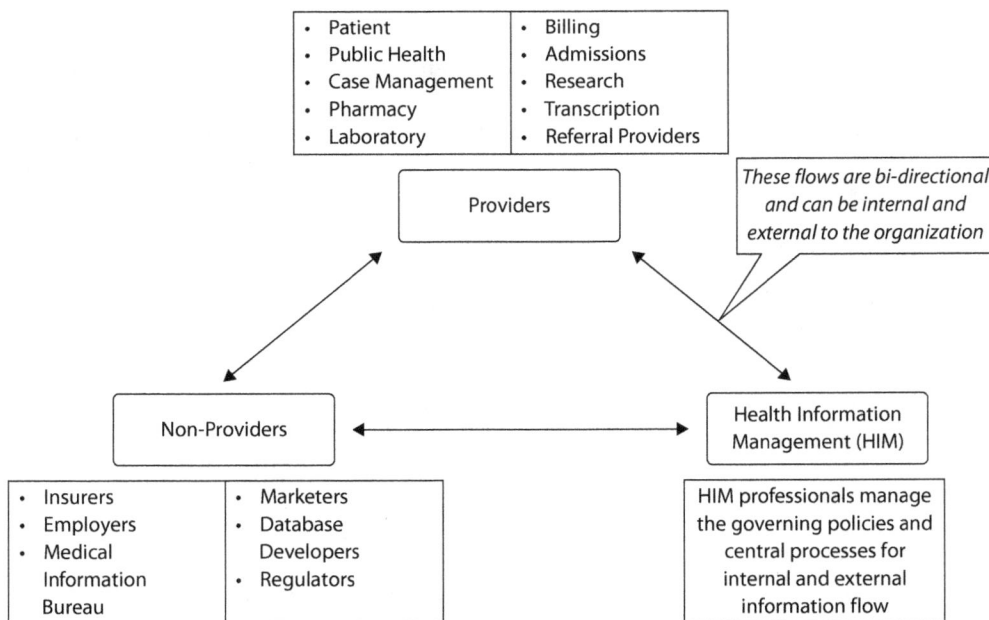

Figure 1-9   Overview of healthcare information flow

information protection professionals must successfully manage and protect this health information as it moves internally within the organization and externally.

Data sharing in healthcare is an essential component of patient care, research, and quality initiatives. Within the organization, providers consider it an imperative to be able to easily access things required for patient care, such as medication lists and laboratory results, precisely when they need it. Even after care is provided, sharing information is important in settings such as peer record review, where procedures are reviewed and measured against organizational and clinical standards. The intent is to discuss best practices, share common experiences, and, in the end, maximize scarce resources by reducing duplication and ineffective processes.

Many healthcare organizations devote a tremendous amount of research and academic training as part of the care they provide. Commonly, these are either purely research providers or teaching hospitals. Enabling these organizations to exchange their findings or even collaborate on research in real time advances medical care. Results become more useful with combining larger data sets on drug responses. Adding genomic data on patients to the clinical trials could really begin to predict exactly what therapies are helpful at an individual level. Data sharing reduces trial-and-error medicine that is costly and may be the source of patient safety risks.

One study has shown that sharing data between provider organizations has saved 92,000 lives and $9.1 billion over four-and-a-half years.[21] Much more impressive numbers result from extrapolating data-sharing benefits across an entire nationwide healthcare system. Improving patient outcomes, streamlining processes, and reducing patient safety risks are all benefits of data sharing.

Enabling one healthcare organization to communicate with others is a challenge, even though healthcare language is based on accepted clinical terminology, standardized code sets, and the same mission of diagnosis and treatment. In addition, the ability to interconnect with other third parties can create administrative and management problems.

For instance, each healthcare organization that uses an information system to automate workflow, an EHR, or a patient administration system probably purchases that system from a commercial manufacturer. Some government healthcare organizations' information systems may be government-developed. Recently, many government healthcare organizations have adopted commercial off-the-shelf EHRs, though the government EHRs may still require interconnection to government-developed business or clinical systems used only within government healthcare organizations. In any case, based on the company that develops the EHR system, interoperability is often difficult. The outcome is that valuable data locked is locked away, unless the systems are from the same manufacturer. As patients typically move from one healthcare organization to another, based on referrals for advanced care, for example, or healthcare organizations desire to submit bills to payers, healthcare organizations must be able to send and receive data no matter what proprietary system they (or their counterparts) use. Throughout the remainder of this chapter, you will be introduced to emerging standards, taxonomies, and interoperability efforts for healthcare information that are intended to improve the secure transfer and use of information between organizations and information systems.

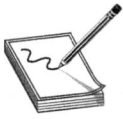

> **NOTE** The interoperability of EHR systems has surfaced as an issue within healthcare organizations as mergers and acquisitions are bringing together multiple providers with different EHRs. It involves standardizing consolidation with different EHR platforms and interconnections through system integrations.[22]

What should be clear at this point is that healthcare information must move along the clinical workflow of patient care, and if the information is not available or reliable, patient care suffers and patient safety may be at risk. Additionally, information has a lifecycle that must be managed to ensure that confidentiality, integrity, and availability are maintained. The goals of confidentiality, integrity, and availability must be aligned with information sharing for patient care. Properly understanding information flow and information lifecycle management (ILM) is essential to reduce costs as well.

The ILM cycle, depicted in Figure 1-10, involves the following phases:

1. **Create** The information must be available, trusted, reliable, and concise, no matter the source of the information—the patient, a provider, or any number of different medical devices and diagnostic tools.

2. **Store** Records must be stored and protected while in the possession of the provider. The value of the information (classification) will determine how long an organization will keep the information. Policies establish the length of time the records are useful and after which outdated records are discarded. The records should be maintained with the same level of availability to providers and with the same level of integrity as long as the information is useful.

3. **Use** Information has to be used in a manner consistent with the reasons it was collected and never for a provider's personal gain. For example, data used for treatment typically cannot be used for published research if the patient did not consent to such use.

4. **Share** Probably the most important feature of use within the information life cycle is protecting the information during transfer. Healthcare organizations use data; that is a given. As the data moves throughout the organization, between organizations, and between providers and payers, safeguards are needed to assure confidentiality, integrity, and availability.

Figure 1-10
Information records management life cycle

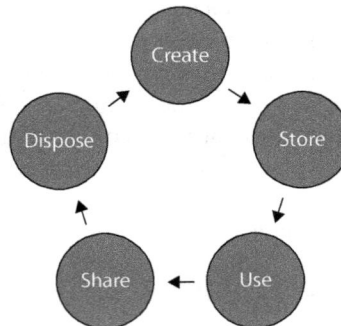

5. Dispose The final step in the process is the most vulnerable. Too many times data is lost or disclosed in an unauthorized manner when the organization no longer deems the information useful. During the transfer of the information for disposal, a data leak or breach occurs because safeguards are relaxed. Until data is destroyed, it needs to be protected.

A key part of any information security strategy is disposing of data once it's no longer needed. Failure to dispose of data properly can lead to serious breaches of data protection and privacy policies, compliance problems, and added costs. Paper records as well as digital information can be lost easily prior to destruction. The essential message to healthcare information security and privacy professionals is this: Data breaches happen, and they can happen to your organization. And they are most likely to happen when you let your guard down at the disposal step in the ILM.

Three common disposal methods are used with paper or digital information:

- **Purging** This is the indisputable erasing of data from the storage device in such a way that the data may never be recovered. It can be accomplished by overwrite, block erase, and cryptographic erasure, using dedicated, standardized device sanitize commands.

- **Cleansing or clearing** The organization can use software or hardware products to overwrite storage space on the media with nonsensitive data, using the standard read and write commands for the device.

- **Destruction** The organization can purge media before submitting it for destruction. There are numerous ways of physically destroying media, including the drive shredders, pulverization, incineration, and acid.

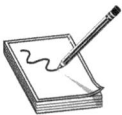

> **NOTE** Data shredding (electronic) should not be confused with the shredding of paper documents; often some confusion occurs when only the term "shredding" is used. Data shredding can be accomplished by destroying the physical media, but there are secure data shedding applications that completely erase the data.

Specific techniques used to dispose of information properly include the following:

- **Zeroing** This process erases data on the disk and overwrites it with all zeros.

- **Degaussing** In this process, the magnetic media is erased and returned to its initial blank state through the use of high-powered electromagnets.

- **Sanitizing** This process purges all identifying data elements from the record or database through data element removal, de-identification, masking, or anonymization.

- **Overwriting** Data is overwritten with random data until the current data is no longer retrievable.

It is common to use several of these methods to destroy data, depending on the value of the data and the media in use. In some cases, the process involves performing the action a number of times to ensure that the data cannot be recovered.

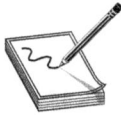

> **NOTE** Publicly available guidance, namely, NIST SP 800-88, *Guidelines for Media Sanitization*, at https://nvlpubs.nist.gov/nistpubs/SpecialPublications/NIST.SP.800-88r1.pdf is a leading source for information sanitization methods.

Data Lifecycle Management (DLM)

DLM concept is different from ILM, though it is similar to ILM as an approach to manage data throughout its lifecycle. DLM is concerned with information at the file level, which is more abstract in nature and less concerned with the use of the data within the file. ILM would deal with the specific information within that file, such as a patient's height, weight, age, and test results. In other words, DLM deals with entire files of data, while ILM deals with the details within the files.

> **EXAM TIP** DLM can be accomplished using a hierarchal storage management (HSM) system, an automated process to move data between high-cost and low-cost storage media options. Each HSM option offers a tradeoff between cost and speed of retrieval.

DLM has sharpened the focus of healthcare organizations and underscored the need for professionals dedicated to managing data and information assets. Proper management includes protection of the assets, but it also incorporates using the data and information to benefit the healthcare delivery system. Health informatics is an activity that has emerged to help healthcare organizations apply a thorough and effective approach to data lifecycle management. Health informatics is information engineering applied to the field of healthcare and deals with the tools and procedures needed for optimizing healthcare information.

Health Data Characterization

Data sharing and interchange typically must be intentional. Based on law, contractual agreements, and technical compatibility, interoperability has to be a premeditated and determined effort. Beyond the concepts of data standards and the languages of healthcare, a couple other topics are important to consider—namely, data classification and data taxonomy. Even if data is technically compatible to exchange between organizations, not all data is equal, and individual organizational policies and procedures must be considered. Attending to health data characterization through proper data classification and data taxonomy makes information exchange feasible. To that end, data analytics is another stakeholder of accurate health data characterization, which relies on correct data classification and taxonomy methods.

Data Classification

ILM requires that a healthcare organization establish a classification system based on the value of the information. It is important to note that this type of data classification differs from that of computer programming, which is also called classification, but relates more to labeling the data to differentiate it into classes and sets. In the ILM context, data classification is required to apply a value relative to the sensitivity and criticality of the information, as defined by the organization. This value will determine what level of information protection controls will be applied to information collected, stored, used, shared, and eventually disposed of.

EXAM TIP   Know the specific types of data classifications. If given a list or a choice of what sensitivity you might apply, you should not confuse data classifications with labels used to designate documents such as For Official Use Only (FOUO) and Limited Official Use.

Your organization must determine what categories to use to classify data. There is no prescribed naming convention and there is no specific number of classification categories you can use. Your choices may be based on regulatory requirements and organizational governance. However, a common structure used by many organizations has four levels of sensitivity and one level of open access:

- **Confidential**   If data in this top sensitivity level is lost, stolen, or compromised in some form or fashion, it is likely to result in significant, long-term harm to the institution or individuals to whom the data refers or belongs.

- **Sensitive**   This level has relative value less than confidential, but it is still important to protect. Losing the data will increase risk to the organization, even if it's just reputational damage. Strategy planning documents or inter-organizational correspondence can be considered sensitive.

- **Restricted**   This may also be termed "private" and includes material that would cause "undesirable effects" if publicly available but may not raise operational risk. Employee retention statistics or salary ranges are often classified as restricted or private.

- **Proprietary**   This is the least restrictive classification but mandates internal company use only and should be based on proprietary use for authorized personnel only. Disclosure outside the company may impact competitive advantage. Many organizational briefings or meeting notes can be classified at this level.

- **Public**   The data is available outside the organization, and the unauthorized disclosure, alteration, or destruction of this classification of data would result in little or no risk to the organization.

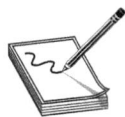

NOTE The "restricted" classification level should not be confused with the term "restricted data" that is used in US government documents, which can be used within government classification levels such as Top Secret, Secret, and Confidential.

Data Taxonomy

Data taxonomy relates to categorizing data into a standardized format with common meaning. Data taxonomy leads to simplicity and facilitates data sharing. As an example, the term "psychologist" can indicate a specialized healthcare provider who is independent of organization and distinct from other provider professions, such as social worker or counselor. Such distinctions help to facilitate appropriate data analysis and information sharing. Having a data taxonomy introduces convenience and reduces wasted efforts in trying to establish common definitions and context. Data taxonomy has also proven effective in streamlining payment and reimbursement activities.

Healthcare Provider Taxonomy Code Set and National Provider Identifier The Healthcare Provider Taxonomy Code Set is contained in HIPAA as a standard. The taxonomy is arranged in a hierarchy of specific codes with descriptions and definitions. Using the taxonomy, you can identify healthcare providers by their type, classification, and provider specialty. The code set comprises two sections—Individuals and Groups of Individuals, and Non-Individuals—and is updated twice a year. Each provider's 10-digit code is structured into three distinct levels: provider type, classification, and area of specialization.

As of 1996, HIPAA requires the adoption of standard unique numbers that identify healthcare providers, as established by the NPI (National Provider Identifier) Final Rule, issued in January 2004. The NPI number is required many health insurance claims and enrollment applications. One of the provisions of the ACA requires all providers of medical or other items or services and suppliers that qualify for an NPI to include their NPI number on all applications to enroll in the Medicare and Medicaid programs and on all claims for payment submitted under these programs.

EXAM TIP Don't be fooled. The Healthcare Provider Taxonomy Code Set and NPI Database are not synonymous, nor are they sources to be used to ensure that providers are credentialed or qualified to render healthcare.

EDI X12 Code Lists Electronic Data Interchange (EDI) X12 is an electronic data format that is governed by standards released by the Accredited Standards Committee (ASC) X12. It is used to exchange specific data between two or more trading partners. A "trading partner" refers to a third-party organization, group of organizations, or some other entity. A trading partner in the US healthcare context is most often a business associate. Some large organizations that act as trading partners impose strict rules and requirements for EDI transactions, which may be in the form of specific data format requirements for some elements, requirements to contain specific segments (segments that are not mandatory in EDI X12 standard being made mandatory), and others. HIPAA recognizes the trading partner and outlines the need to provide requirements in a separate companion guide document. Companion guides are used to inform the user on important interactions with the application, such as access and understanding how to transmit requests and understand responses. It is essential that these documents be followed to the letter when healthcare organizations implement EDI systems.

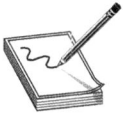

NOTE An example companion document from the Centers for Medicare and Medicaid Services (CMS) is the HIPAA Eligibility Transaction System (HETS) Health Care Eligibility Benefit Inquiry and Response (270/271) 5010 Companion Guide. It defines the Medicare eligibility request sent from Medicare-authorized trading partners and the corresponding response from the HIPAA Eligibility Transaction System (HETS) 270/271 application.

Following are key EDI transactions within HIPAA:

- **837** Medical claims with subtypes for Professional, Institutional, and Dental varieties
- **820** Payroll Deducted and Other Group Premium Payment for Insurance Products
- **834** Benefits enrollment and maintenance
- **835** Electronic remittances
- **270/271** Eligibility inquiry and response
- **276/277** Claim status inquiry and response
- **278** Health Services Review request and reply

Data Analytics

Possibly the most compelling argument for proper data characterization is data analytics. With standard classification and taxonomy, comparative analysis on larger and larger volumes of data becomes a reality at a reasonable cost. Previously, data analytics would be constrained to individual organizations because of incompatibility of policies, procedures, and information systems. At best, data analytics were applicable only to one particular organization. Any comparisons most likely suffered from data latency, because results could not be shared in real time. Today, however, alliances and data analytic firms are able to aggregate and process terabytes and petabytes of data from dozens of healthcare organizations almost instantly and simultaneously to provide outcome measures and lower costs over time.

The evolution of data analytics has information systems able to process more data faster and more economically. As organizational data becomes more compatible and standardized, *big data* has exploded in many industries, including healthcare. Figure 1-11 shows some of the major sources of data that are available to healthcare organizations.

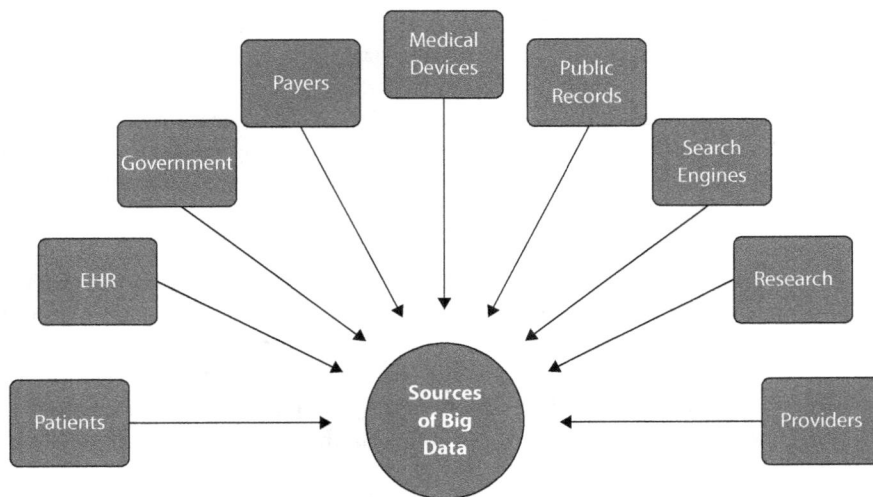

Figure 1-11 Big data sources in healthcare

Healthcare organizations, like other organizations that use data analytics, can be described by measuring against three major levels of capabilities, which explain how organizations use data and analytics to create competitive advantage and become top performers:

- **Aspirational**   A beginning level, focusing on efficiency or simply trying to justify an action. At this point the organization may not have a clear view of how to get value from analytics, and the required level of executive sponsorship may not be apparent. The organization may also have immature or incomplete information retention processes, which would affect the ability of the analytics process to gather, aggregate, and manipulate the information. Decisions are based more on intuition rather than proper data and analysis.

- **Experienced**   At this level, more strategy and business initiatives are enabled by data analytics. The principle benefit is realized in growing revenue through data analysis. There is still a lack of personnel with technical skills to fully leverage the data. These organizations also do not have mature data governance policies, including clear ownership. At this point, the organization can get and use the data, but is not able to reliably and securely share it with other organizations.

- **Transformed**   At this level of proficiency, analytics are used to set a course of action as compared to retrospectively defending an outcome for an organization. And it is at this level that data analytics can provide an advantage over competition. But there still may be problems in exploiting the benefits of the data because the organization can have limited resources or too many priorities to commit to other than more data analytics growth. These organizations continue to mature as they ensure people, processes, and technologies are aligned to maximize data analytics and differentiate the organization from others.

Healthcare as a worldwide industry has a common dilemma: the pressure to reduce costs and improve outcomes. Big data offers many positive impacts fort healthcare, such as facilitating a reduction in fraud, waste, and abuse. From a clinical perspective, big data initiatives have helped reduce medication errors and improve quality healthcare outcomes. The healthcare industry, however, has been slower to adopt the power of data analytics than other industries, such as retail and manufacturing. Stricter regulatory pressures in healthcare may lead to a perception that data analytics would be less effective and possibly illegal in some scenarios.

Healthcare organizations, particularly those subject to HIPAA, must make several considerations with regard to data analytics:

- Third parties that provide or share data analytics technologies or capabilities with healthcare organizations are subject to HIPAA according to clarifications provided by the Omnibus Rule. Before the clarification, healthcare industries were often hesitant to enter into data analytics arrangements with third parties.

- HIPAA prohibits selling of PHI. With large data stores moving from the healthcare organization to third-party organizations that provide analytics, services paid for or reimbursed may be considered marketing or selling of data.

- Allowances are made for compound authorizations in research. It was previously illegal to ask research participants to authorize data collection and add on an authorization to keep the data for future research use after the original study. HIPAA, as amended by the Health Information Technology for Economic and Clinical Health (HITECH) Act, allows for compound authorizations.

- Data de-identification methods such as data masking or anonymization can be used to maintain the usefulness of the data for analytics, and they reduce the risk of unauthorized disclosure of large sets of data.

Data Interoperability and Exchange

Data taxonomy and other standardization methods enable data interoperability and exchange. Interoperability in healthcare refers to the ability of different information systems, devices, or applications to connect in a coordinated manner, within and across organizational boundaries, to access and use data cooperatively among stakeholders, with the intended goal of optimizing health for individuals and populations.[23]

The ways in which health data can be exchanged is governed by standards and enabled by architectures with an objective to effectively and securely transfer the correct information to authorized users when it is needed. Significant numbers of connections and integrations in healthcare settings and information systems depend on an interoperable exchange of data. Beneath the requirement for interconnection and exchange, the importance of usability and reliability of the information is a concern you will address.

Your organization may participate in several types of data exchanges. These components occur with varying degrees of interoperability and may occur simultaneously within a single healthcare setting:

- **Foundational interoperability** There are baseline requirements that must be met for systems to establish basic interconnectivity. These must be in place before any consideration can be made for determining requirements to format what is sent and understand what is received.

- **Structural interoperability** Defines the syntax, structure, and format of healthcare data exchange (the message format standards) that is required for secure transfer of data between systems, maintaining data integrity. It also ensures that there is no alteration or degradation of the data contents that would change the purpose and meaning.

- **Semantic interoperability** This capability is needed to facilitate the exchange of information and to make sense of it so the information is usable. Semantic interoperability relies on common taxonomies and vocabulary to best enable the receiving system to interpret data for the end-user consumption. This high-level interchange of patient information across different healthcare information technology systems is useful in improving healthcare treatment, payment, and operations.

- **Organizational interoperability** Includes technical, policy, social, and organizational elements that enable secure transfer and use of healthcare information by end users located in different organizations. Information transfer must also be on time and unimpeded to achieve organizational interoperability. Beyond the technical specifications interoperability requires, organizational interoperability also elevates the need for underlying ILM and DLM workflows to be aligned and optimized for the best patient care outcomes and provider satisfaction across multiple organizations.

The concept of "meaningful use" in EHRs arose from the implementation of the HITECH Act, which was included in the American Recovery and Reinvestment Act (ARRA) of 2009 that amended HIPAA. The act provided for incentive payments to healthcare organizations that did more than just adopt an EHR. "Meaningful use" means that providers implemented an EHR certified by the Office of the National Coordinator for Health Information Technology (ONC) that demonstrates technological capability, functionality, and security requirements of the US Secretary of Health and Human Services to achieve improvements to patient care. This incentive ended in 2015. After that time, provider organizations that had not implemented an EHR and demonstrated meaningful use could expect to incur penalties from the federal government. Specifically, eligible providers who did not demonstrate meaningful use successfully for an EHR during a specific time period associated with a reimbursement request from CMS will receive a reduced Medicare payment, such as a 3 percent reduction in reimbursement.

The meaningful use program evolved over time to encourage interoperability as well. CMS provides incentives to encourage eligible clinicians to use health IT, most notably certified EHR technology. CMS believes that EHR technology enables clinicians to submit information electronically in a format CMS can process efficiently and effectively. Meaningful use has been replaced by the Medicare EHR Incentive Program. In 2015, the Medicare Access and CHIP Reauthorization Act (MACRA) was passed, and the Medicare EHR Incentive Program became one of the four components of the new Merit-Based Incentive Payment System (MIPS).

Health Level 7 (HL7)

HL7 is a nonprofit, ANSI accredited, international standards developing organization that provides a framework and standards dealing with the exchange, integration, sharing, and retrieval of EHI. The organization aligns its work and standards through ISO. HL7 includes several families of interconnection standards, including Fast Health Interoperability Resource (FHIR); Clinical Document Architecture (CDA); Consolidated CDA (C-CDA); ERH/PHR System Functional Models, Version 2, Version 3; Arden Syntax; and the Reference Information Model (RIM). This organization consists of healthcare information technology professionals, healthcare and health administration professionals, and members of multiple government agencies (CDC, ONC, FDA, and so on). By implementing interoperability standards, healthcare organizations can better deliver patient care and convey clinically significant information that typically would be unavailable because of system incompatibilities.

To help EHRs interconnect, the HL7 has published the EHR System Functional Model, which defines EHRs in terms of important functionality. Using the clinical workflow expected of various patient care settings, the group defined functional profiles with standard descriptions, which are applicable globally. HL7 leads interoperability effort so that providers and manufacturers develop standardized EHR functionality instead of trying to cobble them together after-market.

EXAM TIP HL7 is a central communication protocol in healthcare. Knowing that it supports interfacing between multiple systems without promoting proprietary or vendor-specific protocols should be committed to memory. HL7 follows a philosophy of "open system architecture."

Integrating the Healthcare Enterprise (IHE)

Related to HL7, IHE is an international organization that contributes to the use of standards and protocols to improve interoperability. It promotes the coordinated use of standards developed by HL7 and many other standards development organizations by establishing clinical workflow profiles (such as for cardiology or dental) of existing interoperability standards involving coordinated communication. This enables organizations to purchase systems with tested interoperability capabilities.

IHE creates standards, such as the EHR function standards, and focuses on how organizations implement them. Systems that conform to IHE interoperability specifications are typically easier to implement, easier to interoperate with, and more effectively support provider information use. For example, organizations purchasing any

EHR or clinical information system can refer to applicable IHE documentation, require compliance from vendors, and streamline system implementation and interoperability. Vendors and health systems can claim conformance to IHE specifications following rigorous testing with exchange partners for a given interoperability profile.

IHE publishes standard implementation specifications (profiles) across several domains:

- IHE Cardiology (CARD)
- IHE Dental (DENT)
- IHE Endoscopy (ENDO)
- IHE Eye Care (EYECARE)
- IHE IT Infrastructure (ITI)
- IHE Pathology and Laboratory Medicine (PaLM)
- Merger of IHE Anatomic Pathology and IHE Laboratory domains
- IHE Patient Care Coordination (PCC)
- IHE Patient Care Device (PCD)
- IHE Pharmacy (PHARM)
- IHE Quality, Research and Public Health (QRPH)
- IHE Radiation Oncology (RO)
- IHE Radiology (RAD)
- IHE Surgery

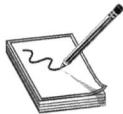

NOTE The IHE Product Registry is a valuable reference guide for healthcare professionals who are charged with buying and implanting systems that must be interconnected. Inside the registry are specifications for interoperability, called IHE Integration Statements. Using these conformance commitments from manufacturers, you can be more certain of IHE capabilities from disparate commercial products.

Digital Imaging and Communications in Medicine (DICOM)

When it comes to information system interoperability, the healthcare industry's reliance on digital images captured from numerous devices, in addition to numerical results and words, creates incredible complexity. Digital diagnostic imaging devices, called modalities (X-ray, ultrasound, computed tomography, and so on), need a standard method for transferring images and information between medical devices and for use in various vendors' EHRs. Each imaging device initially creates the image in a proprietary format. The American College of Radiology (ACR) and the National Electrical Manufacturers Association (NEMA) formed a joint committee in 1983 to develop a standard known today as DICOM. This standard is found in ISO 12052:2017 within the field of health informatics.

DICOM, using ISO 12052:2017, promotes interoperability of medical imaging equipment by specifying the protocols required for transferring digital images across a network. The guidance does not, however, prescribe testing protocols for compliance and does not guarantee interoperability.

Devices used to capture and transfer images can be manufactured by any vendor that complies with the DICOM standard. Images can be stored in databases that can be analyzed using data analysis tools. Leveraging DICOM has resulted in advances in medical imaging and has led to picture archiving and communication systems (PACS), which make up some of the most complex, networked medical devices in healthcare. These can consist of dozens of modalities, set up in a local area networked (LAN) configuration connected to several different types of servers for image processing, demographic patient data integration with the images, and file transfer to end-user viewing stations. PACS is also accessible via the Web when a dedicated web server is added to the architecture. Many healthcare organizations must accommodate a PACS as a LAN within their LAN because its footprint is large. DICOM is an evolving standard that enables the PACS to communicate within its own component and to interface with other systems in the same organization and those outside the organization.

Legal Medical Record

Back when medical records were made up of paper charts, documents, film images, and files, a legal medical record included the entire content related to an individual patient. That began to change with the introduction of paper-to-digital records conversion. Patients have also become more involved with the contents of the records related to regulatory changes, legal issues in healthcare and patient education available on the Internet. The impact of the definition of a medical record is in what is disclosed to law enforcement and for legal proceedings. Only that which constitutes a legal medical record is to be disclosed. The contents of a legal medical record should (at least) do the following:

- **Support patient care decisions** Legal medical records can reduce costs, improve care, and increase efficiency.

- **Full accounting and documentation of the care provided** It is the responsibility of the creator of the record to keep the record in an unaltered form and authenticated by that individual.

- **Serve as evidence in legal proceedings about such care** A healthcare organization must maintain a legal medical record.

Not all health information is digital, and much remains in paper format. Some of the paper information constitute valid elements of a legal medical record. When a healthcare organization defines its legal medical records as having both paper and digital information, the records are called hybrid legal medical records. Along with the location of the various databases where the electronic information resides, a medical record must have references to the sources of the paper-based information it includes.

The security and privacy implications of medical records are significant. The first challenge in defining a legal medical record is that no standard exists.[24] Each organization is required to define the contents for itself. Some components are more obvious and universal than others. For instance, information related to medication orders, pathology reports, and emergency department records would certainly be part of any legal medical record. Administrative data and documents, however, are usually excluded. Other excluded items could be authorization forms for the release of information, incident or patient safety reports, and psychotherapy notes. To identify which documents can be excluded, healthcare organizations typically call these items working documents.

CAUTION A healthcare record, particularly the legal medical record, can often be an important piece of evidence in a legal proceeding. It is imperative that the healthcare organization preserve the authenticity, reliability, and integrity of all healthcare records.

Chapter Review

Healthcare is a dynamic, complex, and highly regulated industry. The computer networks and interconnections are part of the US national critical infrastructure, but the importance and reliance on a safe and secure healthcare delivery system is important worldwide.

This chapter builds a foundation of understanding the organizations in which an information security and privacy professional may work. The start of the chapter includes a general overview and discussion of the various healthcare organizations that make up the industry. The healthcare workforce is diverse and ranges from manual labor trades to highly educated professions. At the center of the healthcare system is the patient. The types of organizations that support the healthcare of the patient are provider, payer, and healthcare clearinghouse organizations. Many external entities also support the healthcare industry. In this chapter, we introduced key stakeholders, such as the surrounding community, that provide sources of labor as well as support businesses not related to direct patient care. Jobs and the local economy may depend on these stakeholders' partnership with the healthcare organization. The impact of information sharing with third parties outside the healthcare organizations is relevant to information protection considerations. For example, vendors, suppliers, and regulators are forces that have impact. Where third parties handle sensitive information on behalf of the healthcare organization, the relationship may introduce risk to each of the organizations that must be addressed.

The healthcare system requires a financial mechanism to allocate resources. In the United States, the financial processes are relatively complex with coding, billing, and payment processing components. It is significant to understand how the US employer-based and private insurance models work. In most other countries, the government (single-payer) model is the predominant model. These differences may present unique challenges for you as a healthcare information privacy and security professional.

To facilitate the general financing models as well as support the delivery of efficient quality of care, the healthcare industry relies on an extensive coding taxonomy of which information privacy and security professionals need to be aware. The chapter continues with a presentation of the categories of foundational health data management principles.

The end product of coding, health data management and delivery of patient care, is a legal medical record that patients, providers, and regulators can depend on to document and communicate the overall events and experiences that are healthcare. Understanding these topics help shape your knowledge and use of information through its lifecycle and help you properly manage products central to healthcare. Whether you work in healthcare already or are just now entering the healthcare workforce to provide information protection services, you will make your work easier if you understand the important points of this chapter.

Very few healthcare organizations can exist independently of third parties that are imperative to business and clinical operations. Many of the external entities that support healthcare organizations are considered vendors, business partners, or suppliers. In the United States, a special affiliation is in place based on prevailing legal guidance, HIPAA. Third parties that handle protected health information on behalf of healthcare organizations are called business associates, and they are also subject to HIPAA. Third parties can also be external stakeholders, such as government agencies, legal authorities, and accrediting organizations. Each of these entities plays a role in ensuring that the healthcare organization operates within established guidelines. In this chapter, we also covered the various information-sharing third parties and healthcare organizations. As information privacy and security professionals, you will need to understand how to share information securely to avoid cybersecurity threats while not exposing your organization to additional risk.

This chapter concludes with an overview of foundational health data management concepts. The understanding of data lifecycle management and classification levels of data are not unique to healthcare, but these and other privacy and security concepts concerning data must be tailored to the healthcare environment to avoid degrading clinical operations or risking patient safety. As the digitization of healthcare information increases, the need for and use of initiatives such as data analytics are introducing challenges for continued protection of large volumes of data that are shared in many new ways with other healthcare organizations and third parties. The standards and formats for data interoperability in clinical operations are important to identify and secure in this emerging data flow, such as DICOM, HL7, IHE, and X.12, to increase efficiency. The end result of the interoperability and data exchange in healthcare is the legal medical record. This central artifact is important to you as an information protection professional because the organization relies so heavily on its contents for healthcare decisions as well as the record's status as a legal document to be used in regulatory matters and litigation.

Questions

1. Which of these types of nurses requires the highest level of formal education?

    A. Licensed practical nurses

    B. Registered nurses

    C. Nurses' aides

    D. Independent duty nurses

2. If a payer is a public source, which of these would be the source of funds?

   A. Employer group

   B. Health maintenance organization

   C. Public health agency

   D. Government entity

3. An inpatient is defined as an individual who

   A. Receives rehabilitation for hip replacement Monday through Thursday, 5 PM to 6 PM

   B. Checks into the emergency room and is admitted overnight for more than 24 hours

   C. Undergoes knee surgery and is transported to assisted-living residence

   D. Is admitted to a sleep study overnight from 11 PM to 8 AM

4. Who is the primary payer in most developed countries for healthcare?

   A. Self-pay

   B. Employers

   C. Government

   D. Military

5. "Per member, per month" is a common way to describe a payment model called

   A. Capitation

   B. Bundled payment

   C. Accountable care

   D. Managed care

6. Reimbursement for healthcare services must be

   A. Unusual, customary, and reasonable

   B. Usual, per customer, and reasonable

   C. Usual, customary, and rational

   D. Usual, customary, and reasonable

7. The standard development organization established to help electronic health records to interconnect is

   A. LOINC

   B. ICD-10

   C. DICOM

   D. HL7

8. A researcher who wants to adhere to Good Clinical Research Practices would be most concerned with

   A. Patient availability

   B. Human subject protection

   C. Informed consent

   D. Notice of privacy practices

9. At what stage of information lifecycle management are you most likely to have a data breach?

   A. Create

   B. Store

   C. Use

   D. Dispose

10. If you were asked to de-identify yesterday's patient appointment list containing medical record number (MRN), patient names, and time of appointment, what action would be most appropriate?

   A. Delete all MRNs and change patients name to "PATIENT."

   B. Change the names to historical figures and delete times of appointment.

   C. Increase each MRN by 15 and use only the last names of the patients.

   D. Only use patients name and times of appointment.

11. A formal, written agreement that describes the access to and expectations for a third party's use of patient information is a _____ agreement.

   A. Service level

   B. Business partner

   C. Liability limit

   D. Data sharing

12. Generally speaking, almost all regulatory guidance allows sharing of patient information without additional patient consent to whom?

   A. Next of kin

   B. Law enforcement

   C. Media

   D. Clergy

13. When a provider is accused of an action such as not properly reviewing mammograms and misdiagnosing breast cancer, they may have committed what?

    A. Adverse event

    B. Practice preference

    C. Case management

    D. Malpractice incident

14. A new data classification technology was purchased by your healthcare organization. One of the features of the tool is the ability to mark data with metadata elements to signify the data protection levels. With this tool, you will begin to identify and classify all protected health information as what?

    A. Private

    B. Sensitive

    C. Confidential

    D. Restricted

15. Bull Run Health Insurer, your employer, has asked for your participation on the committee to establish the organization's legal medical record. The charter of the group clearly states the regulatory obligation that the organization must have a legal medical record. The objectives of the legal medical record are also provided for your review. Those objectives are to reduce costs, improve care, and increase efficiency for clinical and business operations. After a few meetings, you are asked how the new policy can outline delegation for changes to an individual record to increase provider efficiency. What requirement for the legal medical record do you advise the group they are forgetting, if any?

    A. Support patient care decisions.

    B. Include full accounting and documentation of the care provided.

    C. Serve as evidence in legal proceedings about such care.

    D. There is nothing forgotten. There are no agreed upon standards for this action.

Answers

1. **B.** Registered nurses generally require the highest level of formal education completed compared to the other choices. Typically, the designation signifies a baccalaureate degree or completion of a healthcare organization–sponsored curriculum. The other categories of nurses accomplish education and experience requirements as part of applied training or through employment.

2. **D.** An employer group or employer-based healthcare insurance would be considered a private payer. A health maintenance organization can be a method of organizing delivery of care under a government payer plan, such as Medicare, but it is not a public source of funds. A public health agency is unlikely to reimburse

providers for care as part of their surveillance responsibilities. Therefore, the best answer is D, a government entity that uses public tax dollars or other publicly acquired funds to fund or reimburse providers for healthcare.

3. **B.** A recurring appointment each day from 5 PM to 6 PM is an outpatient visit, as are appointments that do not require admissions officially into the hospital. The knee surgery with transportation to an assisted-living residence implies discharging the patient to his or her home. A sleep study, although overnight, is not an admission to a hospital. The emergency room that results in a formal admission into the hospital fits the definition of inpatient care.

4. **C.** The government is the primary payer in most developed countries of the world. Only a small percentage of individuals pay out-of-pocket for their healthcare. While employers are a sizable percentage of health insurance financers in the United States, this far less common internationally. The military, as a portion of government-provided health insurance, is partially correct, but it is not the primary payer.

5. **A.** "Per member, per month" describes capitation. This is a common measurement of what funds are provided to a healthcare organization for the delivery of care. The amount is preset and made available prior to the covered period of time. It has to relate to each individual over that measured period of time. Bundled payment, accountable care, and managed care are all somewhat related to financing healthcare, but none is specifically defined or measured in terms of each covered life over a period of time.

6. **D.** The only correct combination of adjectives is "usual, customary, and reasonable." All of the others are not found within any typical definition of what charges are reimbursable.

7. **D.** Health Level 7 (HL7) is an organization that develops standards for electronic health record interconnectivity. LOINC is Logical Observation Identifiers Names and Codes and is limited to identifying laboratory and clinical observations. ICD-10 is International Classification of Diseases (ICD), 10th revision, and is used to communicate a level of detail for purposes of payment to the payers with a simple number up to six digits long that is internationally understood. DICOM is Digital Imaging and Communications in Medicine and is used to facilitate the transmission of digital images from radiology exams, for example.

8. **B.** Human subject protection is an overall provision that researchers must be concerned with as the concept is central to Good Clinical Research Practices. The other choices are components of protection of the study participants, and each may add to a relevant and compliant human subject protection approach.

9. **D.** Even though any stage of the information lifecycle can have risk of data breach, the create, store, and use stages are not the most likely for data loss. When data is marked for disposal or destruction, either in paper or digital format, it is imperative to continue to apply safeguards against loss, because too many examples exist where data is no longer needed and it is no longer protected, at which point, it is stolen or lost.

10. **A.** The best choice to remove all personally identifiable information and protected health information is to remove the MRN and anonymize all patient names. Choices B and D allow sensitive data elements to remain or do not reduce the chance of easy re-identification. Adding information to the MRN and leaving patient names would have no obscuring or de-identifying impact.

11. **D.** Generally, a data sharing agreement would be used to communicate these expectations and requirements unless another contractual agreement already outlines the same. A, B, and C are documents that serve other purposes that have little to do with information protection.

12. **B.** Most regulatory guidance has provisions for sharing patient information with law enforcement without additional patient consent. A, C, and D would all require additional patient consent.

13. **D.** If they practice with negligence as in this scenario, they will likely endure malpractice lawsuits. A, adverse event, is usually related to a mistake or failure of a process—not necessarily by one person. B is not an official term, but each provider has preferences in how they practice medicine. C, case management, is a general term for nursing and administration staff members who help properly utilize medical resources by managing the care and treatment for patients with extended care plans with referrals to specialists and possibly inpatient stays.

14. **C.** Marking the data confidential affords the highest level of protection category commonly used outside of military and government organizations. In any case, protected health information should be protected at the highest category level even if different terminology is used in an organization. A and D are synonymous. Both are incorrect because protected health information is regulated by government agencies and made publicly available, which would certainly have more than undesirable effects on the organization. While the data is considered sensitive, B is incorrect because sensitive is less restrictive than confidential, and the loss of the data is a significant risk to the organization.

15. **B.** Of the provided options, including a full accounting and documentation of the care provided is most accurate. A legal medical record must be unaltered and accurate. The creator must ensure the integrity of the legal medical record. With that in mind, A and C are more relevant to why you must have a legal medical record that is unaltered and accurate. It is used for patient care decisions and often is a document used in legal proceedings. D has some validity in that organizations have to establish their definition and contents of their legal medical record. In this scenario, it is not relevant because the group has forgotten the need for the record to be accurate with a full accounting and documentation of care provided.

References

1. Nelson, J., B. Sung, S. Venkataram, and J. Moore. 2017. "Transforming care delivery through virtual health." Deloitte Consulting, https://www2.deloitte.com/content/dam/Deloitte/us/Documents/life-sciences-health-care/us-lshc-transforming-care-delivery-virtual-health.pdf.

2. US Bureau of Labor Statistics. 2019. "Occupational Employment and Wages, May 2018; 31-0000 Healthcare Support Occupations (Major Group)." https://www.bls.gov/oes/current/oes310000.htm.

3. Carnevale, A. P., N. Smith, and A. Gulish. 2015. "Nursing: Supply and Demand Through 2020." Georgetown University Center on Education and the Workforce, https://repository.library.georgetown.edu/bitstream/handle/10822/1050292/Nursing-Supply-Final.pdf?sequence=1&isAllowed=y.

4. Rosseter, R. 2019. "Nursing Shortage." American Association of Colleges of Nursing (AACN), https://www.aacnnursing.org/news-information/fact-sheets/nursing-shortage.

5. Miles, S. H. 2005. *The Hippocratic Oath and the ethics of medicine*. Oxford, UK: Oxford University Press.

6. US Department of Health and Human Services Office of the Assistant Secretary for Planning and Evaluation. 2000. "Standards for Privacy of Individually Identifiable Health Information. Final Privacy Rule Preamble. Health Care Clearinghouse." https://aspe.hhs.gov/report/standards-privacy-individually-identifiable-health-information-final-privacy-rule-preamble/health-care-clearinghouse.

7. Stein L. I. 1967. "The Doctor-Nurse Game." *Archives of General Psychiatry*, 16(6):699–703. https://doi:10.1001/archpsyc.1967.01730240055009.

8. Holyoake, D. D. 2011. "Is the doctor-nurse game being played?" *Nursing Times*, 107(43):12–14.

9. The Joint Commission. 2008. "Sentinel Event Alert 42: Safely implementing health information and converging technologies." https://www.jointcommission.org/en/resources/patient-safety-topics/sentinel-event/sentinel-event-alert-newsletters/sentinel-event-alert-issue-42-safely-implementing-health-information-and-converging-technologies/.

10. United States Census Bureau. 2016. "Health Insurance Coverage in the United States: 2015." https://www.census.gov/content/dam/Census/library/publications/2016/demo/p60-257.pdf.

11. Obama, Barack. 2016. "United States Health Care Reform: Progress to Date and Next Steps." *Journal of the American Medical Association*, 316(5):525–32. JAMA Network, https://jamanetwork.com/journals/jama/fullarticle/2533698.

12. Bryan, B. 2016. "Here's how much the price of Obamacare changed this year for every state in the US." *Business Insider*, May 30. https://www.businessinsider.com/obamacare-price-change-for-every-state-in-us-2016-5.

13. US Department of Health and Human Services, Office for Civil Rights. 2013. "HIPAA Administrative Simplification," (45 CFR Parts 160, 162, and 164). https://www.hhs.gov/sites/default/files/hipaa-simplification-201303.pdf.

14. Health Care Industry Cybersecurity Task Force. 2017. "Report on Improving Cybersecurity in the Healthcare Industry." https://www.phe.gov/Preparedness/planning/CyberTF/Documents/report2017.pdf.

15. OCR HIPAA Privacy Rule. 2003. Disclosure for Public Health Activities. [45 CFR 164.512(b)]. https://www.hhs.gov/sites/default/files/ocr/privacy/hipaa/understanding/special/publichealth/publichealth.pdf.

16. Intersoft Consulting. 2016. "General Data Protection Regulation (GDPR): Art. 6 GDPR, Lawfulness of processing." https://gdpr-info.eu/art-6-gdpr.

17. Skipper, J. 2012. "Individuals' Access to Their Own Health Information," ONC Policy Brief. HealthIT.gov, https://www.healthit.gov/sites/default/files/pdf/individual-access-06-03-2012.pdf.

18. Henry Ford Health System. 2019. "Supplier Diversity." https://www.henryford.com/about/supply-chain/diversity.

19. Amatayakul, M. 2002. "United Under HIPAA: a Comparison of Arrangements and Agreements" (HIPAA on the Job series). *Journal of AHIMA*, 73(8):24A–D.

20. National Conference of State Legislatures (NCSL). 2019. "CON–Certificate of Need State Laws." http://www.ncsl.org/research/health/con-certificate-of-need-state-laws.aspx.

21. Monegain, B. 2013. "Data-sharing initiative reduces deaths." *Healthcare IT News*, https://www.healthcareitnews.com/news/data-sharing-initiative-reduces-deaths.

22. Savage, L., M. Gaynor, and J. Adler-Milstein. 2019. "Digital Health Data and Information Sharing: A New Frontier for Health Care Competition?" *Antitrust Law Journal*, 82(2):593–621.

23. Health Information and Management System Society (HIMSS). 2017. *HIMSS Dictionary of Health Information and Technology Terms, Acronyms, and Organizations*, 5th edition. Chicago: HIMSS.

24. AHIMA. 2011. "Fundamentals of the Legal Health Record and Designated Record Set." *Journal of AHIMA*, 82(2):44: expanded online version, https://library.ahima.org/doc?oid=104008#.XjxoojFKhPY.

Information Governance in Healthcare

This chapter covers Domain 2, "Information Governance in Healthcare," of the HCISPP certification. After you read and study this chapter, you should be able to:

- Comprehend the general categories of information governance frameworks
- Differentiate between privacy and security governance components
- Recognize key information governance roles and responsibilities
- Understand the main information security and privacy policies, standards, and procedures
- Recognize and follow a code of conduct or code of ethics as a healthcare information protection professional

The implementation of information governance in an organization is meant to establish and manage clearly defined principles for acceptable behavior for information collection, use, and disposal. The governance process exists to provide structure to help the organization measure good information handling practices as well as manage oversight of any violations. The bottom line is this: governance is the foundation of an organization's comprehensive and proactive approach toward security and privacy efforts protecting information assets. As an HCISPP you are expected to understand and be able to support (sometimes establish) the organization's information governance framework of structure, policies, procedures, and standards.

The need for information governance is established by leading information protection regulations in many countries. Some prominent examples are the US Health Insurance Portability and Accountability Act (HIPAA) and the European Union (EU) General Data Protection Regulation (GDPR). Organizations that have sufficient information governance structures in place for security and privacy functions tend to comply with these regulatory requirements more effectively. Adherence to the information protection guidance through information governance can assist in maintaining high-quality standards for information handling and in maintaining information confidentiality, integrity, and availability.

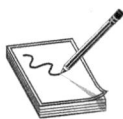

NOTE Information governance has increased the importance of technology such as cloud services. Having solid internal information governance is more important now as the third-party sharing of data may cross geographic borders, jurisdictions, and industries. These are examples of relatively new sources of information risk for healthcare organizations.

Governance is applicable across the entire enterprise and filters down to each individual department. A key outcome of a good governance function is to impose accountability for the management of information assets. There should be an alignment between information governance and the organization's clinical and business strategies. Information governance, when applied, should guide an organization to fulfill its goals. In the healthcare industry, some of the goals are patient-care focused. A governance framework that in practice limits data availability or slows clinical process, for example, must be avoided.

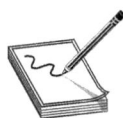

NOTE Governance and management can be confusing concepts. One does not replace the other. Think of management as an application of the governance framework outputs (such as policies, procedures, and standards).

As we move to the next sections of this chapter, we will distinguish between information security and information privacy governance. In many organizations, these governance structures are evolving into a more singular organizational structure, such as information protection governance. This is worth noting because there is overlap and interdependence in privacy and security functions. The primary information security function is focused on defending data and networks. In addition to this function, the effort includes protecting confidentiality (privacy) of sensitive employee and customer information. With the increasing digitization of information and IT capabilities of healthcare organizations, protection of patient privacy is impossible without sufficient information security processes and procedures. For now, we will continue to explore these governance frameworks separately, knowing they work best when they function together. In your organization, you may already see the integration of privacy and security governance into a single enterprise governance structure.

As part of the information governance function, various official groups or teams will be established within the organization. The group may be considered a committee, a council, or maybe a working group. Each comes with a degree of formality. A committee is typically the most formal of these and may require a charter, which is a document that is created at the inception of the committee and updated regularly upon review by committee members. The document outlines the committee's mission, authority and responsibilities, and composition; how and when meetings will be held; as well as how meeting minutes will be written and approved. It also describes any reporting relationships to other organizational management or a board of directors. Having a charter helps to keep the formally established group aligned with its intended purpose. Other less formal groups may use a charter for similar reasons, such as for documenting purposes, but that is an optional step. If a charter is typical for groups identified in this section, it will be noted.

Security Governance

With the evolution from paper-based information to more and more digital data there is the need to have a well-understood structure for information security processes and functions. The security governance in a healthcare organization describes how strategic oversight of information protection happens. The performance of the governance functions is important. Healthcare organizations collect, use, transfer, store, and dispose of sensitive data that could be valuable to criminals and is vital to patient care. The conceptual framework for the information security governance consists of important individual roles and groups.

EXAM TIP   Keep in mind that governance is more than just a best practice. Compliance with regulations is facilitated by implementation of information governance frameworks. For instance, the requirement under HIPAA to implement policies and procedures for authorizing role-based access to protected health information (PHI) makes a committee approach almost essential.

Information security governance is a strategic imperative and needs support from management at all levels of the organization. It requires commitment, resources, and assignment of responsibility for those in key positions. The governance function must also be able to demonstrate that it is effective through measurement and reporting to senior levels of the organization and the board of directors. The likelihood of information security governance being successful is related to the involvement of senior management in areas such as approving policy, providing appropriate oversight, and offering direction when measures and analysis warrant.

At a general level applicable to almost every organization, information security governance is needed for several significant reasons:

- Prepares the organization for potential risks
- Improves coordination and integration at all levels through setting responsibilities
- Protects substantial investments in information technology and data assets
- Supports cultural and organizational factors while enabling business needs
- Establishes and enforces organizational rules and priorities
- Assists in building trust with required supplier relationships and interconnections
- Results in a credible information security program

Healthcare information security is not a concern or a function that can be relegated to IT. Clinical and business leaders throughout the organization must come together to solve information protection issues. When that happens, good governance is a natural outcome of the leadership of the organization's security consciousness and actions. There can be too much governance, however. In an effort to satisfy compliance measures and implement visible information governance teams, process can overtake progress. This happens when governance becomes unidirectional and the system users or information handlers themselves have no input in the process. The number of teams and bureaucracy can become too much to satisfy. The communication loop of sender, receiver, understanding, and feedback underlies the information governance structure in a well-run organization.

EXAM TIP When evaluating exam questions or scenarios, consider information security as a business and governance concern. Sometimes a technology security solution is not the best answer. Address issues using adequate risk management along with reporting and accountability processes, rather than limiting mitigations to technical solutions.

Board of Directors

Governing boards of healthcare organizations may not traditionally be included in discussions about information security governance. Organization management has held the roles and performed the responsibilities of information security governance; however, with rapid increase in the frequency and impact of data breaches and cybersecurity events, more boards are interested and involved in the sufficiency of the information security program. Directors need to understand and approach cybersecurity as an enterprise-wide risk management issue, not just an IT issue. The board should be involved in information security concerns such as organizational risk tolerance, cybersecurity insurance options, and how management is reducing risk for the organization. The high-level information security functions for the board should include the following activities:

- Ensure the organization has information security leadership in positions of authority.
- Review plans for the information security program and receive regular input from the information security leadership.
- Oversee and approve relevant information security policies and evaluate effectiveness.
- Designate a board committee for the responsibility to perform these functions (such as an audit committee).

A principal responsibility for the board of directors is to provide a requirement for organizational management to implement an information security program that is aligned to a risk management focus. The board must also expect management to properly resource the information security program with budget and personnel. The National Association of Corporate Directors (NACD) is a source for board direction. Its handbook specifically mentions the National Institute of Standards and Technology Cybersecurity Framework (NIST CSF) as a favorable option for boards to expect. This is because of the NIST CSF purpose and intent to enable "organizations—regardless of size, degree of cybersecurity risk, or cybersecurity sophistication—to apply the principles and best practices of risk management to improve the security and resilience of critical infrastructure."[1]

Another purview of the directors should be the reporting structure of information security leadership to management and to the board. Many organizations align information security with IT. That may be the right answer for some organizations, but impacts of information security are organization-wide, not just in IT. Information security takes a risk reduction or management focus, while IT has different perspective. Some argue that IT is focused on innovation, advancement, or progress, which may seem like risk-inducing activities. In any case, the skillsets needed to manage risks and deal with issues that are organization-wide need to be independent from those required for organizational reporting structures. Boards are starting to require the senior-most information security professional—in most cases, the chief information security officer (CISO)—to provide a periodic, unfiltered view of the information security maturity of the organization and the information security governance process. Boards are being told by groups such as the NACD that burying information security in IT is a mistake. Without a clear line of communication with the CISO, the board must recognize the risk it faces by being uninformed.

It is not trivial to mention the legal and regulatory liability individual board members and senior management have in the aftermath of information security events. This reality should underscore the involvement of the board in information governance. Directors have increasing ethical as well as fiduciary accountability. Executive management and board members are being held accountable for many high-profile breaches, and in many cases, losing their positions while their companies lose revenue. In 2014, for example, a data breach at retail giant Target cost CEO, President, and Chairman Gregg Steinhafel his job.[2] When Equifax was breached in 2017 and 143 million US consumers' records were potentially compromised, the public backlash and prospect of regulatory intervention resulted in CEO Richard Smith stepping down. These high-profile events, accompanied by very likely civil and criminal liability, easily explain why board members insist on periodic review of comprehensive risk assessments and business impact analyses. Board members should be validating and ratifying the information security governance process for the organization they oversee.

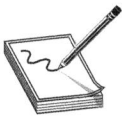

NOTE The accountability of a board of directors stems from its responsibility to uphold a standard of due care for the organization it represents. Due care is measured by the entity providing assurance that governance, risk, and compliance matters are being managed using reasonable measures and efforts to protect assets deemed valuable or assigned sensitivity levels by the organization.

Information Security Program

The first step in applying internal organizational policies against external regulations is to create a robust privacy and security management process. The information security program must be tailored and implemented based on organizational variables such as size, mission, key assets, and risk tolerance. Key elements of the program will be risk analysis and risk management procedures. These are important because standard information security best practices have demonstrated benefits in protecting sensitive information. Healthcare organizations are required to have proactive policies and procedures that implement appropriate information security controls. At the same time, cost and mission requirements must be factored into any information protection efforts. The information protection program will be a component of the information governance framework and will help identify key information security roles and responsibilities. The information security team will influence information security policy development and oversight. Its leadership will monitor ongoing activities and ensure success. Some of the other topics that the information protection program documentation will cover are the continuity of operations, personnel security procedures, and disposal of equipment, to name a few.

Using ISO/IEC 27001 as a guide, we can explore a general framework for an information security program or management system. Figure 2-1 depicts categories of the program along with descriptions of the purpose for the components—in other words, the who, what, how, and why pieces for the program.

The information security program should focus on supporting business processes and initiatives. How the business manages risk, responds to incidents, or assigns responsibility for various information security requirements provides value to the business. The ISO/IEC 27001:2013 standard provides a way for organizations to establish, operate, review, and measure information security management systems (ISMSs).[3] The ISMS includes the information security program and provides guidance for the overall governance. The standard is comprehensive and emphasizes areas such as senior management involvement in the information security program, recommends roles and responsibilities, and underscores the

Figure 2-1
Components of an information security management system

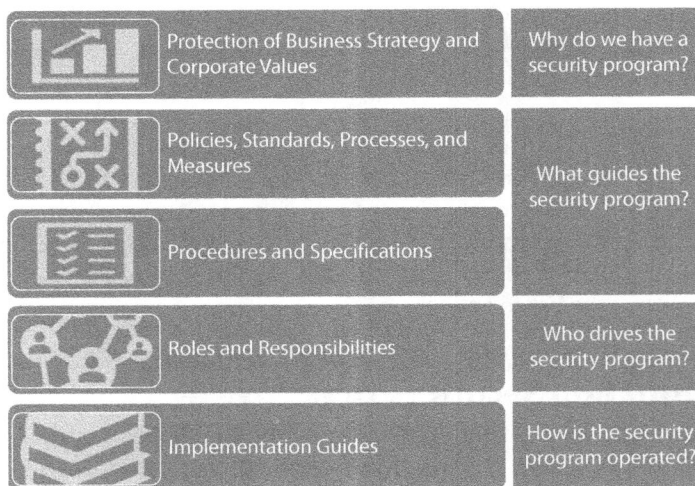

Protection of Business Strategy and Corporate Values	Why do we have a security program?
Policies, Standards, Processes, and Measures	What guides the security program?
Procedures and Specifications	
Roles and Responsibilities	Who drives the security program?
Implementation Guides	How is the security program operated?

need for risk management to support business. It is important to understand the general intent of this standard is to do the following:

- Properly evaluate information risk by considering the interaction of threats, vulnerabilities, likelihood, and impact across the organization.

- Address risks by using a comprehensive approach of security controls tailored to the organization's size, mission, and risk tolerance. Where specific security controls are not reasonable or appropriate, implement other risk mitigation tactics, such as cyber insurance.

- Perform ongoing review of the information security control process for operational effectiveness; continual improvement is a goal and risk levels change.

ISO/IEC 27001:2013 is a proven tool for information security professionals to use to significantly improve the establishment of a proper sense of ownership of both the risks and security controls in an organization. Specific to the information security program, any organization could use the accompanying standard ISO/IEC 27002, *Code of Practice for Information Security Controls*. This standard includes all the security control objectives and recommendations for specific security controls an organization can implement. For healthcare organizations, there are additional considerations: a necessary standard is ISO 27799:2016, *Health informatics – Information security management in health using ISO/IEC 27002*.

Information Security Steering Committee

Creating a culture of security requires positive influences at multiple levels within an organization. This includes an information security steering committee chartered to provide a forum to communicate, discuss, and debate on security requirements and business integration. The committee also encourages colleagues, coworkers, subordinates, and business partners to respect the importance of information security, which is given the same level of respect as other fundamental drivers and influencing elements of the business. It serves in an advisory capacity with regard to the implementation, support, and management of the information security program, its alignment with business objectives, and its compliance with all applicable state and federal laws and regulations. The steering committee also provides an open forum where business initiatives and security requirements can be discussed.

The membership of the committee must include a diverse representation of senior leadership from information security, information technology, business operations, clinical departments, and privacy. The CISO is most likely the most appropriate person to lead the committee. In larger organizations or where information security is more established, the group would benefit from additional members from other parts of the organization like ancillary services, human resources, or public relations. Regular committee meetings can ensure that there is ongoing adherence to the organization's security policies. For example, if a new security policy is created, business unit representatives and/or department heads who are part of the steering committee can make sure their teams implement the policy.

> **EXAM TIP** Remember that a common aspect to leading information security governance teams is participation by representatives from various business and clinical departments; not just IT and information security.

Configuration Control Board

The configuration control board (CCB), aka configuration management board, should play an essential role in how an organization implements and manages its information technology asset. This board is listed as a security control in prevailing standards and policies, such as NIST, HIPAA, FISMA, ISO, and so on. The asset can include the local area network, any endpoint devices (including medical devices), and the various applications that are in operation. The chief information officer (CIO) or another senior information technology official is usually the chair of the group because the CCB focuses on technology. However, having voting members from just about every department in the healthcare organization is crucial.

The CCB is most effective in establishing the baseline configuration of the information asset, but this does not mean the organization must have a standard configuration. Most healthcare organizations have legacy systems (especially medical devices) that cannot meet current standards. Often, the budget does not allow rapid upgrades or modernization to the extent you might desire. Nevertheless, the CCB strives to know exactly what resides on the network. From there, controlling changes through a systematic process will help avoid vulnerability exploitations; whether that involves a patch or an addition of an entirely new system, the CCB is integral in making proper maintenance happen. To that end, the CCB has an eye on security, and members should take every opportunity to address security concerns during every phase of configuration management.

Information Management Council

Information governance is usually managed by an information management council (IMC) chartered to consider management and organizational issues as well as technical concerns. The requirement to have a group like an IMC is something leading auditors and industry evaluators want to see in healthcare organizations. The IMC will have a focus on information use and the impacts that concerns such as privacy and security have. In contrast to groups like the CCB, the IMC will not focus solely on technical issues. As a governance function, the IMC will be a central leadership committee that should have interaction with, and in best cases representation from, other groups such as data governance, the CCB, and enterprise risk management. IMC will concentrate on issues related to the access to information, how technology impacts information use, and the oversight of information policies and procedures. The IMC acts a conduit for senior IT and business leadership on matters of the organization's information assets. It often informs senior leadership groups on use of resources to protect the organization's information by reviewing particular initiatives related to the information security program.

The review of the information security initiatives by the IMC is an example of implementing a culture in an organization in which security is not just the job of IT. All current and planned initiatives, projects, and information capabilities lead by the security team are systematically addressed as enterprise projects. This means the organization realizes there is a shared responsibility for succeeding in the completion of the various projects. Some projects can be conducted within the structure of information technology leadership, but many cannot. Think of a commercially available application that a physician in the emergency room purchases and wants implemented in her department. Imagine, as it turns out, the application is not capable of interfacing with any legacy systems in the hospital. This may be an issue the CCB would address; or, depending on the cost, impact, and perceived value of the application working properly, the IMC could have prevented this scenario by managing it as part of the entire portfolio or list of approved projects. This scenario hints at how culture changes when security is recognized as an enterprise effort. The ability to quantify previously informal efforts based on having the IMC prioritize and value each initiative gives senior leadership an idea of investment and return on investment.

Risk Management Steering Committee

This chartered committee is included in this discussion because it may be the source of governance of third-party information sharing, which incurs a great deal of risk in the healthcare organization. The topic of vendor management may be included in other committee charters, as long as the risks are addressed and governed in alignment with risk tolerance and business strategy. The risk management steering committee is also included here to underscore the integration of governance, risk, and compliance entities with information security and privacy.

The charter and the composition of this committee is selected by senior management. Members represent areas of the organization with significant or impactful risk exposure. The committee reports outcomes to senior management. Some specific components of the committee charter should be the inclusion of specific risks, such as third-party risk, that are within the group's purview. The committee's deliverables include establishing the organization's risk tolerance, which must be approved by senior management and the audit committee of the board of directors. The committee may also create and approve the organization's risk management policy, key performance measures, and its own reporting requirements. A foundational responsibility of the risk management steering committee is to approve results of compliance reviews by internal audits or independent third parties. The committee provides tracking and oversight on remediation of reported deficiencies and provides governance for organizational issues that may unnecessarily increase information security risk.

Data Incident Response Team

Another security control required by various standards and policies such as HIPAA, NIST, ISO, and FISMA, the incident response team should be chartered prior to any data loss or breach occurring. Unfortunately, too many organizations fail to have an active or tested incident response team before an incident actually occurs. According to recent surveys, 77 percent of organizations do not even have a plan for responding to security incidents.[4] Once there is a potential for a breach or an actual breach has happened, there is little time to pull together the right team members and conduct an investigation. Having a team ready to go when needed, with members who know their roles, enables an organization to respond in an accelerated, effective, and organized way when it is needed. Not all reports of data loss are matters that require reporting outside of the organization, such as reporting to government regulators or to patients themselves, but all suspected data losses must be investigated and the outcomes documented. An effective data incident team can prevent a serious loss of profits, public confidence, and/or information assets.

The CISO or senior physical security official likely heads the team. Other members of the team will come from information technology, legal, finance, senior medical representatives, risk management, internal auditing, human resources, and public relations. Of course, based on your organization, it may be important to augment this core group with subject-matter experts in data forensics, health information management, patient admissions, and so on. Ultimately, those who are selected as members of the team must understand their written roles and responsibilities, which should be tested via periodic mock data loss exercises. Prior to actual events, team members must be given the necessary authority to control resources that help them carry out their duties.

Privacy Governance

Personal information continues to be a monetizable asset, identity fraud a profitable crime, and confidentiality a difficult obligation. As a healthcare information security and privacy professional, you must be able to understand and apply governance to protect the privacy of individually identifiable information. Numerous regulatory and organizational implications provide mandates and requirements in this area. Similar to information security requirements, privacy governance can vary depending on jurisdiction per geography or industry.

The governance functions of information privacy within an organization are related and complementary to the information security governance. It is important to note that the relationship is reflective of the evolution of information security and privacy into important disciplines and concerns with increasing overlap. Traditionally, information privacy and security have been siloed. Mature information governance programs are integrating the multiple governance structures, if you include related disciplines such as enterprise risk management, compliance, legal, and audit. Our scope includes only information privacy and security.

Following is the preferred outcome of the integrated governance approach:

- Improved e-discovery, compliance, audit, recordkeeping, and regulatory obligations
- Better data breach prevention, detection, and response
- Enhanced protection of the privacy of employees, customers, and other stakeholders
- Increased linkage with information use and governance, and strategic alignment with business initiatives

Governance promotes and ensures responsible behavior to protect the privacy of all associated individuals. The three lines of defense model, shown in Figure 2-2, can be should be used for information privacy governance and should be tailored to enhance the understanding of information privacy as part of risk management. This framework

Figure 2-2
Three lines of
defense model

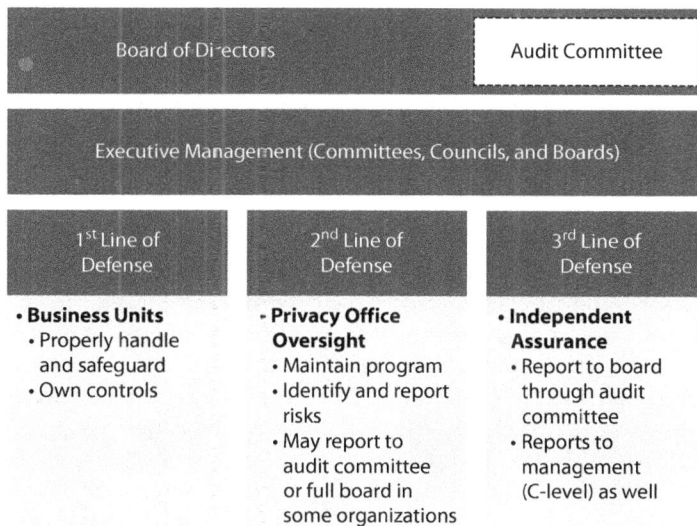

is from an auditing standard, the *Internal Control – Integrated Framework from the Committee of Sponsoring Organizations of the Treadway Commission* (COSO).[5] (In the COSO model for enterprise risk management, a key distinction is the second line of defense, which includes compliance, risk, legal, security, and privacy. This is simplified to use for a privacy governance model. As COSO mentions, "depending on the organization's size and industry, the composition of the second line can vary significantly.") Although many organizations use this model for enterprise risk management, it is applicable to our scope as well. The framework is used to outline and clarify roles and responsibilities. When used for information privacy governance, the model guides oversight of the functions from the board of directors and reduces gaps in roles and responsibilities through layers of oversight, which is required for effective information privacy governance. Figure 2-2 depicts a general structure for the three lines of defense model.

The following provides a brief overview of the three lines of defense structures (they are not prescriptive because organizations may customize them based on unique requirements):

- **First line** This includes the information or data owners who create and use the assets. They are responsive to the data users to make sure data is accurate and complete. They have primary responsibility to ensure the organization meets regulatory requirements.

- **Second line** This includes a centralized information privacy office with chartered committees and groups to create policies and procedures relating to organizational data. These groups also provide oversight and management. Policies or procedures that are not operating effectively are escalated to this line of defense within the governance structure. This function provides strategic perspective for the use of data and investment in information assets.

- **Third line**   This is a final backup mechanism within the organization that has accountability directly to the board of directors (typically through the audit committee) and sometimes directly to government oversight entities. This is usually the internal audit group. Its principal role is the review and assessment of data management and organizational policy effectiveness.

Generally Accepted Privacy Principles

Generally accepted privacy principles (GAPP) are rooted in the principles established by the Organisation for Economic Co-operation and Development (OECD) and by ISO guidance. They attempt to regulate the collection and use of personally identifiable information (PII) in adherence with fair information practices and prevailing laws. One of the biggest proponents of GAPP are Canadian privacy practitioners, which is likely related to the fact that the principles were developed by the American Institute of Certified Public Accountants (AICPA) and the Canadian Institute of Chartered Accountants (CICA).

GAPP is founded on the following privacy objective: "Personal information must be collected, used, retained, and disclosed in compliance with the commitments in the entity's privacy notice and with criteria set out in GAPP issued by the AICPA/CICA."[6]

From that AICPA/CICA guidance, the following are the ten GAPP privacy principles:

- **Management**   The entity defines, documents, communicates, and assigns accountability for its privacy policies and procedures.

- **Notice**   The entity provides notice about its privacy policies and procedures and identifies the purposes for which personal information is collected, used, retained, and disclosed.

- **Choice and consent**   The entity describes the choices available to the individual and obtains implicit or explicit consent with respect to the collection, use, and disclosure of personal information.

- **Collection**   The entity collects personal information only for the purposes identified in the notice.

- **Use, retention, and disposal**   The entity limits the use of personal information to the purposes identified in the notice and for which the individual has provided implicit or explicit consent. The entity retains personal information for only as long as necessary to fulfill the stated purposes, or as required by law or regulations, and thereafter appropriately disposes of such information.

- **Access**   The entity provides individuals with access to their personal information for review and update.

- **Disclosure to third parties**   The entity discloses personal information to third parties only for the purposes identified in the notice and with the implicit or explicit consent of the individual.

- **Security for privacy**   The entity protects personal information against unauthorized access (both physical and logical).

- **Quality**   The entity maintains accurate, complete, and relevant personal information for the purposes identified in the notice.

- **Monitoring and enforcement**   The entity monitors compliance with its privacy policies and procedures and has procedures to address privacy-related complaints and disputes.

Data Governance Committee

Within the organization, the chief data officer (discussed later in the chapter) leads a separate, centralized department that focuses on data governance. Although data governance does concern itself with information privacy and security, there are other important domains in data governance activities: Data governance administers policies and procedures for data usability, consistency, and quality. The function oversees data management practices, strategy, and structure so that the organization can transform data into meaningful information. In today's healthcare organization, the importance of data governance as a component of the information protection capabilities is increasing. To perform data use and analytics functions, the healthcare organization must implement data governance. In fact, healthcare organizations find it difficult to adhere to regulatory guidance and compliance directives across the globe, such as HIPAA and GDPR, without data governance.

A data governance committee will help guide efforts and oversee issues. Membership includes key people often appointed by the CEO or the board of directors. Its charter is to ensure that data is treated like an asset, and that through proper use, it becomes meaningful information. The committee in a healthcare organization should comprise a multidisciplinary group of decision-makers, including a chief data officer, chief analytics officer, chief financial officer, chief medical officer, chief information officer, and chief operating officer. Along with these senior leaders, representation from specific clinical departments, such as radiology or the emergency department, can be valuable. Participants may also come from business and operational areas, at the discretion of the organization. Healthcare organizations can realize a significant benefit from a data governance committee that consists of clinical, operational, and financial leadership, which intends to transform the data asset into a single definition of truth or, again, meaningful information.

The charter of the data governance committee would include some specific technical considerations. The committee establishes and ensures maintenance of metadata definitions that help with data usability. The group also ensures that business rules for access and use are followed. The integration with information privacy and security include ensuring that appropriate levels of data privacy and security audits are conducted.

The responsibilities and charter of the data governance committee extend beyond the data asset itself and include how the data is used. The committee defines and establishes certain roles such as the data steward in the organization. There should be transparency in data flow where data is shared between organizations. The committee has oversight for review and approval of strict data access monitoring as well as reporting policies and procedures. Additional, unique responsibilities include implementing specifications of data extraction, data transformation, and data loads. Of course, the integration of adequate data security and privacy measures is a shared area of responsibility with the types of committees previously mentioned in this section.

Audit Committee (Board of Directors)

As mentioned, the board of directors has a governance role in information protection. It is certainly true that the board's role is not constrained to information security; it also includes information privacy, risk, audit, and compliance. However, depending on the industry, a component committee of the board often has a more specific role in reviewing control effectiveness in information protection. The audit committee of the board is mentioned here because this group has traditionally had purview over information privacy. As data breaches and cybersecurity events have elevated information security to the level of full board concern, the audit committee remains relevant to information privacy governance.

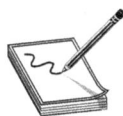

NOTE The audit committee is often chartered with overseeing enterprise risk and other related concerns—in some organizations, the committee may be called an audit and risk committee, for example. In some industries or organizations, the audit committee is actually independent of the full board. The two can share members, but they operate independently in their oversight roles. This fosters additional impartiality in matters of regulatory and compliance issues.

An audit committee is usually appointed by the board and is a minimum of three independent directors with no connection to organization management. The primary charter for the committee is responsibility for internal controls and financial reporting oversight. An example of information shared with the audit committee is a report on data breaches and notifications in a specified period of time. This helps to satisfy the committee's responsibility for overseeing the organization's system of internal controls and compliance with laws and regulations.

Institutional Review Board

If you work in a dedicated healthcare research organization or in an organization that conducts research as part of its academic mission, you will interact with an institutional review board (IRB), also called independent ethics committees or ethical review boards. These are formal, chartered committees that approve, monitor, and review biomedical and behavioral research involving humans. Their primary purpose is to protect human subjects from physical or psychological harm. Much like the first rule of privacy is to determine not to collect information unless you need it, the first rule of research is to determine whether the research should be done. The IRB determines this for the organization through a risk–benefit analysis.

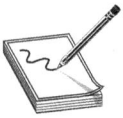

> **NOTE** In the United States, IRBs are accountable for important observation and control functions for research conducted on human subjects that are "scientific," "ethical," and "regulatory." They are empowered by the US Department of Health and Human Services (specifically the Office for Human Research Protections) to conduct research and approve waivers to certain HIPAA provisions such as prior patient authorization to use PHI.

The following are the guiding principles of any IRB according to the Belmont Report:[7]

- **Respect for people** People should be treated as autonomous agents (individuals), and those with diminished autonomy must be protected.
- **Beneficence** The well-being of study participants should be protected by adhering to "do no harm" and maximizing benefits while minimizing potential damages.
- **Justice** Participants should have equal opportunity to be selected, because even if there is a benefit, there is probably a burden some people will have to bear.

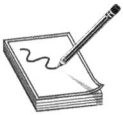

> **NOTE** In the United States, the IRB is governed by 45 Code of Federal Regulations (CFR) part 46 (Department of Health and Human Services regulations for the protection of human subjects) and 21 CFR parts 50 and 56 (FDA regulations on the protection of human subjects). Closely related to IRBs is the provision under HIPAA, specifically the Privacy Rule, which has a provision for a privacy board. Both the IRB and the privacy board are permitted to allow PHI disclosure without additional patient consent for research. This provision is at 45 CFR parts 160 and 164, specifically, section 164.508. Privacy boards differ from IRBs, though. Privacy boards have no other authority within human subject research or FDA-sponsored research like the IRB does.

Information Governance Roles and Responsibilities

The information governance structure in each organization will vary. That is acceptable; drawing from the NIST definition of information governance, you can understand why multiple structures and frameworks can apply to an organization. The purpose of information security governance is to ensure that agencies are proactively implementing appropriate information security controls to support their mission in a cost-effective manner, while managing evolving information security risks. As such, information security governance has its own set of requirements, challenges, activities, and types of possible structures.[8]

Two components of information governance are the definition of key roles and the identification of relevant responsibilities. Common to all information governance structures are activities that support decision-making, defined processes, and personal accountability within the governance framework. This section discusses some common information governance roles and responsibilities you should see in your organization, especially in a healthcare organization.

> **EXAM TIP** You'll see examples of where information governance has improved healthcare in scenarios that describe initiatives such as big data analytics, genomics, personalized medicine, and reduction of medical errors, all within the expanded adoption of electronic health records.

Chief Information Security Officer

It is popular to say that "information security is everyone's job," but in many organizations, leadership and responsibility ultimately reside within the job description of one individual—the chief information security officer (CISO). In larger organizations, the role is likely represented in the senior executive management team. As healthcare organizations evolve to more digital capabilities with numerous interconnections with external partners, the need for a CISO is an imperative. In smaller organizations, the function may be delegated or assigned to an individual who is a non-executive, such as an information security officer (ISO). As the role increases in importance and impact, even smaller organizations should be recognizing the need for specialized, senior-level competence at this leadership level; otherwise, the source of conflict in many companies between IT and information security will continue, and that scenario increases overall information security risk. It makes sense to reiterate that the appropriate segregation of duties for the ISO or CISO is becoming a security standard.[9] In some organizations, the CISO or ISO reports directly to a senior functional executive other than the chief information officer (CIO), such as the CEO, the COO, the CFO, or general counsel. In any case, the senior subject matter expert (ISO or CISO) should be directly accountable to the governing board. Of course, this supposes that the individual has sufficient knowledge, background, and training to be effective and successful.

The role of the CISO is to coordinate and manage security efforts across the company. A CISO also realizes the role includes transforming organizational culture to integrate and engineer information security into business, IT, and clinical processes. The most successful CISOs successfully balance security, productivity, and innovation and act as leaders, teachers, evangelists, and domain experts. The CISO must be an advocate for security as a business executive while being mindful of the need to protect the organization from potential risks; the role comes with opportunities to enable business strategies, but at times, risk management dictates caution. The CISO may not be the most popular executive, and this is why good security decision-making within organizations is not forced on one individual alone: the CISO or ISO must be supported by the governance process consisting of a multidisciplinary committee that represents functional and business units.

Several regulatory requirements relate to the need for a CISO. Although the leading standards stop short of specifying and mandating a CISO, the position satisfies the requirement and is a best practice in these times when information security is paramount for healthcare organizations. Here are some examples of directives drawn from various regulations and standards calling for senior-level information security expertise in an organization:

- **Gramm-Leach-Bliley Act (GLBA)** "In order to develop, implement, and maintain your information security program, you shall (a) Designate an employee or employees to coordinate your information security program."

- **HIPAA/HITECH Security Rule section** "Identify the security official who is responsible for the development and implementation of the policies and procedures required by this subpart [the Security Rule] for the entity."

- **Payment Card Industry Data Security Standard (PCI DDS)** "Assign to an individual or team the following information security management responsibilities: establish, document, and distribute security policies and procedures; monitor and analyze security alerts and information, and distribute to appropriate personnel; establish, document, and distribute security incident response and escalation procedures to ensure timely and effective handling of all situations; administer user accounts, including additions, deletions, and modifications; monitor and control all access to data."

Chief Privacy Officer

The CPO is assigned responsibility for handling and disclosure policies and procedures for personal information, including PII and PHI. CPOs make sure personal information is collected, used, retained, disclosed, and disposed of in conformity with the commitments in the organization's privacy notice and with criteria set forth in best practice, such as GAPP, and in compliance with state, federal, and international law and customs. CPOs also manage organizational processes for identifying data breaches and potential data breaches. They are the central point of contact in providing breach notification and other data incidents to the board of directors, executives, regulators, and government officials. The responsibility extends to reporting breaches that happen at third-party vendors and suppliers as well.

As you can imagine, the impact and weight of these communications have significant impact on an organization. This is one reason why many CPOs are licensed, practicing attorneys with many years of experience, especially in healthcare law. However, a CPO can be successful without being an attorney. In the European Union, a data protection officer (DPO) is analogous to a CPO and is mandated in the GDPR. The GDPR does not specify the DPO's qualifications, but the DPO must have professional expertise in national and European data protection laws and practices and an in-depth understanding of the GDPR.[10]

Privacy law is relatively extensive internationally. To provide evidence of this, consider the following list of leading international privacy laws that some healthcare privacy officers need to discern:

- **Canada** Personal Information Protection and Electronic Documents Act (PIPEDA) governs how you can collect, store, and use information about users. It applies to online information shared in the course of commercial activity. PIPEDA mandates that data collectors disclose privacy policies and make them publicly available to customers.

- **European Union**   The GDPR became enforceable in 2018 and is to date the most robust privacy protection law in the world.[11] The GDPR replaced the Data Protection Directive and has become a model for other nations' legislation concerning individual privacy. Key features of GDPR are the two types of fines it introduces for noncompliance. The first fine is up to €10 million, or 2 percent of the company's global annual revenue of the previous financial year, whichever is higher. The second is up to €20 million, or 4 percent of the company's global annual turnover of the previous financial year, whichever is higher.

- **Hong Kong**   The Personal Data (Privacy) Ordinance (PDPO) applies to public and private entities. It states that users must be informed of the purpose of any personal data collection and with whom the data may be transferred, including third-party vendors and suppliers. PDPO requires that all personal data policies and practices be made publicly available. Those who breach the PDPO can incur financial penalties, which include fines up to HK$50,000 and up to two years in prison. Civil suits by impacted individuals are also permissible against companies that violate the ordinance.

- **India**   Privacy protections are included in the Information Technology Act, which requires every business to have a privacy policy published on its web site. Whether or not the organization collects sensitive data, it is required to have a privacy policy that lists data collected, the purpose of the data, any third parties data might be disclosed to, and what security practices are used to protect the data. Users have to consent explicitly to some types of data use. For example, if the organization is collecting passwords or financial information, consent must be given to the organization.

- **South Korea**   An example of South Korea's national legislation to protect the privacy of citizens is in the telecommunications industry. Communication service providers have to obtain consent before collecting sensitive information to adhere with the Act on Promotion of Information and Communications Network Utilization and Data Protection. The privacy notification must provide the user with information about their rights concerning their own data.

- **United States**   The legislative environment for information privacy in the United States is extensive, but it is regulated mostly at a state or industry level. There are federal laws, but not as many as exist in some other nations. It is valid to conclude that US information privacy laws are a confusing mess of rules and regulations that you must navigate. Following are some pertinent federal and state legislative sources of information privacy protections:

  - The FTC (Federal Trade Commission) regulates business privacy laws. It doesn't require privacy policies per se, but it does prohibit deceptive practices.

  - HIPAA deals with health-related information.

  - The New York State Personal Privacy Protection Law (PPPL) protects individuals from the random collection of personal information by state agencies. The law enables a person to access and correct information on file about themselves. It also regulates disclosure of personal information to persons authorized by law to have access for official use.

- The California Consumer Privacy Act (CCPA) is modeled to a certain extent on the European Union's GDPR. The regulation enhances privacy rights and consumer protection for residents.
- **United Kingdom**   To uphold the information rights in the public interest, the UK Information Commissioner's Office authored the Data Protection Directive. This legislation requires fair processing of personal data. Those who collect personal data must be transparent with regard to the collection purpose and use.

Chief Data Officer

The chief data officer is a senior executive who can support information security and privacy programs through responsibility for the use and governance of data across the organization. A succinct way to think of this important role is as the "voice of the data" for the organization in an era when data is an organization's most valuable asset. The chief data officer oversees a range of data-related functions that may include data management, ensuring data quality, and creating data strategy. Additional roles include oversight of data analytics and business intelligence.

Information System Owner

In the organization, information systems can be centrally managed in IT or decentralized and managed by business and clinical personnel. Some common titles for the information systems owner position are system administrator, product owner, or program manager, depending on how an organization identifies roles and responsibilities. The information systems owner is responsible for applying the principles, policies, and procedures for the overall procurement, development, integration, modification, or operation and maintenance of an information system.[12] This professional is responsible for the security controls needed to ensure the confidentiality, integrity, availability, and privacy of data in all forms throughout the systems development life cycle (SDLC) and data lifecycle for data the system uses.

Data Owner

The data owner helps design policies and procedures regarding how information is used and where it resides. This person oversees information throughout the data's lifecycle and is involved in data-quality management, data security, auditable compliance with privacy and disclosure guidelines, information life cycle management (ILM), and business-continuity planning and disaster recovery. They classify and categorize the information, as PHI or sensitive, for example, because of their knowledge of the assets. This role plays a significant part in safeguarding information assets.

Data Steward

A data steward has a level of responsibility for the quality of data that surpasses that of the data owner. Stewards are not direct owners of the data, but they are selected as caretakers.

Data stewards draft the data quality rules for data, while a data owner approves those rules. Data stewards come from the business side and understand the business, and they are responsible for the data within their area of expertise, which they fully understand. In many cases, a data steward helps with training data owners and users concerning data management and analytics issues.

Data Controller

In the GDPR, data controllers are people or organizations that collect personal data from EU residents. It can refer to an entity located in the European Union or any other country that collects EU residents' data. For example, if a US-based web site is accessed by an EU resident, and the web site collects or tracks personal information through saved cookie files, tokens, or by direct input from the end user, GDPR requirements would likely apply. The data controller role determines the purpose for the information and how it will be used throughout its lifecycle.

Data Processor

A data processor is related to the data controller, but the two are not the same. In the GDPR, the data processor role may be an organization external to that of the data controller and is used to carry out authorized required actions. The data processor cannot change the purpose for which the data was collected. This role is charged with accomplishing data processing activities according to the directions provided by the data controller. Entities such as medical billing companies and cloud service providers may fall into the category of data processors if they are third-party suppliers or vendors for the data collector.

EXAM TIP According to the GDPR, organizations need to understand the difference between data controllers and data processors, and you need to understand the difference as well. The GDPR establishes obligations and limits regarding what you can do with personal data and who is responsible for what.

Data Custodian

A data custodian can be a person or team that owns documents or electronic files. It describes the individuals or entities with responsibility for protecting information through access control and through maintaining administrative, physical, and technical controls for information protection. A key difference between a data custodian and a data steward is that a data custodian is responsible for protection from a technical perspective. A data steward focuses on the business rules or authorized use of the data. A data custodian deals with issues such as security, accuracy, backups, ability to restore, and maintenance of technical standards. The data custodian would provision or deprovision access to data at the direction of the data steward.

End User

An end user of an information system with regard to the governance structure is admittedly a liberal interpretation of guidance on the topic. An end user is any employee or actor, who, on behalf of the organization, creates, transmits, stores, or deletes an organization's information. Add to that definition the policies and procedures we expect end users to know and follow because of end user information protection training. Together, these elements constitute a responsibility for end users that really does integrate into overall information governance. Each end user plays a critical role in protection of information.

Information Security and Privacy Policies and Procedures

Documentation and doctrine for the information governance processes and programs must be in place in any organization that collects data and provides benefits ranging from regulatory compliance to end-user training. The leading information governance programs have documented policies, standards, and procedures that are available for organizations to reference internally as well as to external reviewers, such as auditors, when required. Creating organizational policies that align with well-known standards and procedures provides the following benefits:

- Consistency in structures and procedure to maintain expectations and quality
- Guidance for employee behavior and performance in uncertain processes and scenarios
- Guidance in decision-making in routine situations and clarity during chaotic times
- Fairness and equality demonstrated through adherence to internal regulations
- Just administration of employee misconduct or malicious acts
- A framework for delegation and communication for roles and responsibilities
- The ability to demonstrate a measure of due care and diligence for information protection

It is also important that you align policy and procedures based on relevant national and international laws. On a daily basis, most of us do not refer to national or international laws to do our jobs. It is far more likely that you take actions related to information sharing and protection as a result of what your organization's internal guidance tells you to do, versus citing HIPAA or GDPR. You must be able to determine what internal policies and procedures your organization needs, which must also be consistent with the laws that govern your industry. Lastly, you must be able to apply the internal guidance documents to your daily work while being able to clearly articulate why the proper actions are being conducted.

Although you won't refer directly to national and international law on a daily basis, you can defend the need for organizational policy and procedure on regulations. An overarching control found in almost every regulation is a legal obligation for each healthcare organization to have its own internal guidelines to prevent, detect, contain, and correct information protection violations. Data protection laws mandate that healthcare organizations ensure the confidentiality of its patients. National and international regulations must be customized to reflect your organization's policies and enforcement abilities. You must be able to apply regulation to operations of your organization and assign responsibilities according to various positions in the organization.[13] For instance, the owner of each policy must be identified. That entity, then, will have the responsibility of monitoring the effectiveness of the guidance and making periodic updates as needed. Senior-level officials such as the CIO or CPO may have assigned responsibilities as well. These individuals may enact procedures to commit resources or administer corrective actions when things do not go according to plan.

Policies

Policies offer guiding principles to help in decision-making. These clear, simple, and broad statements regarding how your organization conducts business and healthcare operations can consist of a few paragraphs that cover the various expectations for certain actions. For the most part, organizations use the terms "directives," "regulations," and "plans" interchangeably with "policies." No matter its name, a policy in any form should have the following identifiable elements:

- **Supplemented** Policies tend to be broad statements, so proper implementation usually requires procedures, forms, and other types of direction that can be used by staff to clarify them. Also, rather than reissuing policies, it is often more feasible to supplement a policy with recent improvements or additional parameters using a versioning process. Here's an example: The policy is created and issued as version 1. After reviewing the policy according to how often policies are reviewed for currency (such as every two years), management decides to add responsibilities for a CISO. Rather than completely republish the policy, the relevant information concerning the CISO position can be added as a supplement, or version 2. This also introduces a related element common to all policies: they must be dated.

- **Visible** All policies must be made available, via a web portal or intranet, for example At the least, members of the organization who are responsible in any way for complying with the policies will need to be able to access them. Training related to a policy is also important in making it visible and communicated.

- **Supported by management** This almost goes without saying, but a policy must be supported by management or it will not be followed. More to the point, management must also support the policy by overt action; they cannot circumvent the policy or ignore it and expect hospital staff to comply.

- **Consistent** Unless there is some unique aspect to the healthcare organization, such as its geographic location or community, the likelihood is that any policy will have an origin in a public law or government directive. A policy should not conflict or guide employees to violate these laws. That said, when developing a policy, you should consider references beyond legal ones, such as organizational culture and organizational mission, when writing the expectations.

Your concern is primarily information protection policies. These types of policies will have varying levels of focus within the organization. At one level, a policy is used by management to create privacy and security programs, establish goals, and assign responsibilities. Policies can also be system-specific rules of operation, or they can simply guide managerial decisions concerning one particular issue such as e-mail privacy policy or release of information policy. According to NIST SP 800-15, *Generally Accepted Principles and Practices for Securing Information Technology Systems,* which draws upon the OECD's guidelines for the security of information systems, your organization should have examples of policies at all levels—some governing programs, some system-specific, and some issue-specific.

Procedures

Sometimes called standard operating procedures (SOPs), an organization's procedures describe how each policy will be implemented. These are written instructions, illustrated flowcharts, and/or checklists that cover a routine or repetitive activity. Figure 2-3 illustrates an example of a procedure flowchart for actions that should happen once a data incident or

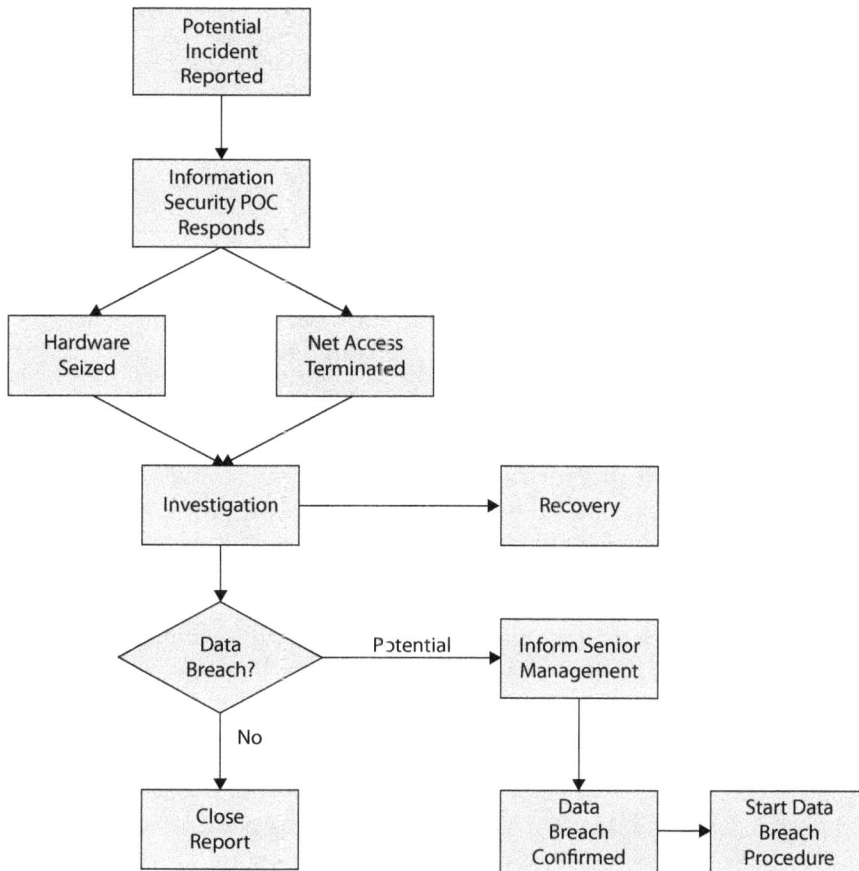

Figure 2-3   Example of flowchart of initial data incident investigation procedure

potential data breach is reported. SOPs should not replace policies but should supplement them, or at least the SOP steps should reference the governing policies. You may encounter terms such as "protocols," "algorithms," "instructions," and "tasks" used in place of "SOP." As long as the content is routine and repetitive and covers how the activity is carried out, these terms are synonymous.

The benefit of having SOPs to clarify policies at the varying levels is to reduce uncertainty and variation in performance. To be most effective, an SOP must accomplish the actions required by the policies, at a minimum. Like policies, SOPs must be visible (maybe even more so), supported by management, and consistent. If they are not or if they seem to contradict the policies, caregivers and business staff will likely create alternative workflows that may or may not be effective and efficient.

EXAM TIP In HIPAA, special considerations are mentioned about all internal guidance and documentation resulting from it (such as a notice of privacy practices form), and you should remember these for your exam. All internal documentation must be implemented with the following:
Time limit You must keep the documents for at least six years (or longer if another requirement exists, such as accreditation).
Availability The organization must make internal guidance available (usually through intranet or printed pamphlets for staff).
Updates The organization must review and update the guidance periodically.

Notable Policies and Procedures

There are almost infinite numbers of policies and procedures that could exist in your organization. Rather than attempt to compile a list, which would ultimately be insufficient, we cover a few important policies and procedures that you will most likely encounter. Keep in mind that this is a small sample, and throughout the text we will address numerous other policies and procedures that are indispensable.

Information Protection Program

The first step in applying internal organizational policies against external regulations is having a robust privacy and security management process. Key elements of the program will be risk analysis and risk management procedures. These are important because standard information security best practices have demonstrated benefits in protecting sensitive information. Healthcare organizations are required to have proactive policies and procedures that implement appropriate information security controls. At the same time, cost and mission requirements have to be factored into any information protection efforts. One of the most important structures established by the information protection program will be an information governance framework that identifies key information security roles and responsibilities. This team will influence information security policy development and oversight. Its leadership will monitor ongoing activities and ensure success.

Some of the other topics that the information protection program documentation will cover are the continuity of operations, personnel security procedures, and disposal of equipment, to name a few.

Release of Information

The need for a policy regarding the release of information is rooted in law. In the United States, HIPAA requires healthcare organizations to have a written policy in place. You will find the requirement internationally as well; for example, the United Kingdom and Australian legislative institutions have ordained laws and policies concerning the disclosure and release of health information.[14] Hospitals in these countries must develop policies and procedures based on relevant laws. The policies need to be consistent with applicable privacy rights for patients. Of course, since the release of information is a common, recurring daily task, a written policy also controls the process so that information is not handled incorrectly.

Although each organization's release of information policy will differ because local workflow is unique to each, every release of information policy should follow these basic principles:

- **Use and disclosure** This includes how the information is normally shared, with whom, and when specific patient consent would be needed. Otherwise, information will be released without requiring a patient signature or additional authorization. You also need to include any situations where information cannot be shared.

- **Minimum necessary rules** Healthcare organizations must make efforts to disclose only what is needed. If, for example, only one specific encounter is under review, the entire legal medical record probably is not needed for disclosure.

- **Patient rights** The healthcare organization must inform patients about what rights they have concerning their information and how it is released to other entities.

- **Organizational controls and safeguards** The release of information policy will include contingency and risk management information concerning how protected health information will be secured during business and clinical workflow interruptions.

- **Right to revoke or opt out** In many countries, the release of information policy must allow the patient to change their disclosure preferences and provide information as to how to indicate their changing preference.

The challenge for you may be in helping your organization keep their release of information policy current against ever-changing standards and regulatory guidance. This can be mitigated by ensuring that this specific policy is created and reviewed by several people in the organization who have privacy and security responsibilities and backgrounds. This is not a policy to be created by one person.

Notice of Privacy Practices

Several laws and regulatory recommendations internationally, including HIPAA in the United States, the Personal Health Information Protection Act (PHIPA) in Canada, and the Organisation for Economic Co-operation and Development (OECD) in Europe, have provisions for notifying individuals of the organization's privacy practices. The notifications should clearly identify collection and use practices and must also cover the privacy rights individuals have with respect to their personal health information.

The notice of privacy practices is similar to the release of information policy, because both include many of the same components. Where they differ is in how they are implemented. To start, there is typically a requirement for the notice of privacy practices to mention specifically that the healthcare organization is obligated by law (if applicable) to protect the information. Under HIPAA and PHIPA, this is the case. Other differences are in data dissemination. Most often, a new patient receives a copy of the notice at the first service encounter or appointment. If the treatment is under emergency conditions, the notice is given to the individual as soon as possible after the emergency is over. The organization must have a notice of privacy practices identified and displayed in their organization for patients to view.

Beyond that, the healthcare organization provides this notice at several times. For instance, in the United States, it is provided at the time of enrollment in a health plan. Every three years, or sooner, the notice is sent as a reminder or upon request. Finally, the notice is to be prominently displayed on the organization's web site for patients to access. As you can see, the notice of privacy practices is not as incident-specific as the release of information policy.

User Agreements

"User agreement" is a general term that you will see in the form of confidentiality agreements, end user license agreements (EULAs), or personal accountability documents. Typically, to instill a level of semiformal accountability in policies and procedures, staff members (users) are required to acknowledge understanding and willingness to comply with training, policy, or other regulatory requirements in a user agreement.

One of the best uses of a user agreement is to authorize a specific user to access an application or clinical system, such as the EHR. In such an agreement, you will find the following general terms and conditions:

- Access to protected health information is intended only for authorized users and for legitimate purposes. All other access is prohibited.

- Users consent to monitoring and auditing of their use of the application or the system.

- Users will protect and not share their access credentials (user ID and password, for example), which would allow someone else to access the system under their login or authentication. Some user agreements specifically mention that users maintain responsibility for any access that occurs using their access credentials.

- If there are specific actions that are worth mentioning concerning user behavior, they can be outlined in the user agreement. Here are examples:
  - Downloading protected health information to external devices may be prohibited.
  - Transporting external media from the healthcare organization may not be allowed.
  - Fully powering off computer systems when not in use to ensure full disk encryption is required.
  - Following data incident reporting procedures according to relative policy is required.
- Users will complete any training that is required prior to accessing the system, and they will provide proof of completion (certificate) to appropriate personnel.

User agreements can certainly include more elements than these. They should be customized based on local requirements, and they can be updated. For instance, leadership may want to allow protected health information to be downloaded by some users on external USB drives (thumb drives). The user agreement can be revised to make this allowance (and perhaps prohibit it for some users).

Incident Reporting Policy

Despite robust prevention and monitoring procedures, data loss can happen. As a point of reference, almost 800 data breaches involving 500 or more individual records have occurred since 2009. This has resulted in a total of almost 30 million records, according to reports received by US Health and Human Services (HHS).[15] It is estimated that all other types of breaches of a single record up to 499 records have accounted for about 80,000 events in the same period of time.

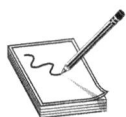

> **NOTE** According to HIPAA, US healthcare organizations are required to promptly report data breaches involving more than 500 individual medical records to HHS.

An organization that is prepared for potential and actual data loss incidents improves its overall privacy and security program, even if it cannot eliminate the risk. Knowing how to handle escalation of events and coordination among the right people is the framework of an incident reporting policy. Incidents are managed according to identified roles and responsibilities. An incident reporting process is required to avoid disruptions in patient care or business processes. In addition, every effort must be made to preserve the evidence of an incidence to allow for proper forensics and analysis. The positive outcome of the policy would be to enable healthcare organizations to improve their information protection based on lessons learned from these events.

The incident reporting policy guides the organization through some general phases. First, the incident is suspected or detected. Here's an example of an incident: An intensive-care nurse notices that his computer has been accessed because he stepped away and left it accessible. When he returns, the screen is on a web site he had never visited. Unfortunately, he was also logged into and using the EHR before he stepped away. Now there is a chance someone else has viewed the record and possibly accessed any number of other records in the database.

Following the detection phase, the nurse escalates the event via the alert phase. This is where the right people are identified for internal notification. This will include the hospital's identified privacy officer and probably the senior information security official. After they are alerted, others who have responsibilities in hospital privacy policy may be included. This action will move the process into triage and response phases.

In leading healthcare organizations, the incident reporting policy enacts a team responsible for conducting actions, including triage and response. The team may include the privacy officer and the senior information security official as well as senior members of the information technology department. Other additions to the team could be the physical security officer, empowered business area leaders, and possibly someone to represent clinical interests. During the triage and response phase, the committee should include interested individuals who have sufficient organization authority to facilitate the completion of the investigation. Keep in mind that as the investigation proceeds, it gets costly, resources may be needed, and senior leadership, including the governing board, may need to be notified.

Once the team confirms the event and takes actions to respond, the goal is to contain the incident and eradicate the cause. From there, the team begins the recovery process and schedules follow-up tasks. These tasks would lead to external notification actions taken by third-party partners that specialize in data loss or breach notification. It may also include making a claim against any existing cybersecurity indemnity insurance the organization may have. In any case, the follow-up actions integrate into additional policies the organization has that are likely outside of the incident reporting policy.

Sanction Policy

In the United States, HIPAA specifically requires healthcare organizations to have and demonstrate how to follow a sanction policy to discipline employees who violate procedures for handling PHI. A sanction policy can be an extension of an organization's incident reporting policy. Once an incident is reported and investigated, data loss is resolved, and any external notification is done, the organization must take the next step and apply the appropriate and consistent discipline.

A good sanction policy will contain two basic components: the type of offense and the type of sanction or punishment. Management would have the flexibility to examine the nature of the offense, any previous offense, or the intent behind the offense. Then management could look at a variety of predetermined discipline actions that fall within a minimum and maximum, depending on the offense. The action could range from a verbal reprimand, to a written admonishment, to suspension and ultimately termination.

In the end, the key points are that this type of policy provides management with a tool to make objective decisions absent of the appearance of impropriety or favoritism. The sanctions provided are not arrived at on a whim or based on emotion. They are included within a written policy, which strengthens the organization against any dispute from an employee who is disciplined. Most importantly, the organization can demonstrate that for particular offenses, equivalent sanctions are applied to all. Of course, organizations do not want to have a lot of sanctions to demonstrate compliance; it's better to have few incidents. Any sanction policy should be communicated to employees during the new-hire orientation process and then annually during retraining. An added measure to gain acknowledgment is to have employees sign a policy document to indicate their understanding of the policy and their obligations to comply.

Configuration Management Plan

In a complex healthcare information technology environment, there must be an organized, coordinated policy and a process to plan, implement, maintain, and decommission information technology assets, including hardware and software. You will find a complex information technology environment in healthcare, where the state-of-the-art medical devices interface with homegrown systems and applications. Often, because of the proprietary manufacturing of certain medical systems, a platform may lag behind the latest supported platform that is preferred. When there is a patient safety risk of replacing the outdated platforms or updating them or when it costs too much to do so, healthcare information technology leaders may be forced to maintain and interconnect the platforms with mitigating controls for privacy and security.

Configuration management is important for information assurance to provide confidentiality, integrity, and availability of data used in healthcare. It is used to manage the security features of hardware and software by controlling changes through the lifecycle of the assets. Not only do the changes need to be managed, but documentation must be updated accordingly. The plan must include provisions for testing proposed changes to the baseline configuration prior to implementation. In fact, many plans include scenarios or regression test cases, which will help ensure that proposed changes, even vulnerability patching, are accomplished safely and efficiently.

You will encounter several common activities in the configuration management process:

- **Planning** The organization will require the objectives and strategies to be documented and available for personnel to use.

- **Classifying and recording** A good configuration management plan (and a good information security program) always starts with a proper inventory to determine the baseline configuration. As the baseline changes, the inventory process continues to document the new normal configuration.

- **Monitoring and control** The change request process must mandate that changes are controlled by a disciplined process of request, testing, approval, and then implementation. Further, those responsible for maintaining the baseline must monitor the process to ensure unauthorized changes are not made.

- **Release management**   Within the control function, release management is the orderly process by which new or modified changes that have been fully tested and approved are installed into the business or clinical system. Releases are classified and recorded based on whether they are major, minor, or emergency releases.

- **Auditing**   To verify that configuration remains at a state that matches the current documentation, you must perform random and routine audits.

- **Preparing reports**   Probably the most important function of the healthcare information privacy and security professional is to communicate results, issues, and recommendations to senior organizational leadership. The configuration management plan must include an expectation for this important function to receive organizational attention.

In healthcare, as most industries, changes to the information systems should never be made haphazardly or without regard to the administrative documentation. Changes must be also tested before being implemented. Otherwise, a change can be dangerous and can impact patient safety—even if the change improves the overall security posture of the information system.

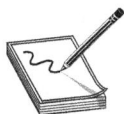

NOTE   Many Department of Defense (DoD) regulations apply to protecting information. Two help to illustrate the connection of internal policies and procedures to national law, international regulations, and industry standards: DoD directive 5410.11, "DoD Privacy Program," and DoD directive 8500.01, "Information Assurance (IA)," shape the military's handling of sensitive personal information. To those who work in the defense environment, these directives are the singular, satisfactory source for protecting information. However, they are really just examples of internal policies and procedures. They are based on US national law, international regulations, and best-practice industry standards. They are tailored to the mission of the DoD and outline the numerous roles and responsibilities of assigned personnel.

Code of Conduct or Ethics in a Healthcare Information Environment

You may work in an organization that has a either a code of conduct, a code of ethics, or both. Keep in mind that these are similar in purpose but differ in how they should be used. A code of conduct can integrate the code of ethics if the organization has both. The code of ethics may encourage employees to foster diversity in the organization. The code of conduct would list relevant regulatory guidance that employees must follow, such as the US Equal Employment Opportunity Act. The code of conduct would also document potential actions the employee may face if the code is not followed. The code of conduct contains employment expectations that are required or prohibited. A code of ethics simply helps guide decision-making toward a preferred, but not mandated outcome. A code of conduct is full of actions that are forbidden and allowed. Ethical guidelines attempt to provide guidance about values and choices. When used together, the organization can provide guidance as to a narrow range of acceptable behaviors from employees and minimize uncertainty.

Computer ethics have been contemplated even as the use of computers became a reality. MIT Professor Norbert Wiener is considered the first to explore this area. His research in 1940 during World War II developed into cybernetics, the science of information feedback systems. He and other, subsequent researchers built upon cybernetics and the increasing use of information technology. These studies revealed that ethical decisions related to computer technology and computer use are subject to three primary influences: the individual's own personal code, any informal code of ethical behavior that exists in the workplace, and exposure to formal codes of ethics. Figure 2-4 offers a view of ethical decision-making related to computer technology.[16] It is important that you know and understand why codes of conduct and ethics are needed. In fact, it is central to certification as a professional (such as HCISPP). You may also find that adherence to your organization's code of conduct and code of ethics is as important to your career as proficiency in your area of expertise.

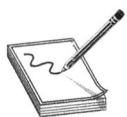

NOTE Wiener authored the book *The Human Use of Human Beings* in 1950.[17] Computer ethics research today is still based on Wiener's foundational work.

Organizational codes of conduct also started to emerge around the 1940s with Johnson & Johnson creating a company credo in 1943.[18] The company's pledge was to maintain corporate responsibility. A founding father of professional conduct, Donn B. Parker, wrote "Rules of Ethics in Information Processing," for the Association for Computing Machinery's (ACM) Committee on Professional Ethics in 1968. Parker's work recognized changes in ethical matters related to the advent of computing technology. He examined the growing incidents of crimes and misuse related to use of computers.

Figure 2-4 Model for ethical decision-making related to computer technology

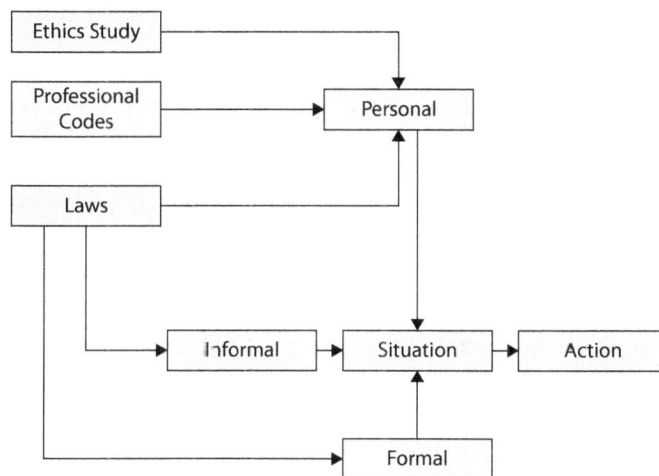

The ACM used his findings and recommendations to create the first Code of Professional Conduct, enacted in 1973.[19] Over the years, this code of conduct has become a guidepost for organizations to operate in a reputable, trustworthy fashion. Legislation and the need for accountability across international borders make the code of conduct an invaluable resource.

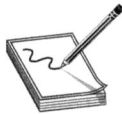

> **NOTE** The term "computer ethics" came from an analysis by computing technology teacher and researcher Walter Maner. He described the ethical problems he observed as early as the 1970s and inspired additional academic studies.

Organizations that rely on information technology and use personal information to provide goods or services for their consumers face a reality described by the Computer Professionals for Social Responsibility (CPSR) in 2007: "Technology is driving the future, the steering is up to us."[20] Although technology has helped us leverage big data, digitize healthcare information, and improve patient care using advanced medical devices, we cannot ignore the significant ethical considerations associated with access to technology. Technological advances have introduced new and expanding risks. We must know and understand how current uses of technology can result in identity fraud, individual right to privacy, and disruption to the system. Then we can understand that protecting personal information is more than a legal obligation; it is a moral imperative.[21]

Organizational Codes of Conduct in Healthcare

As a future HCISPP working in the healthcare industry, you need to understand the common components of a healthcare organization's code of conduct and code of ethics. Many codes of conduct establish compliance as an obligation for employees. Although relevant laws may not obligate the organization to comply with such a code, organizational management determines which rules are important enough to ascribe a mandate. Many organizations use words such as "commitment," "integrity," and "honor" in their codes of conduct to underscore the sincerity of the code. The code of conduct is also meant to apply equally to relationships with all stakeholders—patients, visitors, physicians, third-party payers, contractors, vendors, and each employee as they work together.

Several common tenets are specifically relevant to a code of conduct in healthcare:

- **Patient rights** Patient rights are central to a healthcare organization. Within patient rights is the requirement for the security and privacy of their personal information.

- **Accurate and honest billing** Many healthcare business practices must be conducted within strict compliance or fiscal guidelines.

- **Legal compliance** Healthcare organizations are subject to numerous laws, and an explicit directive to obey such laws is important.

- **Marketing practices**   These practices relate to patient rights as well as modifying behavior. Most healthcare organizations encourage channels of communications and various means for providing patient education, but there are prohibitions against marketing to patients without their consent or sharing PHI with third parties.

- **Fundraising and philanthropy guideline**   Healthcare organizations may use a foundation or equivalent to raise funds to be used for the benefit of their patients. The intention of such fundraising must be a commitment to the public good with accountability to the public.

- **Harassment and workplace violence**   Employees must have respect for one another and treat co-workers professionally at all times.

- **Conflicts of interest**   An employee may have investments or outside employment that conflicts with organizational goals or are deemed illegal by regulators.

- **Political and community involvement**   Although we want to be part of the community in a positive way, some activities may reflect badly on the organization.

Of course, this is not a complete list of all potential components of a code of conduct in a healthcare organization. It is important that you know and understand the code of conduct for your organization, which will contain these, and possibly additional, components.

Organizational Codes of Ethics in Healthcare

A code of ethics for a healthcare organization, like the codes of ethics for other industries, is similar in some ways to a code of conduct. Let's look at some ethical considerations that are included in healthcare organizations' codes of ethics as well as some general differences from codes of conducts:

- **Social responsibility**   Know the community's healthcare needs and provide adequate access that is affordable and convenient.

- **Multi-disciplinary clinical review and ethical decision-making**   Commit to involving patients, family, and other healthcare professionals in significant consultation rather than supporting a unilateral determination.

- **Sanctity of life and compassion**   Many healthcare organizations are faith-based. Your organization may state some ethical considerations that relate to beliefs or religion that shape employee expectations.

- **Personal conduct**   This concept is also covered in the code of conduct, albeit it a level at which conduct violates a law. A healthcare organization may also have unwritten standards for engagement, collaboration, cultural fit, and inclusion in a code of ethics.

- **Accountability**   This is important in situations where self-reporting or self-regulation is needed. It is expected that employees take responsibility for their work on behalf of the organization.

(ISC)² Code of Ethics

Earning a credential from (ISC)², including HCISPP, consists of three main components: passing an exam; being endorsed by a current, certified member in good standing; and adhering to the (ISC)² Code of Ethics. You can lose your certification and member status if you fail to live up to the (ISC)² Code of Ethics. A credentialed healthcare information security and privacy professional is also expected to recognize ethical infractions made by fellow HCISPPs and report any issues to (ISC)² through the ethics complaint procedures.

EXAM TIP Before you take the HCISPP exam, visit the (ISC)² web site at https://www.isc2.org/Ethics to review the exact and latest contents of the (ISC)² Code of Ethics and complaint procedures.

This section includes excerpts and summaries of the (ISC)² Code of Ethics Preamble and canons, which all associates, credential holders, and HCISPPs must follow. Compliance with the ethical standards is not optional. (ISC)² states the following in the Preamble section of the code: "The safety and welfare of society and the common good, duty to our principles, and to each other, requires that we adhere, and be seen to adhere, to the highest ethical standards of behavior." As with other codes of ethics, these requirements are meant to guide professional actions, interactions, and decision-making while working with colleagues, your employers, and the public in general. An (ISC)² credential indicates that you are of solid character, ability, strength, and truthfulness, and that you deserve professional standing in your dealings with your peers, your organization, and the public.

Four mandatory canons act as an action plan for the code, as listed next. (ISC)² contends that the canons are not equal, and if you encounter any conflict, you should resolve the issue using the canons in order, because they are listed in order of importance. (ISC)² provides guidance and details on the meanings and applications of the canons.

- *Protect society, the common good, necessary public trust and confidence, and the infrastructure.*
  - Promote and preserve public trust and confidence in information and systems.
  - Promote the understanding and acceptance of prudent information security measures.
  - Preserve and strengthen the integrity of the public infrastructure.
  - Discourage unsafe practices.
- *Act honorably, honestly, justly, responsibly, and legally.*
  - Tell the truth; make all stakeholders aware of your actions on a timely basis.
  - Observe all contracts and agreements, express or implied.

- Treat all members fairly. In resolving conflicts, consider public safety and duties to principals, individuals, and the profession, in that order.

- Give prudent advice; avoid raising unnecessary alarm or giving unwarranted comfort. Take care to be truthful, objective, cautious, and to work within your competence.

- When resolving different laws in different jurisdictions, give preference to the laws of the jurisdiction in which you render service.

- *Provide diligent and competent service to principals.*

  - Preserve the value of their systems, applications, and information.

  - Respect their trust and the privileges that they grant you.

  - Avoid conflicts of interest or the appearance thereof.

  - Render only those services for which you are fully competent and qualified.

- *Advance and protect the profession.*

  - Sponsor for professional advancement those best qualified. All other things equal, prefer those who are certified and who adhere to these canons. Avoid professional associations with those whose practices or reputations might diminish the profession.

  - Take care not to injure the reputation of other professionals through malice or indifference.

  - Maintain your competence; keep your skills and knowledge current. Give generously of your time and knowledge in training others.

EXAM TIP   Imagine scenarios where you can apply the canons. You'll probably be asked to do more than identify one or more of them in the exam.

(ISC)² Ethics Complaint Procedures

In the unlikely event in which you observe a fellow HCISPP breaking the code of ethics, you will need to know how to file a complaint. Those who do not follow the code risk losing their credential. Keep in mind that failure to file a complaint could result in losing your credential as well. The (ISC)² web site provides a very specific set of procedures you must follow to file a complaint. You should be aware of the following general expectations:

- *Ensure that you are eligible to file the complaint.* The answer comes from the canons. Anyone can file an infraction for canons one and two. Only employers can submit a complaint based on canon three. The fourth canon requires that a fellow certified (ISC)² member register a complaint. If these criteria are not met, the (ISC)² Ethics Committee will probably not agree to hear the complaint.

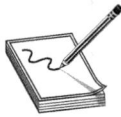

> **NOTE** The Ethics Committee is established by the (ISC)² board of directors and serves at the convenience and discretion of the committee chairman. The committee chairman is selected by the board chairman every year.

- *Don't expect (100 percent) confidentiality.* (ISC)² will give your name to the person against whom you brought the complaint. Beyond that disclosure, all parties are expected to maintain the confidentiality of the complaint outside of the proceedings.

- *Be as specific as possible: identify the specific canon being violated.* (ISC)² will not be able to conduct an exhaustive investigation and will rely on accurate and detailed reports from you. Make sure you have clear, undisputable evidence.

- *Put it in writing: complaints must be submitted using an official (ISC)² affidavit.* You must submit your complaint in writing. In a written affidavit, you will provide a list of identifying facts concerning the situation (names, dates, places, and so on). This is followed by further facts, documentation, and/or evidence of the infraction. In addition, the complaint must be notarized before you mail it to the (ISC)² corporate office in Clearwater, Florida.

When a *prima facie* case has been made, meaning the evidence presented is considered sufficient to pursue by the Ethics Committee, the committee will provide a recommendation to the (ISC)² board. If the evidence is in dispute about facts or details, the committee can choose to hear more evidence. The additional input can be additional facts, corroboration from witnesses, or rebuttals to get clarity on the situation. The committee may choose not to refer the matter to the board and may instead dismiss the complaint. If the Ethics Committee refers the matter to the board, it will do so with a recommendation. (ISC)² states that the recommendation will always be the "most limited and conservative" action available. If the board takes up the case, both parties can make comments concerning the potential board action during a 14-day period. Board action is discretionary and can entail the revocation of certification. Both parties are notified within 30 days of the decision, and decisions of the board are final and cannot be appealed.

Chapter Review

In this chapter, we covered the general categories of information that governance frameworks within organizations should establish and manage. We also defined principles for acceptable behavior for the collection and use of sensitive information. The protection of sensitive information is regulated by national and international laws, such as HIPAA and GDPR. Within those laws and others, the requirement for information governance is established. Information security and privacy are closely related and interdependent concerns in an organization, and there is a significant overlap in the governance of each. The governance structures require multidisciplinary groups within the organization to oversee the proper information protection standards. However, some distinctions apply to information security and privacy individually. For example, information security governance includes some technical security control oversight, such as a configuration control board. Information privacy governance tends to be focused more on legal perspectives, as the privacy controls in healthcare, at least, have deeper roots in legislation than do those of information security.

The implementation of information governance requires assignment and accountability for various roles and responsibilities in the organizations. Here again, there are many similarities between information security and privacy. Each discipline has a need for a senior-most individual subject matter expert to be identified in the organization, such as a chief information security officer or chief privacy officer. It is important to understand the roles and responsibilities individuals have as well. Data owners, information system owners, and end users all have day-to-day duties that are imperative to protecting information. In a digitized healthcare system, an employee today can handle, and mishandle, an unprecedented amount or information in an instant. Extending accountability and capability to the end user is a vital component of your information security and privacy governance.

Although information governance is steeped in national and international laws, you will not refer to those laws as much as you refer to your organizational policies and procedures. Policies and procedures are required by national and international information security and privacy legislation as administrative controls. They also must be aligned to prevailing national and international laws. Each organization must tailor what the law requires to its specific operational and governance models. In this chapter, you learned about variations with regard to how an organization complies with laws that require governance committees; laws do not prescribe what specific committees must exist or their specific names, such as information protection committee, configuration control board, and so on. Implementation of policies and procedures must be relevant to local conditions. Policies and procedure are more often written for local decision-making and guidance purposes, rather than to meet the requirements of national and international laws.

This chapter concludes with an introduction to organizational code of conduct and ethics and a specific overview of the (ISC)² Code of Ethics. No law can completely cover all personal behaviors and expectations. Organizations, specifically healthcare organizations, typically have additional sets of values or ideals that help guide decisions and choices. The contents of these codes are usually not concerned with illegal actions. For example, a code of conduct and ethics may include a provision for ensuring that the organization is patient-focused, but the lack of patient focus may not be a legal issue. Making decisions based on profit or making something easier for the organization, short of patient abuse or malpractice, is not a legal concern but can be considered unethical. As a healthcare information security and privacy professional, you are expected to adhere to a code of ethics for an organization to which you belong and for the (ISC)² Code of Ethics. Four straightforward canons make up the (ISC)² Code of Ethics, and each has several detailed statements to help explain expected behavior of credentialed HCISPPs. Keep in mind that HCISPPs are expected to adhere to the standards and to hold one another accountable. Where an infraction is observed, (ISC)² expects credentialed members to file a complaint. The (ISC)² Code of Ethics outlines the process for how to do that and what each party can expect.

Questions

1. Which of the following would be an expected responsibility for a healthcare organization's board of directors?

    A. Ensure the organization has information security leadership in positions of authority

    B. Select key leadership positions because of fiduciary obligations of the directors

    C. Act as official communication contacts for healthcare organizations during a data breach

    D. Create information security programs once the board established risk tolerance levels

2. What governance board oversees protection of human research information?

    A. Information management council

    B. Configuration control board

    C. Incident response team

    D. Institutional review board

3. If internal organizational policy requires that the chief information officer of the healthcare organization lead the incident reporting team, which of the following could be said of this policy?

    A. Supported by management

    B. Visible

    C. Consistent

    D. Supplemented

4. Which of these apply to the privacy officer position?

    A. Must be a lawyer

    B. Must report to the senior information technology officer

    C. Must be designated in writing

    D. Must oversee third-party partner negotiations

5. Which is true concerning notice of privacy practices?

    A. Once the notice is reviewed by the patient, there is no need to send another copy within three years.

    B. It is a specific requirement applicable to US healthcare organizations only.

    C. Because the notice contains personal information, a copy cannot be disclosed to the general public.

    D. If a patient receives emergency treatment, the patient can review privacy practices after treatment is received.

6. When should training for sanction policies, like most information protection policies, be provided to employees?

    A. At hire with signature acknowledgement

    B. Annually with assessment of understanding

    C. Ad hoc periodically on specific topics

    D. All of the above

7. An internal policy requires that employees obtain patient consent for use of the patient's personal information. The stated intent is for purposes of billing for services. However, the healthcare organization also uses patients' personal information to send invitations to the organization's charitable foundation events. This internal policy violates which element?

    A. Visible

    B. Consistent

    C. Supported by management

    D. Supplemented

8. A good sanctions policy will contain which two basic components?

    A. Names of person responsible and person reporting

    B. Alternative punishments considered and precedents

    C. Type of offense and the type of punishment

    D. Amount of fines allowed by law and criminal penalties prescribed

9. As a newly certified HCISPP, you have a renewed focus at your healthcare organization. You now notice areas of improvement that you learned to identify in preparation for your exam. You also begin to notice that the person who endorsed your HCISPP candidacy, your colleague, is possibly violating the (ISC)² Code of Ethics. You ask him about his actions and he denies he is doing anything unethical. What is your most appropriate next step?

    A. Collect any evidence.

    B. File a complaint with (ISC)².

    C. Report him to his supervisor.

    D. Nothing; it is unethical to accuse fellow (ISC)² members without evidence.

10. A third party handling sensitive health information for a healthcare organization, such as a company that handles payroll functions, is called what?

    A. Data processor

    B. Data subject

    C. Data controller

    D. Data supervisory authority

Answers

1. **A.** The board of directors would be expected to ensure the organization has information security leadership in positions of authority. Of the other choices, the board would likely not select the key leadership positions, act as a communication point during data breaches, or create information security plans, as these are functions of organizational management.

2. **D.** The institutional review board (IRB) is the only choice that is relevant to human research. When information protection in healthcare research with human subjects is referenced, there must be a governing IRB in place. Although the other choices are legitimate groups of internal staff members and leadership in a healthcare organization with information protection responsibilities, none is specifically required for the research of human subjects.

3. **A.** The policy is supported by management. Only this answer relates to the leadership of the chief information officer. The other answers are best practice elements of internal policy but describe different actions.

4. **C.** Most frameworks and laws stipulate that a privacy officer must be designated in writing. A is incorrect because although privacy is steeped in legal guidelines, the privacy officer does not have to be a lawyer. B is incorrect because there are many reporting relationships for privacy officers in an organization, and the relationship in B is not common let alone mandatory. D is incorrect because it is not necessarily required for the chief privacy officer take part in all third-party negotiations, especially if information sharing is not part of the agreement.

5. **D.** In emergency situations, patients may not be able to give consent or be advised on the privacy practices of the organization. After the patient care is provided and the patient is stabilized, it is still required to inform the patient after the fact. A is incorrect because even if nothing changes, the notice should be disseminated to patients periodically. B is incorrect because international healthcare organizations also require similar notices. C is incorrect because the notice does not contain personal information.

6. **D.** All of these answers are appropriate. When it comes to training, communication, and awareness policies, there is no such thing as too much. Using all resources available at every opportunity keeps employees focused.

7. **B.** A consistent policy element ensures that internal policy is derived from external laws and regulations. Policy should not conflict or guide employees to violate these regulations. A is not at issue in the scenario, because the policy is visible to the employee, even if not to the patient. C is incorrect because management may be supportive of the internal policy, but the scenario does not examine that requirement. D is not applicable to the scenario because the policy does not appear to be supplemented with any notice about use of information for fundraising or marketing for the patient to give consent.

8. **C.** A good sanctions policy would include type of offense and the type of punishment outlined. A is incorrect because people's names would not be included in the policy; instead the policy may indicate personnel only by their department. B is too prescriptive for a good policy because management discretion is important. D is not applicable to internal policies.

9. **A.** Based on the scenario, the next step is to observe his behavior, and if you can collect evidence, you can take appropriate steps after that. B, filing a complaint, may be an appropriate step, but only after you have collected sufficient evidence. Otherwise, (ISC)² will likely dismiss the complaint. C is not appropriate because the (ISC)² Code of Ethics requires confidentiality in the process. D is incorrect because you are required to report infractions by fellow credential holders when you have evidence to support your complaint.

10. **A.** Under GDPR, this describes a data processor. B, C, and D have different roles as defined in GDPR and other privacy regulations.

References

1. National Association of Corporate Directors. 2017. *NACD Director's Handbook on Cyber-Risk Oversight, Directors Handbook Series.* https://insidecybersecurity .com/sites/insidecybersecurity.com/files/documents/jan2017/cs2017_0014.pdf.

2. Isidore, C. 2014. "Target CEO out." *CNN Business*, May 15, https://money.cnn .com/2014/05/05/news/companies/target-ceo-out/index.html.

3. International Organization for Standardization. 2013. *ISO/IEC 27001: 2013 Information Technology – Security Techniques – Information Security Management Systems – Requirements.* Geneva, Switzerland: International Organization for Standardization.

4. Forest, C. 2018. "Report: 77% of companies don't have a consistent cybersecurity response plan." *Tech Republic,* March 14, https://www.techrepublic.com/article/ report-77-of-companies-dont-have-a-consistent-cybersecurity-response-plan.

5. Anderson, D. J., and G. Eubanks. 2015. *Leveraging COSO across the three lines of defense.* Committee of Sponsoring Organizations of the Treadway Commission, https://www.coso.org/Documents/COSO-2015-3LOD.pdf.

6. From the GAPP, written by the American Institute of Certified Public Accountants and the Canadian Institute of Chartered Accountants in 2009. See https://www.cippguide.org/2010/07/01/generally-accepted-privacy- principles-gapp/.

7. US Department of Health, Education, and Welfare. 1979. *The Belmont Report: Ethical Principles and Guidelines for the Protection of Human Subjects of Research*. Part B: Basic Ethical Principles. https://www.hhs.gov/ohrp/regulations-and-policy/belmont-report/read-the-belmont-report/index.html.

8. Goodman, S. 2018. "Aligning Privacy and IM Within the IG Framework." *Information Management Journal*, 52(2), 30–35.

9. Shayo, C., and F. Lin. 2019. "An Exploration of the Evolving Reporting Organizational Structure for the Chief Information Security Officer (CISO) Function." *Journal of Computer Science and Information Technology*, 7(1):1–20, http://jcsitnet.com/journals/jcsit/Vol_7_No_1_June_2019/1.pdf.

10. General Data Protection Regulation (GDPR). 2016. *Article 29 Data Protection Working Party, Guidelines on Data Protection Officers ('DPOs')*. http://ec.europa.eu/information_society/newsroom/image/document/2016-51/wp243_en_40855.pdf.

11. Price II, W. N., M. E. Kaminski, T. Minssen, and K. Spector-Bagdady. 2019. "Shadow health records meet new data privacy laws." *Science*, 363(6426):448–450.

12. Bowen, P., J. Hash, and M. Wilson. 2007. *Information Security Handbook: A Guide for Managers*. National Institute of Standards and Technology Special Publication 800-100. https://nvlpubs.nist.gov/nistpubs/Legacy/SP/nistspecialpublication800-100.pdf.

13. National Institute of Standards and Technology (NIST). 2011. *Managing Information Security Risk: Organization, Mission, and Information System View*. NIST Special Publication 800-39. https://nvlpubs.nist.gov/nistpubs/Legacy/SP/nistspecialpublication800-39.pdf.

14. Yarmohammadian, M. H., A. R. Raeisi, N. Tavakoli, and L. G. Nansa. 2010. "Medical record information disclosure laws and policies among selected countries; a comparative study." *Journal of Research in Medical Sciences*, May–Jun, 15(3):140–149.

15. US Department of Health and Human Services. "Health Information Privacy. Breaches Affecting 500 or More Individuals." www.hhs.gov/ocr/privacy/hipaa/administrative/breachnotificationrule/breachtool.html.

16. Pierce, M. A., and J. W. Henry. 1996. "Computer ethics: The role of personal, informal, and informal codes." *Journal of Business Ethics*, 15(4):425–437.

17. Weiner, N. 1950. *The Human Use of Human Beings: Cybernetics and Society*. Boston: Houghton Mifflin Co.

18. Johnson & Johnson. nd. "Our Story: Living Our Credo." https://ourstory.jnj.com/living-our-credo#our-credo-ch-3.

19. Bynum, T. 2015. "Computer and Information Ethics." *The Stanford Encyclopedia of Philosophy Archive,* Summer 2018 Edition. Edward N. Zalta, ed. https://plato .stanford.edu/archives/sum2018/entries/ethics-computer/.

20. Computer Professionals for Social Responsibility. 2007. "What is CPSR?" http:// www.cpsr.org/.

21. Franklin Jr., C. 2019. "Cybersecurity's 'Moral Imperative.'" *Dark Reading, The Edge,* October 30, https://www.darkreading.com/edge/theedge/cybersecuritys-moral-imperative/b/d-id/1336206.

Information Technologies in Healthcare

This chapter covers Domain 3, "Information Technologies in Healthcare," of the HCISPP certification. After you read and study this chapter, you should be able to:

- Comprehend the importance of healthcare information technology (HIT) tools
- Understand the privacy and security implications for HIT
- Recognize regulatory and legislative impacts on HIT secure use
- Describe the major benefits and challenges for HIT secure interoperability
- Know the components of data lifecycle management
- Identify and apply models and standards for third-party connectivity

Healthcare information technology (HIT) includes all the computer, digital, and electronic hardware and software used in a healthcare organization to collect, use, transfer, and store information. This technology can differ distinctly from other forms of IT used in business, industrial control, financial, or telecommunications, for example, though many of the IT components are the same across these industries. You would recognize operating systems, databases, hardware, and mobile platforms in all of them, for example. The difference with HIT that you, as a healthcare information security and privacy professional, need to be aware of is in the function and purpose of HIT compared to the other forms of IT. HIT can be directly central to human life and safety issues as well as being critical to very complex medical procedures, where precision is required. The security implications for HIT used in medical devices and electronic health records, for example, are equally critical.

This chapter focuses on special-purpose computing resources used to conduct healthcare operations or support patient care. When we cover privacy and security in healthcare more in depth in Chapter 5, you will gain more insight into the frameworks, regulations, and responsibilities that come with health information privacy and security obligations.

As you understand how these technologies are used in the healthcare environment, you will realize that the implementation of privacy and security controls must be tailored to each situation. In many cases, the best security practices used in other industries and IT protection specifications may not operate efficiently or effectively in a patient care environment. In fact, these privacy and security controls can actually introduce unintended consequences leading to patient safety and quality of care issues.

Fostering Privacy and Security with HIT

To review, the term "privacy" in a healthcare context refers to processes and safeguards put in place to protect the confidentiality of certain personal health information. The definition of "security" is the means and methods used to control access, collection, use, storage, transfer, and disposal of an individual's sensitive information. By implementing privacy and security correctly, we foster patient trust in our organizations. The advent of HIT has had a positive impact on patient care. State-of-the-art imaging systems, monitoring devices, and robotic surgical tools are all examples of HIT that have improved provider practices and saved lives. Throughout this chapter, we will examine areas where HIT has impacted privacy and security in ways that require us as information protection professionals to design and implement controls to safeguard digital healthcare information.

Before we begin that discussion, it would be worthwhile to mention how HIT has actually improved healthcare information privacy and security concerns. For example, the implementation of electronic health records has improved the secure availability of medical information. Traditionally, medical records were kept in paper documents that were immediately available only in one office or organization. Information sharing for continuity of care or public health surveillance, while protecting the privacy and security of such information, could be very difficult. Transferring a digital patient record across a network to authorized providers and public health officials, on the other hand, can be a more confidential process that enables the right information to be available at the right place when needed. Remember that availability is one of the components of the information security triad of confidentiality, integrity, and availability.

Another example of a positive impact from HIT is that data integrity is vastly improved. The complex algorithms and data analytics that are sometimes inherent to a medical device make possible important data integrity capabilities. Medical errors such as drug-to-drug interactions or dosage mistakes have plagued healthcare. Using an advanced medical device in patient care may enable providers to collect and analyze information, and these devices may alert providers to various potential problems. Imagine, for example, a provider authorizing a dosage of Warfarin through an infusion pump. The device may alert the physician to the patient's earlier doses of Warfarin or other drugs, and this could help avoid overdoses or negative interactions. The implementation of HIT in such cases not only improves data privacy and security, but also improves patient care and safety.

EXAM TIP HCISPP candidates must be able to consider the impacts that implemented controls will have on patient care. Be ready for scenarios that suggest safeguarding access to information or implementing technical controls and how those may change healthcare delivery.

Increased Exposure Affecting the Threat Landscape

Confidentiality, integrity, and availability—the CIA triad—must be addressed in every healthcare environment. The privacy and security controls we implement and monitor are intended to protect one or more facets of the CIA triad.

- **Confidentiality** Protects information from disclosure to unauthorized parties
- **Integrity** Safeguards information from unauthorized alteration or modification
- **Availability** Ensures that authorized parties have access to the right information when needed

The introduction of HIT has increased exposure to information security and information privacy threats. You must constantly assess these threats and the impact on the CIA triad relative to HIT systems while managing and using sensitive information. When security or privacy risks are realized, they can cause adverse effects or problems for patients. To avoid these problems, HIT engineers are responsible for working with security professionals to design, build, and implement systems that integrate information protection and risk management. This results in more trustworthy systems that include privacy and security as integral attributes. In selecting and securing HIT, you should use the following three design attributes with regard to protection of sensitive information:

- Knowledge of what data is collected and used
- Support for restricted access by enabling granular controls
- Ability to limit authorization based on operational requirements

Lines between information security and information privacy can be blurred. The context of these information protection concerns offers an opportunity for you to recognize the boundaries and overlaps. You must determine when existing security risk models and security-focused guidance can be applied to address privacy concerns in HIT. Where there are gaps, security engineering must be added to achieve an approach to privacy.

Figure 3-1 depicts the entwined relationship between privacy and security. A key point to remember as we explore HIT is the relationship between these disciplines that is best served by managing the material distinctions and leveraging the overlaps. Security risks arise when sensitive information is not handled appropriately. Privacy risks, however, arise when sensitive information is disclosed in an unauthorized manner and exposes the data (confidentiality failure) to potential problematic actions.

Figure 3-1
The overlapping relationship between information security and information privacy

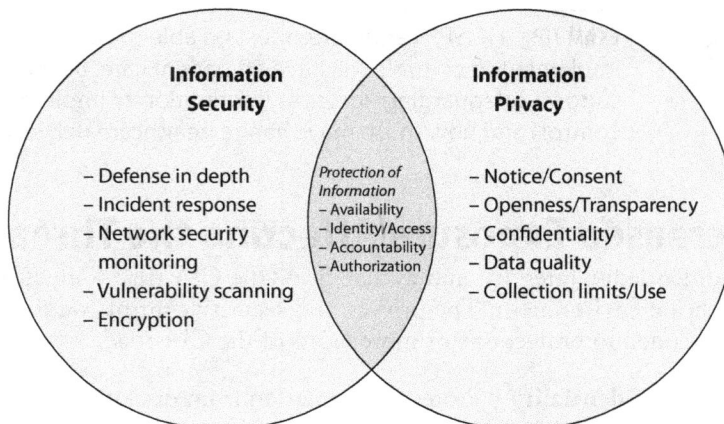

Internal Threats to HIT Privacy and Security

To begin the examination of how HIT increases exposure to threats, we need to start with how internal actions are part of the risk profile. Remember that HIT systems that are designed to make our patient care processes safer, more efficient, and more effective can also pose privacy and security risks. Because HIT operations usually depend on human interaction with the technology, errors can result with unintended consequences, such as unauthorized disclosures or exploited vulnerabilities, leading to privacy or security issues. In fact, in some cases, an internal error or mistake could result in a patient safety issue.

The Emergency Care Research Institute (ECRI) highlights the privacy and security threats introduced by HIT. This industry group focuses on helping healthcare organizations use healthcare technology that is effective and safe for use with patient care. Each year, the ECRI assembles a top 10 list of healthcare technology hazards that cause the most incidents that impact patient safety. Relevant to internal incidents, in 2019, ECRI listed mistakes such as entering the intended flow rate into an infusion pump's dose rate field as a leading privacy and security problems that can result in dangerous medication administration errors.[1] This is an example of wrong-field programming, and even sophisticated medical devices can be misconfigured and operated in an insecure or unsafe manner. The problem is that these errors often go unnoticed by the clinician because of their assumption that the HIT is working correctly.

External Threats to HIT Privacy and Security

Addressing the threats from another perspective, the growing numbers of IP-enabled HIT systems are imperative to clinical operations and patient care. Initially, manufacturers paid little attention to protecting their equipment from external attackers possibly targeting their HIT systems. However, with embedded software in many products, ranging from health-tracking wristbands to cardiac-monitoring undergarments, regulators and manufacturers are becoming increasingly concerned about the potential threat to poorly secured devices.

Threats to Medical Devices

This concern is not new, yet it is very real—witness the issue in 2013 with former Vice President Dick Cheney and his defibrillator, or a recently sanctioned medical device–hacking challenge at an industry security conference in 2019.[2,3,4] Internet-enabled medical devices and electronic databases for clinical and administrative operations are networked technology that provide greater connectivity, but they increase HIT exposure to cybersecurity threats. HIT device manufacturers, hospitals, and other healthcare providers must evaluate and manage a new set of risks. Connected medical devices—like other computer systems—can be vulnerable to security breaches and have a potential major impact on the safety and effectiveness of these devices. Specifically, in a healthcare environment, this vulnerability increases as medical devices and medical equipment are becoming more connected through the Internet to other medical devices, patients, and/or to hospital networks (also referred to as the Internet of Medical Things, IoMT).

In 2017, the FDA issued a safety communication, noting that cybersecurity vulnerabilities in St. Jude's Medical implantable cardiac device, the Merlin@home Transmitter, which sends and receives radiofrequency signals wirelessly to the pacemaker, could pose a serious problem. The FDA determined that this transmitter was vulnerable to attack and noted this in its 2017 press release:

> The FDA has reviewed the information concerning potential cybersecurity vulnerabilities associated with this transmitter and has confirmed that these vulnerabilities, if exploited, could allow an unauthorized user, i.e., someone other than the patient's physician, to remotely access a patient's RF-enabled implanted cardiac device by altering the transmitter. The altered transmitter could then be used to modify programming commands to the implanted device, which could result in rapid battery depletion and/or administration of inappropriate pacing or shocks.[5]

Fortunately, according to the FDA, no adverse events, including death, have resulted from the vulnerability. The FDA later noted that St. Jude Medical issued a patch that fixed the vulnerability and was quick to issue a statement taking the appropriate remediation actions by patching its systems against cyber risks.

This was not the first FDA comment on cybersecurity issues, however. In December 2016, the FDA issued a recommendation that both hospitals and medical device manufacturers implement a proactive, comprehensive risk management program that includes the following:

- Implementing the National Institute of Standards and Technology (NIST) Framework for Improving Critical Infrastructure Cybersecurity
- Establishing and communicating processes for vulnerability intake and handling
- Adopting a coordinated disclosure policy and practice
- Deploying mitigations that address cybersecurity risk early and prior to exploitation
- Engaging in collaborative information sharing for cyber vulnerabilities and threats

Hospitals must make medical device security a central component in their entire risk management and business resiliency programs. The FDA also called for manufacturers to increase their attention to medical device security and connected cybersecurity with regard to current safeguards to ensure device quality and patient safety.

Threats Related to Cloud Computing

Cloud computing has introduced new threats to healthcare information security. The increase in protected health information (PHI) and personally identifiable information (PII) in cloud environments brings new concerns. Cloud computing is being increasingly adopted by healthcare because it offers benefits such as improved access to data and cost efficiency. There are, of course, risks as well. Processes and techniques used to protect data within the cloud can be different from those required for data located in a data center under the direction of the healthcare organization. In the cloud, data loss prevention monitoring and vulnerability management scanning may be the responsibility of the cloud service provider alone. The configuration of security technology in the cloud may also be a risk undertaken by a third party, rather than by the healthcare organization.

To illustrate, consider the 2019 Capital One data breach incident that potentially exposed the data of 100 million of the bank's customers. Capital One, like many users of cloud technology, relied on internal employees as well as third-party contractors to protect its cloud-stored data. Potential vulnerabilities the criminal attacker exploited may have included misconfiguration of assets in the cloud and disregarded authentication protocols.[6] Who was at fault is not important to this discussion; what is important is that the use of the cloud, as is clear in the Capital One report, introduces the organization to new sources and types of threats to its data. While Capital One is not a healthcare organization, the example is relevant because cloud use of and reliance on third-party contracted support are a shared reality among all industries using the cloud.

What is also shared are the risks to information privacy and security of which this scenario illustrates but one example. Depending on the type of service model you have with a cloud service provider, you will have different responsibilities. With a Software as a Service (SaaS) cloud agreement, you will likely have responsibilities for access and authentication. The cloud service provider is responsible for maintaining the hardware and software; particularly vulnerability management and security monitoring. In comparison, an Infrastructure as a Service (IaaS) cloud service vendor would likely be responsible for overall security of the facilities and possibly disaster recovery capabilities, but your organization would remain responsible for maintenance of the hardware and software resources you are leasing for use within the cloud service provider's environment. We will explore the shared security concerns and the variety of cloud service provider models in greater depth in Chapter 7.

Figure 3-2 illustrates some categories of information privacy and security threats that are relevant to using cloud computing models.

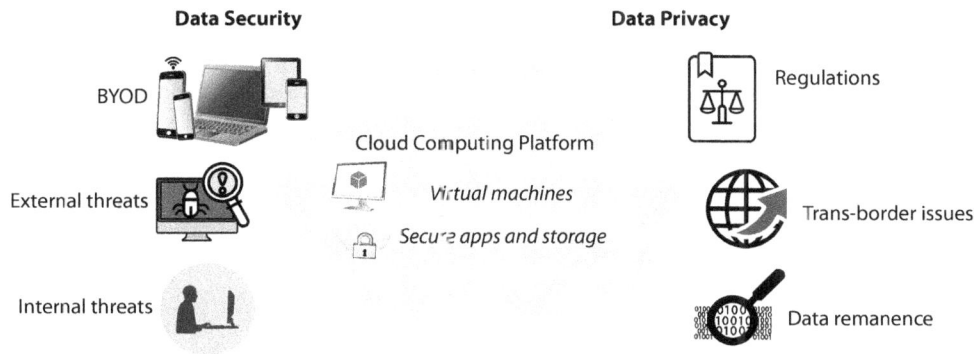

Figure 3-2 Major categories of information privacy and security threats to cloud computing environments

Software-Initiated Threats (Malware)

Additional cybersecurity threats for connected HIT, including computer viruses and malware, also have the potential to jeopardize a patient's treatment and privacy. It is important to recognize the threats to HIT that can come from simply being connected to a network.

A case in point is Bayer, a medical device manufacturer, which confirmed in 2017 that the company had received reports from customers in the United States that their computers had been targeted by the WannaCry ransomware attack.[7] This compromise happened because some medical devices were connected to a network and used a commercial software operating system (Microsoft Windows).

To prevent such attacks, our roles and responsibilities as healthcare information security and privacy professionals is to have a thorough and well thought out cybersecurity management policy that incorporates software threats to HIT, including medical devices. This is critical today for both healthcare organizations and medical device manufacturers.

E-iatrogenesis

The internal and external threats that have emerged from increased use and reliance on HIT has concurrently introduced a new concept into the healthcare information security lexicon: *e-iatrogenesis* refers to any patient harm caused by the application of HIT (and, by extension, healthcare information security efforts).[8] The term evolves from *iatrogenesis*, which is an inadvertent adverse effect or complication resulting from medical treatment or advice from a healthcare provider.

For example, suppose a doctor writes a prescription for a patient but does not cross-referenced this medication with the patient's current medication list; an adverse reaction happens when the new drug negatively reacts with the medications the patient currently takes. Table 3-1 highlights some real-life examples of episodes of e-iatrogenesis that have occurred at various engineering stages of HIT, specifically relating to medical devices.

Engineering Stage	Adverse Event	Contributing Factor
Requirements specification	Radiation therapy machine: Patients died from massive overdoses of radiation.	An FDA memo noted that an apparent lack of documentation on software specifications and a software test plan contributed to this issue.
Design	Pacemaker/implantable defibrillator: Implant can be wirelessly tricked into inducing a fatal heart rhythm.	Security and privacy were not part of the product's early design process.
Human factors	Infusion pump: Patients were injured or killed by drug overdoses.	The software did not prevent a key bounce that misinterpreted keypresses of 20 mL as 200 mL.
Implementation	Infusion pump: Under-dosed patient experienced increased intracranial pressure followed by brain death.	A buffer overflow (programming error) shut down the pump.
Testing	Ambulance dispatch: Emergency calls were lost.	Ambulance workers accused the computer system of losing calls and claimed that because an acute number of deaths occurred when calls were lost, the computer system was withdrawn. The ambulance company attributed the problems to "teething troubles" with a new computer system.
Maintenance	HIT devices: Computer systems were globally rendered unavailable.	An antivirus update misclassified a core Windows OS component as malware and quarantined the file, causing a continuous reboot cycle for any system that accepted the software update. Numerous hospitals were affected, and the problem affected thousands of computers, forcing hospitals to postpone surgeries and stop treating some patients in emergency rooms.

Table 3-1   Some Adverse Events Resulting from Medical Device Software Issues

Even if an incident does not actually harm the patient, the healthcare organization may face consequences. The Joint Commission, a nongovernment organization in the United States that inspects, accredits, and certifies hospitals, requires reporting of a *sentinel event,* in which death or serious physical or psychological injury, or the risk of either, was the result of prescription drug administration.[9] A drug reaction scenario would be considered such an event. Another example, having a medical device reboot in the middle of a patient procedure, can certainly be considered a near-miss event. It is also easy to imagine how the process or procedure could go wrong and cause a serious adverse outcome for the patient. In sum, the best information security practices, as applied to the healthcare industry, must include a risk-reward consideration with the number one rule of healthcare at the core: first, do no harm.

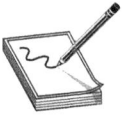

> **NOTE** Although the Joint Commission is US-centric, it has peer organizations in most advanced nations. In fact, the Joint Commission itself has had an International component since 1994, with almost 700 organizations—certified in South Korea, Italy, Spain, Turkey, and Brazil, to name a select few.

Oversight and Regulatory Challenges

The healthcare environment has evolved into a highly interconnected system of systems that depends on the exchange of digital information. Increasingly, many agencies and entities have varying degrees of authority to improve healthcare quality, safety, and efficiency through the promotion of health IT, including electronic health records and private and secure electronic health information exchange. They may be government organizations or private governing bodies made up of volunteers. The work that they do results in guidance, standards, or even laws that impact the usability of HIT, for the benefit of information security and privacy. These oversight and regulatory activities should encourage secure and authorized interoperability and information sharing using HIT is an imperative to quality patient care.

HIPAA and HIT

The US Health Insurance Portability and Accountability Act (HIPAA) has a material impact on HIT. HIPAA is a collection of multiple rules and amended guidance consisting of the following:

- **HIPAA**   The original intent of HIPAA included significantly more regulatory intent than just protection of patient information. The first iteration in 1996 was aimed at clarifying the portability of health insurance so that people were able to change health insurers without disruption. The law also contained administrative simplification to begin to address issues that result in waste, fraud, and abuse in the healthcare system. That effort continues today.

- **Privacy Rule**   This major addition was enacted in 2002 and addressed the specific requirements to protect the confidentiality of patient information. To that end, the law described safeguards such as restrictions for authorized use and limits on the disclosure of protected information. Informed patient consent for information use was included in this law. It also outlined patients' rights with regard to reviewing records and requesting corrections to their records.

- **Security Rule**   This 2004 law addressed the evolution of healthcare information to more electronic formats, as HIT increased in healthcare organizations. This law required that healthcare organizations safeguard electronic healthcare information that they collected, and use reasonable and appropriate administrative, physical, and technical controls.

- **HITECH**   This act, formerly known as the Health Information Technology for Economic and Clinical Health Act, was passed in 2009 and focused on the implementation of electronic health records (EHRs) in healthcare organizations. HITECH was part of the American Recovery and Reinvestment Act of 2009 (ARRA), and together they offered financial incentives for EHR adoption in an initial phase. The act had to also address some security requirements, including evidence of an enterprise risk assessment completed by healthcare providers. After an initial adoption phase, the ARRA and HITECH removed the incentives and introduced penalties for not meeting EHR implementation targets. HITECH included harsher penalties for healthcare organizations that failed to protect information, such as those that experienced data breaches or had findings resulting from federal audits.

- **Omnibus Rule**   This rule organized and combined some interim final rules that were in various phases of authority and effect. In 2013, a major component of the rule was the clear definition of who was subject to HIPAA by defining the conditions for being a business associate.

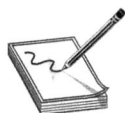

NOTE   In the foundational law, HIPAA or Public Law 104-191, the original purpose of the act included the phrase "and for other purposes." As the Privacy Rule, the Security Rule, HITECH, and the Omnibus Final Rule have emerged, most of the "purposes" have made HIPAA synonymous with the privacy and security of health information.

We'll examine HIPAA in more depth in Chapter 4, with additional regulatory sources that impact healthcare. The introduction of regulatory sources is meant to highlight how laws are designed to motivate healthcare organizations to improve the healthcare system by implementing HIT that can reduce costs, enhance quality, and improve the delivery of care. For example, HITECH helped in this regard by making Medicare and Medicaid incentive payments available to healthcare organizations that adopted HIT. Those organizations that could demonstrate they were meeting established workload targets and transactions with electronic health records earned reimbursement from the US government. HIPAA has affected HIT in the following ways:[10]

- **Encryption services**   These have advanced because of requirements for PHI to be made unreadable, unusable, or indecipherable to unauthorized persons.

- **Employee training**   This emphasizes that awareness and training of personnel are central to the regulations.

- **Risk management**   This mandates assessment, evaluation, and reduction of risk across the organization as well as per HIT system or application.

- **Cloud service providers**   Specifically, the Omnibus Final Rule helps clear the way for healthcare organizations to enter into contractual agreements with cloud providers.

- **Electronic health records** HITECH provided reimbursement, which catapulted implementation rates for digitized record use.
- **Access and authorization** The ability to limit and monitor access to information is improved by HIT because logging and auditing enables the accounting of disclosures and data forensics.

The use of HIT regulated by HIPAA can be exceptionally beneficial to a healthcare organization. The implications of information privacy and security are important for you to understand and leverage on behalf of patient care and patient safety.

Office of the National Coordinator for Health Information Technology

An influential source of HIT guidance is the Office of the National Coordinator for Health Information Technology (ONC) located in the US Department of Health and Human Services (HHS). Established by HITECH, the ONC aims to provide information to clinicians to help them connect using HIT. Its goals include making healthcare more individualized, which will also improve outcomes for the community. Success with the ONC relies on input and assistance from many private-sector experts or practitioners to develop communication standards, software, hardware, and training for those who use HIT. ONC provides recommendations for strategies that will result in a US HIT infrastructure based on standards and policies that support the exchange of health information. To recommend standards, the HIT Standards Committee provides implementation specifications and HIT certification criteria. It also tests and ensures consistency with privacy and security guidance.

GDPR and HIT

The EU General Data Protection Regulation (GDPR) was created and adopted in April 2016 and has been enforced since May 2018. The law explains and increases privacy rights in light of the growing use of the Internet for commerce in the EU and globally. The GDPR is a single set of rules on data protection. A single market is established to reduce administrative complexity, costs, and burden to member states. However, each EU nation has an autonomous national protection authority.

The following GDPR items highlight HIT:[11]

- The regulation strengthens individuals' rights so that the collection and use of personal data is limited to the minimum necessary.
- The GDPR defines rights to data portability to ease the transfer of personal data from one service provider to another.
- The "right to be forgotten" is explicitly recognized. The previous privacy law limited the processing of data unless specific criteria were met; the GDPR expanded that to include individual rights, to enable a patient to demand removal of his or her information.
- GDPR rules have clarified and strengthened data breach notification requirements.

The GDPR has more of an impact on health data than HIT. This does not minimize the law's regulatory impact, but clarifies and focuses its attention. For example, the GDPR continues the previous privacy law's approach to treating health data as sensitive personal data. The GDPR, however, has added emphasis and requirements for genetic data and biometric data as sensitive personal data that should be classified more restrictively. Member states are permitted to introduce stricter conditions beyond the GDPR with regard to the processing of biometric, genetic, or health data.

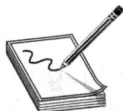

> **NOTE**   With GDPR, the government is looking at applications and systems that implement "privacy by design"—in other words, privacy and security controls are integrated and engineered into their original frameworks or architectures.

Interoperability

Interoperability refers to the availability of data with regard to its ability to be transferred between connected systems and applications. Several conditions establish interoperability:

- The HIT must be able to share information securely with other HIT systems without the need to create custom configurations or require manual interventions.
- The interchange of information needs to be comprehensive and must support authorized access and use.
- Systems should not introduce information blocking, a problem characterized by proprietary HIT systems purposely not supporting interoperability with systems from other manufacturers.

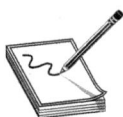

> **NOTE**   The ONC has initiated a Shared Nationwide Interoperability Roadmap and Interoperability Standards Advisory to establish a collaborative public agency and private sector partnership to develop and achieve shared, comprehensive interoperability agenda and action plans. For more information, visit https://www.healthit.gov and read "Connecting Health and Care for the Nation: A Shared Nationwide Interoperability Roadmap."

Interoperability in HIT is important, because data sharing in healthcare is an essential component of patient care, research, and quality initiatives. Within the organization, providers consider data sharing an imperative that enables them to access things easily, such as medication lists and laboratory results, precisely when they need it. Even after care is provided, sharing information is important in settings such as peer record review, where procedures are reviewed and measured against organizational and clinical standards. The intent there is to discuss best practices, share common experiences, and, in the end, maximize scarce resources by reducing duplication and ineffective processes.

When HIT systems and applications cannot send and receive information, you can imagine the resulting delays and frustrations.

> **EXAM TIP** Remember three key qualities of HIT interoperability: it improves patient outcomes, streamlines processes, and reduces patient safety risks. Your role is to enable secure connections and facilitate data sharing to achieve these benefits.

Given the imperative for data sharing, enabling one healthcare organization to communicate with another is a challenge. We covered data interoperability and exchange in Chapter 1 and introduced the primary data standards. You'll remember that the use of common standards and taxonomies makes interoperability possible. Impediments can exist even though the language of healthcare is based on recognized clinical terminology, many standardized code sets, and a mission of diagnosis and treatment. You may find challenges in your organizations ability to interconnect with suppliers, payers, and other stakeholders (including government agencies) that result in administrative and management problems.

Such communication breakdowns are not always technology-based impasses. Sometimes overcoming political and personal hurdles resolves disconnects. For instance, each healthcare organization that uses an information system to automate workflow, an EHR, or a patient administration system probably purchases that system from a commercial manufacturer. In the case of some government healthcare organizations (the military or Veterans Administration), the information systems may be government developed. In any case, based on the agency that develops the system, interoperability may be limited. As you investigate the reasons why systems are difficult to connect, you may discover proprietary interconnection requirements or a lack of standards-based interfaces. The outcome is valuable data locked in seemingly impenetrable silos. We know this is counter to interoperability, because it creates information blocking. We also know this can be a huge problem as patients typically move from one healthcare organization to another based on referrals for advanced care, for example. Or, as healthcare organizations desire to submit bills to payers, the organizations must be able to send and receive data independent of what proprietary system they (or their counterparts) use.

Figure 3-3 shows a high-level view of the entities that are present and dependent on system interoperability.

Software and System Development

Software and system development, in a generic sense, are important with respect to HIT and interoperability safeguards in that too often information security is "bolted on" at the end of development and during implementation. Referencing the concept of "security by design," a focus on integrating secure interoperation is needed for the identified phases of HIT development. Software and system development lifecycle management is akin to the configuration management process, but the former is more focused on

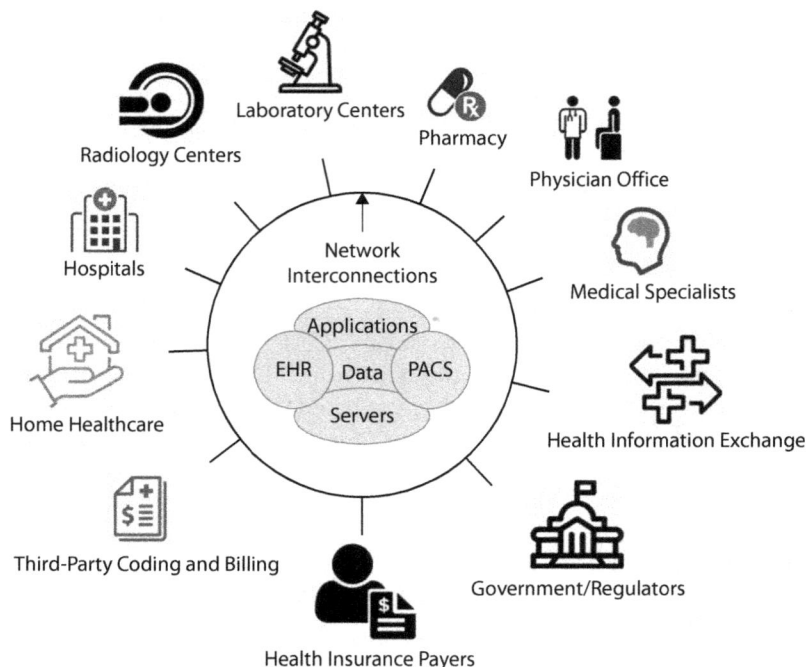

Figure 3-3 Interoperability of healthcare systems between interdependent entities

systems or software as it is being engineered before implementation. Generally speaking, development lifecycles have four development phases, which are listed next. To build-in information security and privacy properly, all phases have relevant inflection points for your involvement.[12] The relative milestones for information security and privacy are listed in italics corresponding to the appropriate development phase:

- **What** Specification of WHAT the product is to do

  Initiation: An initial threat and risk assessment to provide input for IT security requirements

- **How** Specification of HOW the product does it

  Initiation: Assessment for awareness of potential engineering challenges of implementing security controls and interoperability requirements to include identification of secure integration and reuse of proven strategies and tools

- **Build** Development or BUILD of the code or components that implement HOW

  Design and development: An appropriate balance of technical, managerial, operational, physical, and personnel security safeguards that will help to meet the requirements

- **Use**   Operational deployment or USE of software or system that performs WHAT

  Implementation: Design documentation, acceptance tests, and certification and accreditation to be performed

  Operation: System security monitoring and maintenance to aid in the evaluation of modifications for interoperability that could affect security

Levels of Interoperability

According to the Healthcare Information and Management Systems Society (HIMSS), interoperability is the technology antidote for the lack of communication among disparate systems. Three levels of interoperability should be addressed.

- **Foundational interoperability**   An HIT system is able to send information to another. This level does not include concern for the receipt of that transmission.

- **Structural interoperability**   Data must be structured and constructed in standard, meaningful ways and formats to be useful by other systems.

- **Semantic interoperability**   At this level, the initial system successfully sends the message, the message is structured appropriately, and the receiving system is able to receive and understand the information.

EXAM TIP   Expand your understanding of interoperability as more than a connection of two or more HIT systems. You may be presented with examples of information exchange, but unless the systems can use the information and the information has value, the systems are not truly interoperable as defined by the ONC.

Within many organizations and between HIT systems, you may find that interoperability is more an issue about bridging cultural, social, policy, or economic concerns. The technical obstacles may be relatively straightforward to address. There are valid reasons for not making systems interoperable, such as when the receiving entity has a suspected or known information security problem that makes data transfer a high risk. You will have to determine through risk assessment when those situations exist. In general, however, health information blocking is an impediment to achieving interoperability, and we should do our best to establish and support secure, meaningful information exchange between systems to maximize benefit from the HIT.

Medicare Access and CHIP Reauthorization Act of 2015

As a part of this comprehensive act, MACRA, nicknamed the Permanent Doc Fix, is legislation intended to incentivize healthcare that demonstrates value and achieves outcomes. It established an important reimbursement program, called the Quality Payment Program (QPP). Healthcare providers could participate in QPP through the Merit-based Incentive Payment System (MIPS) and Advanced Alternative Payment Models

(Advanced APMs). Relevant to our discussion on interoperability, QPP promoted the increased use of certified HIT that supports interoperability and advances the criteria that came from meaningful use (which were introduced as part of ARRA earlier in this chapter). QPP, in fact, took the place of meaningful use as healthcare providers were now measured against a "promoting interoperability" framework of standards and measures. Meaningful use encouraged digitizing healthcare information, and QPP advances the concept to include meaningful exchange and use of health information across multiple systems to provide complete and high-quality healthcare. Providers have to provide evidence that they satisfy QPP guidelines, which could include demonstration of electronic exchange of health records, test results, or physician consults from one organization to another in providing patient care.

Information Technologies

The healthcare and medical industries have witnessed an increasing amount and reliance on HIT. HIT supports health information management across computerized systems and the secure exchange of health information between consumers, providers, payers, and quality monitors. The systems also integrate with many traditional business and office automation systems, such as human resources or financial platforms. When used appropriately, HIT is helpful in improving the overall quality, safety, and efficiency of patient care and clinical operations. The electronic interchange of information has also shown reductions in medical errors and better accuracy in procedures. This section highlights some specific examples of information technologies unique to healthcare providers and payers.

Electronic Health Records

An EHR is basically one or more electronic files that has replaced the traditional paper medical chart. That may not be the best description, but it does acknowledge that the information that was once collected on paper is now digitized in EHRs. This information includes hand-written physician notes, images, audio, and prescription orders. The EHR has made gathering and organizing diverse types and formats of information easier, and, if properly secured, the information can be safely stored and made available without delay.

A better description is that EHRs are a system of HIT systems that house a comprehensive amount of patient and business data to help healthcare organizations deliver patient care. You will find them as central HIT systems in doctors' offices, hospitals, and healthcare payer organizations. Here are some of the common components of EHRs:[13]

- Medical histories, diagnoses, medications, treatment plans, immunization dates, allergies, radiology images, and laboratory and test results
- Connections to diagnosis and treatment applications and tools to support evidence-based decisions by providers for patient care plans
- Automated and streamlined provider and information workflows

EHRs have ushered in an era of expanded connectivity and interoperability between healthcare systems and providers. EHRs provide immediate access to extremely important patient information, without the physical separation that existed in the predigital world, when data was stored on paper in file cabinets. EHRs are the core of quality patient care and bring together valuable clinical information from internal and external caregivers. The ability to share information securely and quickly between organizations is illustrative of the transformative power of EHRs. Figure 3-4 shows how EHRs store and distribute healthcare data, including imaging, scanning, analysis, pathology, observations, and more. EHR implementation has transformed not only healthcare data storage, but its use has resulted in a reduced risk for medical errors.

Although the EHR has created efficiencies and gains for healthcare organizations, it has also experienced some unintended consequences, including the threat to patient privacy and the increased potential for data misuse. Your role as an information security professional is important because healthcare organizations have obligations, both legal and ethical, to establish security measures and safeguard sensitive information entrusted to them. Ensuring the privacy and security of health information, including EHR, is the key component to building the trust required to realize the potential benefits of electronic health information exchange. If individuals and other participants in a network lack trust in the electronic exchange of information because of perceived or actual risks or the accuracy and completeness of such information, it may affect their willingness to disclose necessary health information and could have life-threatening consequences.[14]

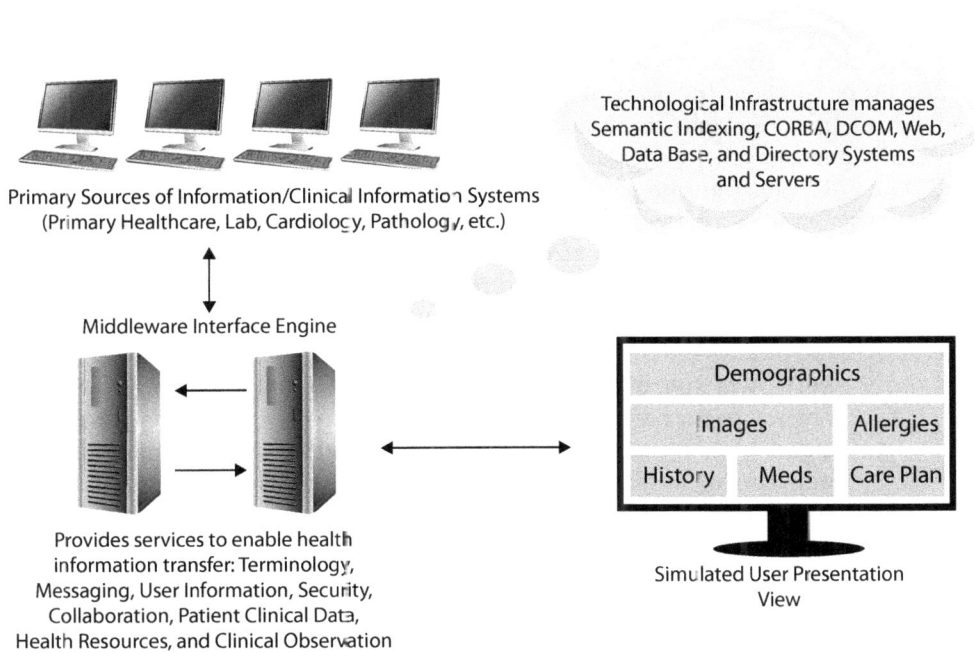

Figure 3-4   EHR is a system of HIT systems

A subcategory of EHR you need to be familiar with is the *legal medical record*, a set of particular patient data that is part of the entire patient record. Although there are no regulations specific to a defined legal medical record, federal and state governments have offered guidelines regarding legality. Simply put, a legal medical record is an official patient record recorded and stored by the healthcare organization that can be used as evidence in a court of law. A legal medical record is connected to revenue, because it supports reimbursement payments to the relevant third parties. The organization must meet baseline requirements for content and disclosure to authorized recipients in support of legal proceedings or in response to patient requests for release. Above these baseline requirements, each organization can make an assessment regarding what is and is not appropriate to reveal. Keep in mind that the components of the legal medical record may be located in multiple HIT systems, and the organization must be able to find and assemble the record when needed.

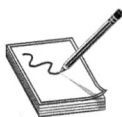

> **NOTE** A legal medical record may include some paper-based documentation that is combined with the electronic or digital information.

Another subset of medical records is the *designated record set* (DRS). HIPAA distinguishes the DRS as a set of records that include PHI and that is maintained, collected, used, or disseminated by or for covered entities for each individual who received care from a healthcare organization. The DRS normally contains more information than the legal health record. It may include patient medical and billing records; the enrollment, payment, claims, adjudication, and cases or medical management record systems maintained by or for a health plan; or information used to make care-related decisions.[15] Individuals have the right to obtain a copy of their DRS, request amendments, and set restrictions and accountings of any information used to make decisions about their care. The DRS can comprise paper records, film images, electronic data, and any other medium used to store a patient's healthcare data. You can think of the difference between a legal health record and the designated record set like this: direct patient care is recorded in the legal medical record; the designated record set includes that information, plus all the business information unrelated (but important) to patient care.

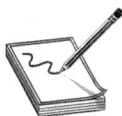

> **NOTE** A feature of EHRs is electronic prescribing (e-prescribing), or e-order entry. A paper prescription can get lost or misread. E-prescribing enables a doctor to communicate directly with a pharmacy, lab, or radiology department, as examples. The prescription or order is entered and sent securely without a paper copy and poses less risk of errors due to handwriting illegibility.

Another form of EHR is the personal health record (PHR), an electronic application through which patients can maintain and manage their health information (and that of others for whom they are authorized) in a private, secure, and confidential environment.[16] Sometimes called a patient portal, a PHR is a lot like an EHR, except that patients themselves can control what kind of information goes into it. Patients can use a PHR to keep track of doctor visits, but it can also reflect a patient's life outside the doctor's office and can include health priorities, such as tracking eating and exercise habits and blood pressure. A PHR may be linked to the doctor's EHR. When used effectively, PHRs can help patients focus on managing their health information and controlling, to varying extents, who can access that health information.

EXAM TIP Security professionals should know that audit logs and revision histories for EHRs are generally not mandated to be included in defined legal medical record sets. These are examples of numerous types of information that do not constitute either the legal medical record or the DSR.

An EHR uses a mix of security controls to keep patient health information confidential, to provide data integrity, and to assure availability. Technology also brings new responsibilities for safeguarding patients' health information. Widespread adoption of EHRs in healthcare occurred only after the US government provided reimbursement for their adoption as a result of the American Recovery and Reinvestment Act (ARRA) of 2009. Although, prior to that date, some healthcare data was being collected in digital format, electronic order entry and digitization of most of the patient record was still the exception, not the rule. Post-ARRA, in the United States, the EHR is very common.

Next, we will examine a few privacy and security concerns that EHR implementation introduces in access management and data management categories.

Access Management Concerns

Identity, access, authentication, and authorization within the context of information security controls are important in any information technology that handles sensitive information. This is especially true for EHRs, which must be protected by appropriate administrative, physical, and technical controls. For EHRs, patient rights concerning viewing, writing, and otherwise editing access permissions must be protected. In a healthcare environment with physicians, nurses, and clinicians filling multiple roles, often based on temporary responsibilities, we can expect a highly dynamic access management environment around the EHR. Consider the example of a cardiologist who wants access to a pediatric record. If the cardiologist is not currently treating that patient, she should be denied access to the patient's records. If, however, the cardiologist was serving on a peer review panel or as the CMO in the hospital, access to the record may be authorized for purposes of fulfilling those responsibilities. Just because the EHR is a medically unique application or system, it is not unreasonable or even unusual to implement certain specific access control management methods.

To begin with, access can be controlled by physical safeguards. Never overlook or underestimate the use of locked doors, surveillance cameras, or even security guards to augment other controls. Ensuring that resources are not physically available to those who are not authorized to access the systems is imperative. With the proper credentials, unauthorized users may be able to access digital and physical information and network resources unless they are physically prevented from doing so.

In addition to physical barriers, security must include active and continuous monitoring processes to help control access. The process may start with coworkers who are vigilant in monitoring who is accessing systems in their view or work area. Questioning people who are not known or do not behave normally (for example, someone who seems nervous and rushed) is the first line of defense. Next, EHR administrators should maintain an up-to-date access list with designated roles or levels of access specified. The individuals who are on the list should be supplied with unique IDs and mandated to create strong passwords or personal identification numbers (PINs) unless another form of multifactor authentication is available.

An often-overlooked control that can help prevent unauthorized access is an automatic shutdown routine. When an authorized user is done working or simply walks away from his or her access point (for example, a desktop, laptop, smartphone, or medical device), the device should log off or shut down after a short, but reasonable, amount of time. This forced termination of access can reduce the likelihood that someone who is not authorized could piggyback or continue the session under the authorized user's credentials. In fact, even if the second person is authorized, conducting business on the network under another person's credentials is not acceptable, because it violates the information security principles of authentication, authorization, and nonrepudiation.

A final consideration for healthcare organizations relative to access management is to audit access and user activity logs periodically. Having an active monitoring process that is reviewed and analyzed can help prevent and detect security incidents. Additionally, when it comes to providing data subjects or patients an accurate history of who has accessed their data or what actions were taken, the access management process can support that disclosure, which is required by privacy and security frameworks. In the United States, this disclosure supports a healthcare organization's obligation to provide, upon request, a full accounting of the use of a patient's PHI upon request.

Data Management Concerns

EHR data management is the process of storing, protecting, and analyzing data pulled from the multiple HIT systems that support patient care. Managing the wealth of available healthcare data helps healthcare organizations develop processes and approaches to improve care for their patients and their health status. Effective data management in a digitized healthcare organization can be a daunting task, and protecting that data is the purview of the HCISPP. A key consideration involves identifying and knowing use and demand requirements for authorized EHR users.

As an HCISPP, you will design and implement security and privacy solutions for specific components of EHR data management, including the following:

- **Data sharing** Providers cite data security and privacy concerns as reasons for not sharing data, but regulations generally support interoperability. HIPAA, for example, permits the use or disclosure of health information for treatment, payment, and healthcare operations, which includes disclosure to another healthcare organization for the continuum of treatment, payment, and operations for the recipient organization.

- **Data at rest**   Healthcare organizations must protect health information confidentiality. Regulations require that organizations safeguard information, through means such as encryption of data at rest, to protect against threats or hazards to the security, unauthorized use, or disclosure of the information. Proper encryption procedures render sensitive health information unreadable and unusable against unauthorized access.

- **Data mining and analysis**   Healthcare organizations must protect sensitive patient data from unauthorized use or use without patient consent. One way to accomplish data mining and analysis that falls outside of acceptable treatment, payment, and operations, such as selling data to a company to conduct risk of illness analysis on a patient population, is to offer patients options to opt-in or opt-out of such information sharing during treatment. Another tactic is to apply de-identification or data masking processes to databases to remove identifying information but keep relevant health information unaffected.

- **Retention and recovery**   Central to EHR data management is the ability of the organization to enable full restoration of data from frequent backups that is stored in a separate location. The same safeguards that are appropriate during normal operations are required during recovery mode. Data retention must be governed and limits must be established and followed based on regulatory guidance to minimize risk of exposure to unauthorized disclosure.

- **Privacy**   Healthcare organizations must realize that patient privacy regulations generally give patients the right to view their medical records on demand within a reasonable period of time, such as 30 days. Patients must be informed through notice of privacy practices and offered consent documentation that informs them of relevant health data management practices, particularly in the organization's use of the EHR. Management of the data outside of these stated uses requires additional permission from the patient.

- **Availability**   If patient care is disrupted when data is not available, because of a successful malware attack or denial of service, the healthcare organization may face fines and penalties. This is in addition to the operational, clinical, and financial risk present when patients cannot receive the standard of care that is expected when there is access to data.

In summary, healthcare organizations must administer proper health data management security and privacy procedures when collecting, using, storing, and transferring patient data. Marketing and other business departments must adhere to patient privacy and security considerations as well when using health data that may be outside of treatment, payment, and operations beyond which the patient consented. As an HCISPP, you will play a lead role in ensuring that the organization satisfies all requirements, but many stakeholders in the organization will have a responsibility in proper health data management.

The Ease of Data Collection and Storage Creates Substantial Security Issues

Many organizations may tend to relax controls on the amounts of data collected or maintained as they convert to digital information. This may occur because organizations do not need to procure rooms or buildings to house the information to the extent they had to with paper records. But the ease of data collection and storage that an EHR provides is also a glaring vulnerability. To put it simply, the ability for a healthcare organization to lose more than 500 individual medical records at one time has increased immeasurably. Whereas 500 medical records may have taken up an entire small records room, floor to ceiling, when all records were paper-based, today that same amount easily fits on a USB thumb drive. The 500 individual medical records is the threshold at which a data breach requires increased levels of government notification under HIPAA. This number illustrates how easy it is to have significant data breaches with electronic health information. While paper-based records would have to be transported in numerous (and noticeable) trips in and out of the records room, 500 digital records can be downloaded and transported out of the hospital door in mere minutes, completely undetected by onlookers. Therefore, with the implementation of EHRs, information security and privacy professionals must continue to educate and communicate the importance and proper management of sensitive PHI and PII data.

Internet of Medical Things

Modern healthcare systems now rely on advanced computing methods and technologies, such as Internet of Things (IoT) specific to healthcare devices, or the Internet of Medical Things (IoMT). IoMT is a category of medical devices and applications that are HIT systems or that connect to HIT systems through Wi-Fi, online computer networks, and cloud platforms. IoMT leverages machine-to-machine communication to collect, store, analyze, and transfer personal health data at an unprecedented scale and depth. Patients, healthcare providers, and researchers use information derived from such data sources to monitor patients remotely, diagnose diseases earlier, and find personalized treatments and medications. Without appropriate privacy protection, however, IoMT introduces potential security and privacy nightmares:[17]

- **Volumes of data**   IoMT devices significantly increase the volume of data, and you must know where your sensitive data is located. Inventory and protection around new sources, locations, and computing infrastructures may not be thoroughly vetted. Another issue is the scalability of current encryption capabilities at large data volumes.

- **Quality of data**   With IoMT, the devices that collect, store, and transfer sensitive information may be used for personal reasons, such as a fitness watch or a voice-activated digital assistant. These are vulnerable to security breaches that could lead to data quality issues based on how the information is gathered and transferred.

Such issues could result from a cyber attack or something related to device misuse. For example, a patient may give the device to a friend, and you may not have the ability to regulate the friend's data input. As a result, analysis and outputs may be flawed. Without proper security safeguards, such personal use could jeopardize the quality, security, and confidentiality of sensitive data.

- **Sharing of data** Many privacy and security professionals identify the potential for information leaks that IoMT can introduce. For example, cloud providers that manage digital personal assistants may have access to PHI that should be protected. The ability of devices such as Alexa and Google Home to process and understand human voice can also lead to collection and transfer of data. When devices are used for healthcare monitoring or consultation, the sharing of data over the devices requires information protections.

- **Data accuracy** Data analytics are often performed on samples, not full volumes, of data. As IoMT devices collect large volumes of data, the accuracy of data is a consideration. In many cases, the data is gathered using input from devices outside of the organization's control. Controls that help assure data integrity, such as sensors and telemetry, help to minimize manual input to IoMT.

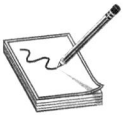

NOTE Cybersecurity for IoT is an emerging and dynamic area. A developing resource for privacy and security concerns is the NIST Cybersecurity for IoT Program. For more information, visit https://www.nist.gov/programs-projects/nist-cybersecurity-iot-program.

Medical Devices

Medical devices are central to our concern with ensuring information security and privacy in a healthcare environment. Medical devices can range from a thermometer to a digital X-ray machine. Networked medical devices are special-purpose computing systems and instruments, apparatuses, and implants that are intended for use in the diagnosis of disease or other conditions; in the cure, mitigation, treatment, or prevention of disease; or to affect the structure or any function of the body.[18] Increasingly, medical devices are networked (to each other or to larger networks), and they are continuously communicating, which presents a unique challenge to securing them within a healthcare environment. An increasing number of devices are connected to the hospital network or use network resources to operate.

It will be helpful for you to identify and learn about the various medical devices that are used in your organization. In some cases, the number of medical devices connected to the organization's network may equal or outnumber business systems. There are several basic types of medical devices

- **Diagnostic equipment** Medical imaging machines such as ultrasound and MRI machines, PET and CT scanners, and X-ray machines

- **Treatment equipment** Medical treatment devices, including infusion pumps, medical lasers, and LASIK surgical machines

- **Life support equipment** Medical devices used to maintain a patient's bodily function, such as medical ventilators, incubators, anesthetic machines, heart-lung machines, extracorporeal membrane oxygenation (ECMO), and dialysis machines

- **Therapeutic devices** Physical therapy machines such as continuous passive range of motion (CPM) machines

- **Medical monitors** Monitoring devices used to view and assess a patient's medical state or vital signs, including electrocardiogram (ECG), electroencephalogram (EEG), and blood pressure monitors

- **Medical laboratory equipment** Analytic devices that automate or help analyze blood, urine, genes, and dissolved gases in the blood

- **Home health devices** Diagnostic and treatment equipment used outside the healthcare environment for certain purposes, such as the control of diabetes mellitus or congestive heart failure

Although these devices are typically built upon standard IT operating systems and run well-known applications, their special-purpose natures mean that the normal operational safeguards that would be appropriate in office automation IT could cause patient harm when indiscriminately applied to medical devices. In the future, more types of medical devices will be developed to wear on the body, with some devices implanted or ingested; many already exist and are providing patient care today.

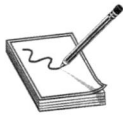

NOTE The growing field of clinical engineering that covers wearable, implantable, and ingestible types of networked medical devices is called *biomedical telemetry*. The leading professional organization governing this technology is the Institute of Electrical and Electronics Engineers (IEEE). For more information on this topic, visit https://www.ieee.org.

Medical devices entered the medical marketplace under the purview of the US Food and Drug Administration (FDA). Figure 3-5 depicts some important events in the history of medical device privacy and security.

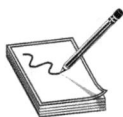

NOTE The FDA hosts the MedWatch web site, at https://www.accessdata.fda .gov/scripts/medwatch, where anyone—including healthcare organizations and patients—can submit a complaint about the potential misuse or faulty operation of a medical device. In the past few years in which cybersecurity concerns have begun populating the MedWatch database, the FDA has recognized the impact of malware on medical devices.

For several years, the FDA has provided urgent warnings and updates to the field concerning medical device cybersecurity vulnerabilities. This forward-thinking approach recognizes the growing reality that medical devices are targets for attackers. The FDA has assured healthcare organizations that these vulnerabilities have not resulted in known patient harm. However, the FDA is taking a proactive stance against vulnerabilities that could allow unauthorized users to remotely access, control, and issue commands to

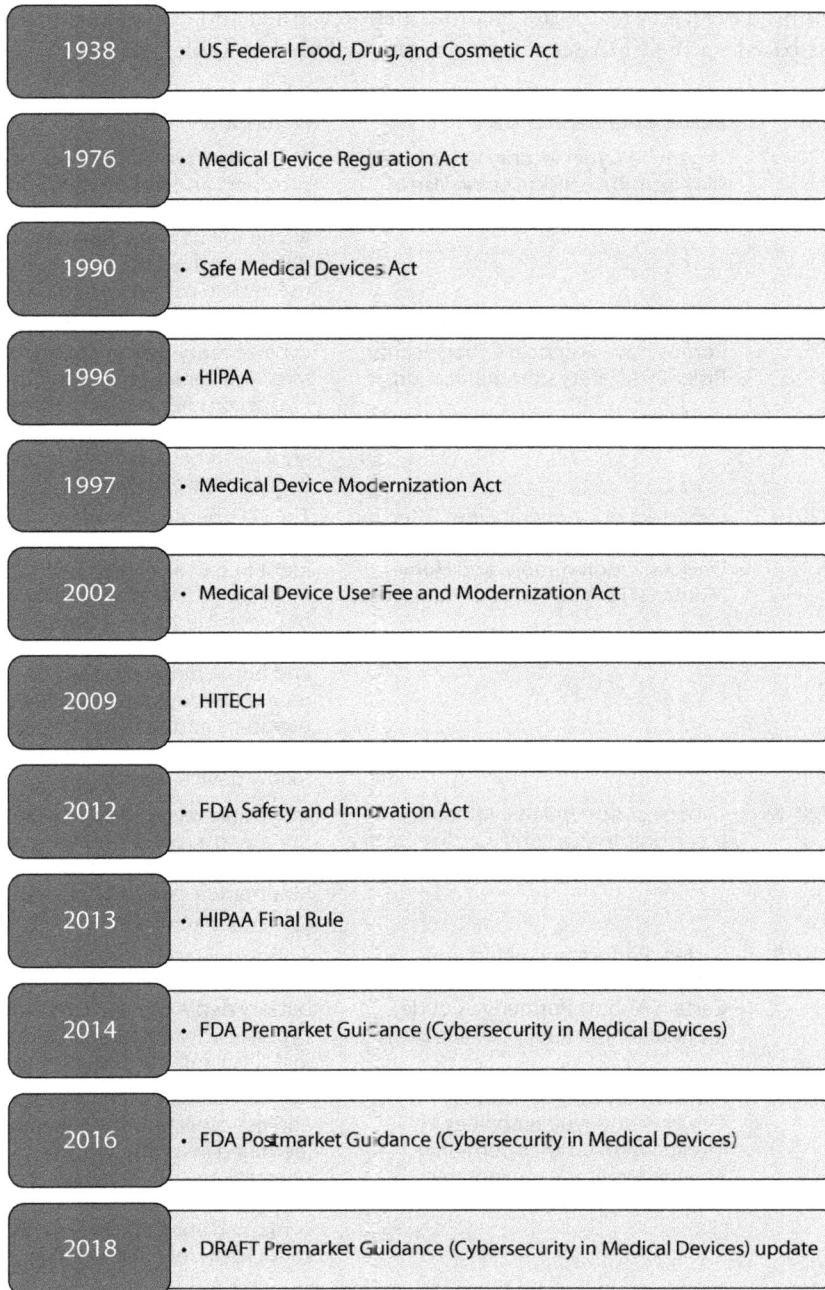

Figure 3-5 A brief history of medical device law and associated privacy and security guidance provided by the FDA

compromised devices. Healthcare facilities are forewarned and can take action to reduce the risks based on the FDA recommendations included in Table 3-2.[19]

Date	Safety Communication	Description
10/01/2019	Urgent/11 Cybersecurity Vulnerabilities May Introduce Risks During Use of Certain Medical Devices	The FDA informed patients, healthcare providers and facility staff, and manufacturers about cybersecurity vulnerabilities for connected medical devices and healthcare networks that use certain communication software.
06/27/2019	Certain Medtronic MiniMed Insulin Pumps Have Potential Cybersecurity Risks: FDA Safety Communication	After becoming aware of potential cybersecurity risks in Medtronic MiniMed Paradigm insulin pumps, the FDA recommended patients replace affected pumps with models that were better equipped to protect them from these potential risks.
03/21/2019	Cybersecurity Vulnerabilities Affecting Medtronic Implantable Cardiac Devices, Programmers, and Home Monitors: FDA Safety Communication	The FDA became aware of cybersecurity vulnerabilities identified in a wireless telemetry technology used for communication between Medtronic's implantable cardiac devices, clinic programmers, and home monitors. The FDA recommended that healthcare providers and patients continue to use these devices as intended and follow device labeling.
10/11/2018	Cybersecurity Updates Affecting Medtronic Implantable Cardiac Device Programmers	Medtronic released a software update to address the cybersecurity vulnerabilities associated with Medtronic's cardiac implantable cardiac device programmers.
04/17/2018	Battery Performance Alert and Cybersecurity Firmware Updates for Certain Abbott (formerly St. Jude Medical) Implantable Cardiac Devices	Abbott released an additional firmware update to address premature battery depletion and confirmed cybersecurity vulnerabilities identified in its implantable cardiac devices.
08/29/2017	Firmware Update to Address Cybersecurity Vulnerabilities Identified in Abbott's (formerly St. Jude Medical's) Implantable Cardiac Pacemakers	Abbott released a firmware update to address cybersecurity vulnerabilities identified in its implantable cardiac pacemakers. The firmware update continued Abbott's efforts to mitigate confirmed vulnerabilities discovered by an independent research firm in 2016.
01/09/2017	Cybersecurity Vulnerabilities Identified in St. Jude Medical's Implantable Cardiac Devices and Merlin@home Transmitter	The FDA became aware of cybersecurity vulnerabilities in these devices after an independent research firm released information about these vulnerabilities.

Table 3-2   FDA Cybersecurity Safety Communications

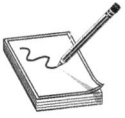

> **NOTE** Cybersecurity issues and the relevant governance published
> by the FDA are applicable to an international audience of privacy and
> security professionals. Here are two terrific references for those who have
> responsibility for managing the cybersecurity of medical devices: "Guidance
> for Industry - Cybersecurity for Networked Medical Devices Containing
> Off-the-Shelf (OTS) Software" (http://www.fda.gov/MedicalDevices/
> DeviceRegulationandGuidance/GuidanceDocuments/ucm077812.htm),
> and "Content of Premarket Submissions for Management of Cybersecurity
> in Medical Devices" (https://www.fda.gov/media/119933/download).

In the pursuit of implementing good privacy and security practices, unintended consequences can occur with networked medical devices. These devices are essential to direct patient care and are highly regulated by the FDA. If a device fails to perform or performs in an unsafe manner, it can mean patient injury or death. If privacy and information security practices exclude medical devices, vulnerabilities can evolve, and this can introduce patient safety risks. The proper way to address the privacy and security of medical devices is to implement, whenever possible, practices that understand and account for special considerations relative to each device. These devices may have IP addresses, operating systems, and relational databases, but they are not identical to office automation endpoints or servers performing office automation tasks or business functions. If a prescribed information security control may cause unintended issues, security professionals must seek out alternative controls and tailored safeguards. For instance, a medical device may use an operating system that is no longer supported by the software manufacturer, yet the device manufacturer can't upgrade the software unless it upgrades the device to the next model. Because a new model may be too expensive for an organization, the current model may work sufficiently for its intended clinical purpose.

Upgrading to a newer model simply because the operating system cannot be updated with future vulnerability patches likely is not justified from a cost–benefit perspective. A better control is to segment the device into a separate enclave that is firewalled (quarantined) from the rest of the network but still able to access the network. In these types of cases, the required skill for an HCISPP is having the savvy to know when to implement the prescribed control (for example, upgrading to new operating system) and when to seek a compensating or alternative control (for example, quarantining the device).

Here is another scenario to help illustrate the concept: Imagine your job is to configure and perform periodic software vulnerability updates to your local area network (LAN). Typically, once a prescribed update is tested against your standard computing configuration for endpoints (desktops, laptops, and so on), you are authorized to perform the update through automated routines across the network. The efficiency and effectiveness of this pushbutton approach are clear industry best practices. Now imagine that some of those endpoints are in a cardiac catheterization lab. Sure, they look like desktop computers running standard operating systems, and they have a network IP address assigned to them. However, these special-purpose computers also run medical applications that serve up diagnostic-quality (high-resolution) video and imaging that enable physicians to perform complex cardiac procedures. If, in the middle of such procedures, your automatic push of a software vulnerability patch causes the system to reboot involuntarily (as patches often do), that unanticipated downtime may cause a patient safety issue.

Following are the main concerns about integrating networked medical devices into an overall information security program without much regard for their unique characteristics:

- *Medical devices are used in direct patient care scenarios.* Medical devices that malfunction can put patients at risk and impede diagnosis or treatment by clinicians.

- *Medical devices depend on special applications with unique protocols and standards.* Although most devices run on known operating systems and use common database technologies, they also depend on or use special-purpose applications and use distinctive protocols. The use of Health Level Seven International (HL7) data transfer protocols and Digital Imaging and Communications in Medicine (DICOM) as an imaging standard are just two examples.

- *Medical device manufacturers play a major role in ensuring safety.* Unlike other computing device manufacturers, medical device manufacturers retain a great deal of responsibility for their devices even after they are sold to a healthcare organization. The reason for this has to do with safety rather than cybersecurity, and this responsibility can actually introduce security risks. Because medical devices are FDA-regulated and patient safety is a concern, medical device manufacturers must test and approve all third-party software before a healthcare organization can update a medical device. This process can, at best, delay the software vulnerability patch management process; at worst, it can cause medical devices to remain unpatched and vulnerable to exploit on the hospital LAN.

- *Medical devices often exist on legacy operating systems and sunsetted applications (those no longer supported by their developers).* The cost of upgrading a medical device to a newer model simply because the operating system or database application is no longer supported, for example, is sometimes cost prohibitive.

The point of discussing medical devices and their privacy and security implications is not to say that medical devices cannot or should not be fully integrated into the overall information security program. In fact, the opposite is true. If medical devices are not part of the enterprise information security program, it is certain that the LAN will be extremely susceptible to attack. In 2015, the FBI published a public service announcement regarding its investigations of healthcare organizations in the United States. The FBI identified some profoundly disturbing levels of vulnerability related to poorly managed medical devices.[20]

Medical devices offer information security and privacy professionals an opportunity to protect information by developing appropriate compensating or tailored controls. Here are some of the approaches you should consider:

- *Include the medical devices in the information security program.* Medical devices are often managed by biomedical technicians, and sometimes the department is completely outsourced to a third-party management team. Proper communication and coordination must include these devices in the overall asset inventory and vulnerability management process. According to the 2015 FBI report, simply knowing which devices have up-to-date software configurations and which do not is a big first step toward solving security problems.

- *Segment the LAN.* Quarantining medical devices or segregating them in a defense-in-depth architecture in a firewalled enclave, for example, is helpful. Because software vulnerability patch management can be on a compliance schedule that differs from one that the medical devices can support, segmentation not only provides a series of subnets and an additional line of defense from external infiltration, but it also protects the rest of the organization's network from these vulnerable devices while the testing and approval steps are taken and the manual patching process is completed.

- *Ensure that medical devices are included in the organization's data incident response policy.* When a medical device malfunctions or its performance degrades, it may not be obvious that the cause is related to malware or security. As repair actions are taken, a data security incident must be considered as a potential source of the problem. Additionally, the data incident policy must allow for biomedical technicians to report potential and actual issues. This also means that the healthcare organization will notify the medical device manufacturer and the FDA as part of normal data incident processes. Make sure that you use the FDA reporting channels.

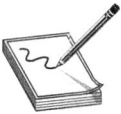

NOTE Bots are a very common type of malware found on infected medical devices. Bots (short for robots) refer to software applications with an ability to function automatically. One automated function is to seek other vulnerable devices and spread itself to other machines. When several bots operate across the Internet from separate devices it is known as a botnet. In medical devices, bots lodge inside the computer and communicate back to command-and-control (C2) servers. They can act immediately or wait for a specified period of time to begin sending spam or conducting other types of attacks on a medical device across the botnet. Often the goal of a specific bot is to establish a botnet and attack other networked resources on the healthcare organization's network. The initial medical device serves as the launching pad.

Classification of Medical Devices

FDA classification is an important privacy and security component of medical devices. The FDA uses classifications categories for approximately 1700 different generic types of devices and groups them into 16 medical specialties, or panels. Each device is typed into one of the following three regulatory classes based on the level of control necessary to assure its safety and effectiveness:

- **Class I** General Controls (defined in the Note that follows) must be applied. Almost half of all medical devices are in this category, which includes enema kits, elastic bandages, manual stethoscopes, and bedpans. Almost none of these devices undergoes a premarket regulatory process or evaluation by the FDA, but the devices still must register with the FDA before being marketed in the United States. Class I devices present low to moderate risk to the patient or user.

- **Class II** General Controls and Special Controls (defined in the Note that follows) are implemented for this classification. About 43 percent of medical devices are Class II devices. The risk level to the patient or user is considered to be moderate to high. Examples include powered wheelchairs, biological indicators, X-ray systems, gas analyzers, pumps, and surgical drapes.

- **Class III** General Controls apply and the devices must go through a process of scientific and regulatory review to evaluate the safety and effectiveness called FDA Premarket Approval. These devices usually sustain or support life, are implanted, or present a high risk of illness or injury. Heart valves, implantable pacemakers, silicon-based breast implants, and cerebellar stimulators are a few examples of Class III medical devices. These devices make up about 10 percent of the medical devices in use and present the highest level of risk to the patient or user.

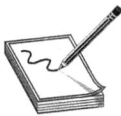

NOTE General Controls are the basic provisions expected from manufacturers to ensure medical device safety and effectiveness. General Controls apply to all medical devices and include provisions that relate to adulteration; misbranding; device registration and listing; premarket notification; banned devices; notification, including repair, replacement, or refund; records and reports; restricted devices; and good manufacturing practices.

Special Controls are relevant to Class II medical devices. They are added to General Controls when basic provisions alone are considered insufficient to provide reasonable assurance of the safety and effectiveness of a device, and for which there is sufficient information to establish special controls to provide such assurance. Special Controls include performance standards, postmarket surveillance, patient registries, special labeling requirements, premarket data requirements, and device-specific guidelines.[21]

Device classification depends on the intended use of the device and upon indications for use. For example, a scalpel's intended use is to cut tissue. A subset of its intended use could be a more specialized indication included in the device's labeling, such as, "for making incisions in the cornea."[22] The most relevant impact of device classification to an HCISPP is the other reason devices are classified: classification is based on risk. The level of risk the device poses to a patient or the device user determines its classification. Class I includes devices with the lowest risk and Class III includes those with the greatest risk. As you implement privacy and security controls that may impact medical devices, the classification will influence how you evaluate information risk reduction against patient care and patient safety concerns.

Cloud Computing

In an effort to increase efficiency, reduce costs, and garner expert HIT support, healthcare organizations are rapidly moving toward the cloud. In cloud computing, resources, software, processing power, and storage are shared and accessible via the Internet. In short, in cloud computing, HIT services are delivered much like utilities such as electricity are delivered. As with many other industries, healthcare organizations are moving to these virtual computing environments and away from the traditional on-premises IT environment, which suffers from single-purpose server and storage resources. In traditional HIT environments, IT costs can be prohibitive, and this can often result in low device utilization, gross inefficiency, and inflexibility in responding to changing organizational initiatives. By contrast, the return on investment with cloud-based, HIT-as-a-service arrangements are promising. Because future HIT costs seem to be boundless, potential savings and efficiencies gained from initiatives such as cloud computing are very attractive to the healthcare industry.

According to leading sources such as the NIST Cloud Computing Program (NCCP) and the Cloud Security Alliance (CSA), the benefits offered by cloud computing in healthcare organizations include the following:

- EHR technologies
- Improved data exchange or sharing
- Availability of large amounts of data for analytics (big data)
- Patient enrollment
- Home health, telehealth, and picture archiving and communication system (PACS) technology

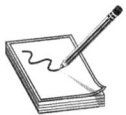

NOTE   For more about the NCCP, visit https://www.nist.gov/programs-projects/nist-cloud-computing-program-nccp. For more on the CSA, visit https://cloudsecurityalliance.org.

Moving healthcare data to the cloud introduces concerns relative to privacy and security, however. Some of these concerns involve general privacy laws, and others are unique to healthcare. All organizations, including healthcare organizations, face many concerns with regard to cloud computing. Among the most prevalent concerns that impact healthcare are multiple tenants, trans-border concerns, and third-party risks. Figure 3-6 provides a visual representation of the cautionary tale for those that ignore guidance

Figure 3-6
Plan for privacy and security before you implement cloud computing solutions.

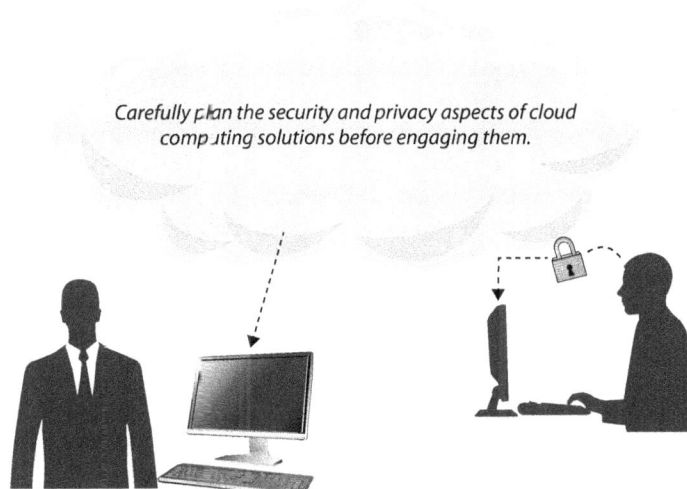

Carefully plan the security and privacy aspects of cloud computing solutions before engaging them.

such as that found in NIST SP 800-144, *Guidelines on Security and Privacy in Public Cloud Computing.* Leading cloud security sources caution that including proper privacy and security safeguards is necessary to prevent adversaries from gaining access, because adversaries also see the cloud as a terrific business opportunity—for a very different and untoward purpose.[23]

EHRs in Multitenant Cloud Environments

By definition, in a cloud computing environment, many different customers intermingle within the same cloud service provider's architecture. These customers can come from banking, retail, and academic organizations, as well as healthcare. Each industry may have varying mandatory information security requirements—for example, the US healthcare industry must abide by HIPAA data storage regulations, while a retail organization may be affected by the Fair and Accurate Credit Transaction Act (FACTA) and the Red Flags Rule. For instance, under HIPAA, disclosure of healthcare information is prohibited outside of treatment, payment, and operations. HIPAA prohibits health data from being accessible by other cloud tenants, because that would be unauthorized disclosure. Cloud service providers, therefore, must provide extra technologies to segregate health data properly within shared virtual machines (VMs) and physical servers with multiple clients.

Under HIPAA, healthcare data in the cloud must be secured in the same way it would be secured in an in-house data center. Some cloud providers may not have the ability to meet stringent HIPAA requirements, and some providers may not be able to accommodate security policies and procedures required by a healthcare organization. Healthcare organizations should therefore use only cloud providers that are equipped to handle healthcare data specifically.

With regard to identity and access management, the healthcare organization must be able to restore or delete its cloud-stored data on demand. Cloud providers that want to support healthcare organizations must also be able to provide networks that are logically partitioned enclaves with segmented database and storage layers. If the data is not properly segmented, restoration or data disposal will be difficult or impossible.

Mobile Device Management

Bring your own device (BYOD) is a popular strategy that end users are embracing and organizations are trying to adopt. The positive aspects of BYOD, including reducing inventory costs and maintenance for the organization's IT department, are evident. End users like the flexibility of using a device that they can personalize and customize (for improved productivity). These BYOD environments typically include laptops, tablets, and smartphones that run operating systems and mobile applications the organization cannot provide resources to support.

Because of the information privacy and security implications with BYOD, a mobile device management (MDM) process must be in place. The MDM policy will include access management, user rights and responsibilities, as well as what actions the organization can take with respect to BYODs. A growing number of healthcare providers are realizing improved productivity by accessing the organization's EHR and ordering tests and medication by using computerized provider order entry (CPOE) via their own personal mobile devices. Because healthcare organizations are required to protect PHI and PII, they will need to address mobile device management to protect their patient's data.

BYOD presents unique challenges in healthcare, in that any PHI or PII located on a BYOD is beyond the information-protection reach of the organization. An organization has little control over third-party software, including malware, that is loaded on a personal device. Further, mobile devices can be easily lost or stolen. If a device is not encrypted and contains PHI or PII, the data loss may require patient notifications as well as government intervention. In addition, the economic costs of data loss from personal devices can be significant. According to research conducted by the Ponemon Institute, "Just one mobile device infected with malware can cost an organization an average of $9485."[24]

Healthcare organizations can implement network access control (NAC) to identify an end user's device when it's being used to access the healthcare organization's network. Prior to allowing the device any level of access, the device can be scanned for compliance with the latest antivirus version and up-to-date vulnerability patches. NAC technologies can support all brands of mobile devices, including medical devices.

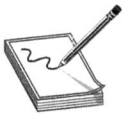

NOTE There is a significant overlap among mobile device management, BYOD, and medical devices. For instance, handheld ultrasound machines are commercially available that include smartphones, medical applications, and scanning peripheral devices with Wi-Fi capability, all wrapped in one device. For an example of such a device, visit http://www.mobisante.com/products/product-overview.

Another architecture solution that is facilitating mobile device management is the implementation of the virtual desktop interface (VDI). This configuration, relying on VM equipment and software, basically enables an authenticated user access to network resources without delivering and storing those resources on the end device. In the past, "dumb terminals" were used to access mainframes in a mainframe computing environment, which bears some similarity to how mobile devices now access VDIs.

Health Information Exchange

We are in an age in which the digitization of patient information has made sharing the information much easier. This makes security constraints with regard to using sensitive health information more important than ever. Hospital A cannot freely share patient information with Hospital B unless the use is for treatment, payment, operations, or if the patient gives informed consent for the sharing. However, advantages exist for sharing health information beyond treatment, payment, and operations; these are the basis of health information exchange (HIE). Healthcare organizations see value in HIE in that it can improve access to clinical data by providing safer, timelier, and more equitable care, with better outcomes. Sometimes HIE is part of treatment, payment, and operations; other times, it can occur for research, public health, or another valid clinical reason. HIE introduces its own privacy and security concerns—namely, the creation of multiple copies of data. Decentralized database locations with overall system awareness can help keep control localized and safeguarded.

Before we go further, rest assured that HIE is not just a US-centric phenomenon. Although US healthcare organizations are implementing HIEs, their global use is increasing annually by 10 percent. An estimated $2.21 billion will be spent on HIEs by 2024.[25] The global demand for HIEs is based on motivating factors similar to those in the United States: cloud computing, mobile devices (BYOD), and emerging global economies. With rising economic levels, EHR implementation is spreading; thus, so is information sharing through HIEs.

For the most part, HIEs provide healthcare providers across the same or multiple organizations almost real-time access to clinical information, reducing the delay in information transfer that occurred with traditional, paper-based record systems. Built into the HIE is the ability to ensure information integrity if operational safeguards are integrated. Because of the availability of PHI, HIEs may also provide a way for healthcare organizations to accomplish public health reporting, measure clinical quality, conduct biomedical surveillance, and perform advanced population health research. But this is true only if the element of trust is present and the PHI is deemed reliable from each perspective: the patient, the provider, and the HIE activity.

HIEs are also subject to HIPAA rules. Patients have specific rights regarding how their health information is used and disclosed. HIEs are required to publish their practices and inform participating patients of their individual rights. The only way to build trust is to communicate these terms and conditions clearly. The ONC has outlined a privacy and security framework that, when used, constitutes good data stewardship and forms a foundation of public trust in the collection, access, use, and disclosure of PHI by HIEs.[26] Along with the ONC framework, the US Department of Education's Office for Civil Rights (OCR) has provided an expectation for HIEs using principles from leading privacy frameworks to increase individual control over the collection and use of PHI while limiting and securing the sharing between healthcare organizations to specific scenarios.

If HIEs are implemented correctly, with protection of properly collected PHI or PII, their international evolution will give healthcare organizations unprecedented access to public health reporting, outcome measures, biomedical surveillance capability, and research. However, patients and regulatory authorities will be the judges when it comes to determining whether or not the HIEs can share information safely and securely.

Data Lifecycle Management

Secure data lifecycle management must be a priority as healthcare organizations make the shift from paper to digital records, as data is shared more easily, and as methods for data storage change. Healthcare organizations must establish governing principles for the useful life of healthcare and business data.

Chapter 1 introduced and differentiated DLM from information lifecycle management (ILM) and information flow within a healthcare organization. You'll remember that although DLM is similar to ILM, DLM is concerned with information at the file level, which is more abstract in nature and less concerned with the use of the data within the file. ILM deals with specific information within that file (patient height, weight, and so on). This section provides an overview of the specific components of the data lifecycle and how to manage its privacy and security impacts.

Figure 3-7
Data lifecycle
components

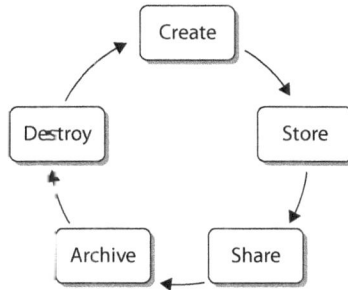

The data lifecycle begins with a creation (create) phase and ends with the secure disposal (destroy) of data that is no longer needed. This section discusses the major components of a data lifecycle as shown in Figure 3-7.

EXAM TIP A simple definition of "information" is "data with meaning." This perspective may help you recognize the difference between DLM and ILM. DLM addresses creation to deletion of data, while ILM uses measures of relevancy and accuracy to determine the position of information in the lifecycle.

Phase 1: Create

Healthcare organizations create, or collect, a tremendous amount of data. An incredible amount of patient healthcare data is required for treatment, payment, research, and quality improvements. Storage manufacturers (such as DellEMC)[27] have estimated that we will have about 2314 exabytes of stored healthcare data globally by this year (2020). In fact, the healthcare industry has the highest compound annual growth rate (CAGR) of any industry at 36 percent through 2025.[28] The explosion of data sources is the result of multiple innovations and advanced HIT as the healthcare industry has evolved from paper-based data storage to digital storage. The proliferation of data collection and storage has come in part from the incredible abilities of medical devices that connect directly to the patient or are ingested. This data can inform providers of more information in an instant about the patient than was ever possible before.

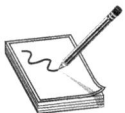

NOTE With IoT and IoMT, data collection in a big data context involves a concept known as *signal reception*. Medical devices with telemetry and sensors are collecting volumes of data without requiring human interface or input.

Massive amounts of collected and stored data have ushered in the era of "big data."[29] The promise of big data is that healthcare providers, payers, and researchers will have ready access to relevant information to use and share. The goals are to improve healthcare practices, enhance the quality of patient care, and reduce healthcare costs over the long run.

While big data may provide deep statistical and analytical insights that benefit patient care, safety, and reimbursements, significant concerns for privacy and security are a constant. Because the sensitivity and criticality of the data created or collected is important, the regulatory environment is constantly working to keep up with the pace of progress. Updates to HIPAA, state laws, the EU GDPR, and other laws and standards have published substantive new and adaptive changes that acknowledge the amount of data collected and stored and how much control individuals have in determining the information's use by the healthcare organization. A proven practice during the creation phase is to ensure that data classification is applied here to identify data as public, internal, sensitive, or restricted.

Phase 2: Store

As data is collected, it has to be processed and stored. At first, the organization does not yet gain any value from the data, because it is simply moved into the environment to be entered into the data repositories and applications. At that point, the data begins to be manipulated to start becoming valuable.

In this phase, the data is copied from one or more sources into a destination system, known as the extract-transform-load (ETL) processes. Data governance policies and procedures, which you will help support and enforce, will have primary focus in this phase. Roles and responsibilities for moving data to authorized users are also relevant. The aim is to prevent problems such as sprawl of data to unauthorized locations or reduction of numerous copies of databases that diminish the data source.

Data storage across the lifecycle employs a hierarchical approach to support secure lifecycle management. In hierarchal storage, data is stored based on operational considerations, such as how frequently the data is used. The same volumes of data may move between high-cost and low-cost storage media. Speed and access come with higher costs: high-speed storage devices such as solid state drive arrays cost more than the slower storage options, such as hard disk drives, optical discs, and magnetic tape drives. Use of high-speed storage is appropriate for data that is frequently retrieved and provides low latency. Secure movement of records to slower storage media according to the organization's record management schedule supports the progression of data to future steps of the data management lifecycle.

EXAM TIP In addition to understanding the accessibility options for stored data, you should also understand the concepts of storage volatility and mutability. Volatile memory requires power to maintain the data. The data is lost if there is no power supply to the media. It is most often the fastest form of storage. Mutability refers to the read/write properties of the storage media. For example, full read/write properties mean the storage device can have data copied to it, and the data can be overwritten many times. Some storage is write once read many (WORM), which allows one copy to be written, but no subsequent copies of data can be overwritten; the device can be accessed to read the data, however.

Phase 3: Use

At the point of data use, meaningful information is generated from the data. At this phase, the collected data is used in support of the healthcare organization to conduct analysis or support decision-making.

As an HCISPP, one of your concerns is defining and administering permitted use of data guidelines and controls. The permitted use of data is a crucial concept that refers to how a company manages and uses individuals' data. The concept is defined in many international privacy laws. Under the GDPR, organizations are required to be open and transparent about their data collection and use policies. Consumers have to provide consent to those collection and use policies before the organization can use the data for those stated purposes.

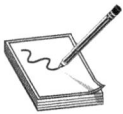

NOTE   For an example demonstrating how permitted use was not followed by a company, refer to the scandal of Facebook and Cambridge Analytica, where as many as 87 million Facebook user profiles were used in an unauthorized manner without the individuals' consent.[30]

Along with rules for obtaining consent and openness and transparency for how the data is going to be used, organizations must create and abide by a strict process for sharing sensitive data along with access and authorization rules. By committing to proper data use policies and procedures, a healthcare organization will not only adhere to regulatory guidelines but will also maintain the trust of its patients.

Phase 4: Archive

Data may have a long life span in an organization and may be used for a variety of purposes. When data is no longer useful, it is retired or moved to an archival location. Data archival becomes relevant as the need for routine or quick access begins to decline, as the data is less likely to be used or shared. However, because of retention requirements such as legal discovery or regulatory guidelines, a healthcare organization may need to archive patient data for a specific amount of time.

The key point at this phase is that although the data is no longer available routinely within the active production environments, it can be accessed if necessary. While the data is in archival status, it is no longer accessed for day-to-day use, and additional processing in the data's storage phase is halted.

Traditionally, paper documents and physical media required sufficient storage space. Because securing rooms in buildings can be an expensive endeavor, organizations were motivated to save costs by archiving data for only as long as it was needed. Of course, data archival had to adhere to regulatory guidelines for minimum retention periods.

The transformation of data from paper documents and physical forms of media to digital formats has not removed the need to retain data safely during its lifetime. The fact that digital archival costs and space requirements are far less than traditional paper-based technology and methods does not lessen the need to employ proactive and mandatory archival policies for electronic data. Because digital archival requires so little space, many organizations have not set boundaries on how and when data will be moved from normal storage to archival. To underscore this point, imagine the amount of space required to store 5000 medical records comprising paper-based images, charts, notes, and print-outs. The ability to provide access to data and long-term archive requirements could easily command multiple rooms filled with medical files. With EHR today, thousands of records can fit on an inexpensive USB thumb drive.

CAUTION Medical and legal liability issues must be addressed in data retention policies. Whether an organization is a provider solely in the United States or has international reach, it may be affected by financial implications if, due to lack of retention compliance, records are not available when they are supposed to be. Conversely, records that are maintained longer than required remain discoverable in judicial proceedings. This can add unnecessary cost, delay, and liability to the discovery process.

Some organizations are opting to archive their on-premises data in cloud computing solutions, even where the source data is not stored and used on a day-to-day basis. The benefits of cloud storage include a high-availability environment that is kept current with security patches and technical support. Compared with the costs incurred by an organization trying to archive within their own data center, the cloud solution helps defray infrastructure and time expenses.

Phase 5: Destroy

Simply put, when a healthcare organization has no business, clinical, legal reason or obligation to maintain data, it needs to securely dispose of it. The destruction of data must be guided by organizational policy and relevant regulations, both local and national. In the United States, data retention is not prescribed by HIPAA, but some state laws provide governance. The governance is important to establish a minimum amount of time that data elements must be maintained. A maximum limit should also be established, with a caveat that allows longer limits if the information is determined to be valuable to business processes or clinical treatment. There are international standards, too. The Canadian Privacy Act is not prescriptive in that it does not mandate how long the government must store personal information; however, if the act charges government data collectors with retaining the information for a minimum time period, set by additional regulation. This time period must be sufficient for the data subject to have access to the information. Because healthcare is funded by the Canadian government, this provision can mandate longer retention periods. In the European Union, the GDPR also has a provision that describes maximum limits for how long the information should be retained, so that it is kept no longer than necessary. At the same time, GDPR allows member states to establish longer retention periods if they have historical, statistical, or scientific uses for the information that are valid and otherwise permitted by the GDPR.

Data destruction is important for you to master. One major reason is because data users often relax controls for protecting sensitive data when it is no longer needed.

When computing equipment is decommissioned from production, a common reuse is to donate it to charity organizations. But if hard drives are not sanitized, the goodwill of a donation can be ruined by a data breach.

With the advent of data collection and storage of petabytes of data, the impact of losing data is significant enough. But when the story also includes acknowledgment that the breached data was no longer needed by the organization, but kept anyway, the impact is magnified. Consider the case of US company InfoTrax that found hackers had compromised its servers, and that customer data, including sensitive information, had been accessed by the attackers. Over one million accounts with Social Security numbers, payment card information, bank account information, and usernames and passwords in clear text were potentially leaked—information that, by the company's own admission, was kept longer than it needed to be.[1] Maintaining privacy and security vigilance throughout the entire data lifecycle, especially at the data destruction phase, will help you keep your organization and patients safe.

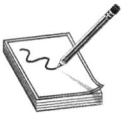

> **NOTE** Disposal and destruction methods apply to paper-based sensitive records as well as electronic records. The available methods for paper-based disposal aren't covered in depth in this text, but shredding and incinerating documents are commonly accepted procedures. The key is protecting the information as the paper-based records are transported from storage to a destruction site.

You will need to know and use appropriate methods for securely disposing of data. Again, in this stage, the information remains sensitive, whether it is payment related or contains health data for an individual. Proper disposal and destruction methods, collectively called "sanitization methods," are needed to prevent unauthorized disclosure. There are two general approaches to data destruction. The first approach is to render the actual device containing the media useless. Physical destruction of the media, electromagnetic degaussing, and incineration are common tactics. If the organization intends to repurpose the device after destroying the sensitive data, these approaches would not be appropriate. If the media is not rewritable, physical destruction is the best method to ensure the information is destroyed.

The second type of data disposal is by cleansing or sanitizing the media/drive. The physical media can therefore be reused, but there is no trace of data on the media after the data-wiping action, which can occur when data destruction efforts are insufficient to prevent data reconstruction. There are numerous validated processes for this objective. The techniques outlined in Chapter 1 for information sanitization would also apply here. Keep in mind that data sanitization is usually considered a minimum standard because of the risk of data remanence.

The best methods use both approaches as needed based on the level of sensitivity of the information and the possibility of reusing the media. The goal of sanitization as an information security control is to render the data so that it is impossible or impractical for someone ever to retrieve it.

Physical Media Destruction

Somewhat analogous to physical destruction of paper-based records, media that contains sensitive data can be destroyed completely as opposed to removing the data securely while leaving the physical media asset (backup tape, hard drive, and so on) intact. The processes for physically destroying the media are not very technical or elegant, but they are highly effective. For instance, drilling holes into a hard drive through the spinning disk is effective. This method may not actually destroy the data, but the data will become unreadable or unrecoverable. Large shredders can also be used to shred the physical assets into small pieces. Some other methods that can be used are disintegration, incineration, pulverization, melting, sanding, and treatment with chemicals.

Secure Overwriting   Secure overwriting renders data unusable by destroying just the data. Other methods render the drive completely unusable, even those that do not destroy the physical asset. If an organization wants to reuse storage assets, such as expensive storage area network components, it can overwrite the data. The secure overwriting process consists of writing meaningless data over and over onto each of the sectors on an asset's hard drive. The meaningless pattern typically consists of combinations of 1's and 0's. The number of times this process must happen to be effective varies across a number of standards. Probably the most often referenced standard is the NIST SP 800-88, *Guidelines for Media Sanitization*, which calls for multiple overwriting passes to overwrite the data completely.

Degaussing   Degaussing is a process used to erase all data on magnetic field types of media, such as backup tapes or hard drives. The device used to degauss the media generates a magnetic field that completely randomizes the 1's and 0's on the media with no preference to orientation, thereby rendering previous data unrecoverable. This process is useful in sanitizing large amounts of data quickly. It is also very effective to use when the media is damaged and is inoperable. Many argue it is impossible to remove the magnetic field completely and thereby fully randomize all the 1's and 0's. A remnant can remain, making it theoretically possible for some of the data to be recovered. For this reason, much like secure overwriting, information security best practices require multiple degaussing for each piece of media. NIST recommends multiple degaussing passes. Degaussed media cannot be reused.

Third-Party Connectivity

Because many healthcare organizations have implemented EHRs, the work required to connect any existing data systems, engineer the local area network, and prepare physical environments to house the equipment may require additional support from external organizations. Other types of third-party entities may require access to your organization's data to accomplish the duties they are contracted to do. If the third party works at a location away from that of the healthcare organization, they made need to make remote external connections into your computing environment.

The operations of healthcare organizations extend well beyond the clinical care settings to include a new type of supply chain between the healthcare organization and vendor suppliers. This supply chain must be managed as a valuable asset to be protected and shared securely according to organizational, regulatory, and legal requirements. In international terms, data controllers rely on partners who are data processors and, in many cases, have other data processors that must be approved to handle the sensitive information. In the United States, this relationship is called the *business associate* and can include all of the downstream business associates as well (that is, the business associates of the business associates). The traditional vendor relationship has moved from contractual relationships to include various. complicated interconnection agreements. As you would expect, there are several considerations for privacy and security of information related to third-party connectivity.

There must be a chain of trust between the healthcare organization and its third-party vendors. Imagine the complex relationship between third-party organizations that manage an HIE process for exchanging relevant healthcare information between (often competing) healthcare organizations that have patients in common. This may involve a data center or cloud provider contracted as a third-party vendor to host the data from the healthcare organizations. This third party would have access to healthcare information, with statutory and contractual responsibilities to protect that information.

One reality is constant across the globe: no matter who is the third party for the healthcare organization, data controller, or covered entity (synonymous depending on country of origin), accountability for the loss of sensitive data is always the healthcare organization's responsibility. Although the regulatory or legal liability can fall to the third party, this is of little benefit. The patient may not understand the complexity of the third-party relationship and will lose trust in the healthcare organization. After all, the healthcare organization collected the information and made promises to the patient to protect personal information (and use only as much of it as needed for intended purposes).

Although contractual agreements and business relationships do not change this, the healthcare organization must implement controls to outline expectations, define procedures, and identify matters of redress relevant to any third party's use of protected information. Failing to take these interconnection actions represents a lack of accountability to regulators. The absence of such may result in the healthcare organization facing additional civil and even criminal penalties. Keep in mind that even if an organization is found to have done everything reasonable and appropriate to prevent data loss (due diligence), civil and criminal penalties are a possibility—including fines and penalties incurred by not properly attending to third-party relationships.

EXAM TIP   Grasp the complexity of the relationship with third-party entities. No matter how comprehensive the healthcare organization's risk assessment and oversight actions may be, the ultimate responsibility for properly handling sensitive healthcare data remains the legal and ethical responsibility of the healthcare organization. That cannot be outsourced or fully transferred away based on contracting or insurance.

Trust Models for Third-Party Interconnections

Starting with an understanding of regulations and laws for data use outside of the healthcare organization, you will have a role in establishing third-party interconnections. You should expect to design, implement, and enforce technical solutions as well as administrative controls such as contracts and data-sharing agreements to support external connections. As you work within that role, you will be required to define privacy and security parameters, such as minimum data sets and least privilege levels for access. You will outline third-party on-boarding, credentialing, and termination processes to make sure these parties are properly cleared to use the healthcare organization's network and applications. Another responsibility you will have in this area will be in securing data transfer capabilities, such as encryption, for safeguarding information. Communication of these processes and many others must be done within the healthcare organization and to third parties before contracts are signed and work begins.

After considering the complexity, magnitude, and nature of the arrangement and associated risks with the third-party connection, the healthcare organization should decide how to manage interconnections and data sharing. A trust model, or a selection of connection controls, is important. A quick look at some technical controls of the third-party trust model is helpful. Such models and tools are important to help formalize a level of trust with third-party organizations that provide a service. To formalize the chain of trust and to gain the satisfactory assurances required, you can expect to see these technical trust models in practice. By no means comprehensive, here are some leading examples:

- **PKI certificates**   Public-key infrastructure (PKI) certificates are used to support the encrypted transfer of healthcare information. PKI is a collection of hardware, software, organizations, policies, and procedures that work together to facilitate the appropriate use of digital certificates, which make encrypting information possible. Within PKI, each user has a unique identity validated by a trusted authority. The transfer of information between two individuals with an established trust relationship under PKI is secure, and the sender and recipient have assurance that each is who they say they are (nonrepudiation).

- **Transport Layer Security (TLS) and Secure Sockets Layer (SSL)**   TLS and its predecessor, SSL, are security protocols that enable the secure transport of information across protected network tunnels on the Internet. The X.509 class of certificates are used (PKI, for example). Like PKI, the use of certificates allows nonrepudiation and the data is encrypted. Several versions of these protocols make possible secure applications in web browsing, e-mail, Internet faxing, instant messaging, and Voice over IP (VoIP).

- **Virtual private networking (VPN)**   Through a user-created connection, remote access is made possible by a combination of passwords, biometrics, two-factor authentication, or other cryptographic methods. The remote user establishes a secure connection that extends a private network across the Internet. Data is shared just as it is all within the organizational domain or private intranet. Logically, the connection is a virtual point-to-point connection using dedicated connections, encryption, or a combination.

- **Virtual desktop interface (VDI)**   Because external vendors may need access via mobile endpoints, a VDI may be a preferred, secure solution. VDI is remote access to a virtual desktop and is enabled through client software on the remote endpoint. The client system presents the remote computer desktop image to the remote user on his or her mobile device. The remote user can manipulate and access the client's system. VDI adds data security because it can be configured to make it impossible for data to leave the organization's network.

Not only should interconnection terms be spelled out in contracts and agreements, but it is also incumbent upon the primary entity to ensure that termination actions are carried out. Appropriate activities must all be taken into consideration, such as removing access to the data; appropriately destroying, disposing, and/or returning the data; terminating network connections; and ensuring that files are no longer exchanged.

Technical Standards: Physical, Logical, Network Connectivity

The process of interconnecting third parties to the healthcare organization network could open the organization to various information risks. It is imperative that entities take appropriate steps to implement effective security controls. This will start with ensuring that current controls are configured correctly and any gaps are addressed using new controls. Technical security controls will be a combination of firewalls, identification and authentication mechanisms, logical access controls, encryption devices, intrusion detection systems, and network behavior monitoring systems. Technical standards will include physical, logical, and network connectivity components, as shown in the following list. Objective standards can easily be found in leading information security guidance and risk management frameworks such as the NIST Cybersecurity Framework, ISO 27001, and the HITRUST Common Security Framework.

Physical Controls

Physical control considerations include the physical environment in which the vendor's computing network resides as well as the physical architecture of the computing environment itself. You need to collect information about the data center or facility that houses equipment that collects, stores, or transfers your organization's sensitive data. Such external assessments are considered necessary. An example of such an assessment is SOC 2, an auditing procedure developed by the American Institute of CPAs (AICPA) that can be used to evaluate the management of customer data based on five "trust service principles": security, availability, processing integrity, confidentiality, and privacy. SOC 2 assesses the effectiveness of physical controls in place.

The physical technical standards relate to the hardware, software, and pathways that must support and conform to industry regulations, relevant law, and your organization's policies and procedures. These standards must consider a third party's system architecture and the interconnection components that will provide access to your organization and support data sharing. You may require documents that show the technology used by the vendor, such as firewalls, IDS, data loss prevention, and VPNs. You can also review relevant system and security logs as well as audit reports. Information should also include ports through which network traffic travels as well as protocols used.

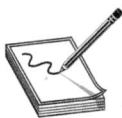

NOTE To gain a deeper understanding of which physical architecture technical standards are appropriate, organizations and frameworks such as SABSA (Sherwood Applied Business Security Architecture) outline the best enterprise physical infrastructure architecture approaches. For more information on SABSA, visit https://sabsa.org/.

Logical Controls

Technical standards for logical security refer to the controls the third party will have and use to grant access and limit authorization to data. Your role will be to review and enforce the use of acceptable logical security technical standards based on interconnection requirements. These logical security controls include systems used to manage user profiles, privileged access, and passwords. Advanced technical standards for logical security controls are tokens that generate one-time use codes to enable multifactor authentication and identity systems that enable biometric access control methods. In addition to reviewing the identity and access management tools, you'll need to understand the vendor's policies and procedures regarding granting access and credentials for employees. This will include an assessment of the vendor's process for termination of employees' access when that access is no longer needed, such as after an employee's contract terms expires.

Network Connectivity Controls

Technical standards for network connectivity will involve an evaluation of how the vendor's network is configured, protected, and monitored. This evaluation will confirm whether or not the third party has sufficient network controls in place to prevent, detect, and respond to unauthorized attacks or intrusions. Network connectivity must also consider mobile and cloud connectivity if applicable. Additionally, network connectivity technical standards will outline the only approved methods and technologies a third party may use to connect to the healthcare network. For example, approval may be granted for solutions using VPN or SSH tunnels. If the organization's risk levels are high enough to warrant the additional costs, some interconnections may be established with direct, dedicated circuits, such as ISDN, T1, or T3 connections.

Connection Agreements

To support the physical and logical controls, organizations must use a number of administrative controls to implement and sustain information privacy and security for third-party interconnections. Connection agreements contain relevant terms and conditions that establish interconnections, with details, specifications, expectations, and responsibilities outlined within the documents. These agreements help healthcare organizations communicate requirements, evaluate performance, and hold all parties accountable for compliance. The more comprehensive the connection agreement, the better job the organization can do monitoring and enforcing the interconnection over time. Connection agreements are also helpful when a healthcare organization's expectations and requirements exceed those of the third party's other customers.

Memorandum of Understanding

A memorandum of understanding (MOU) contains business and legal requirements, including purpose and rules of engagement, necessary to support the interconnection between the healthcare organization and the third party. A good MOU clearly lists areas that both sides must abide by, such as confidentiality of data. Technical configurations are not part of the MOU, however; those are covered in accompanying interconnection security agreements (ISAs). Although not a legally binding contract, an MOU is a formal agreement and is often created before a contractual relationship is formed. The document establishes an outline of how the two organizations will work together based on roles and responsibilities. An MOU is often used in conjunction with a service level agreement (SLA).

Service Level Agreement

Healthcare organizations may choose to require a written SLA before hiring a third party. These can be legal contracts with binding conditions enforceable in court, or they can represent informal obligations between the two parties. Either way, an SLA will cover important, measurable performance expectations and the responsibilities of the provider as well as the customer. An SLA also covers how problems will be handled. When a disaster happens, the SLA will guide actions and obligations for the recovery of systems covered by the agreement. Finally, the SLA must include terms and conditions for ending the agreement, including what happens in data disposal.

The most effective SLAs include scheduled times in which the customer and service provider meet to discuss ongoing operations. This communication may integrate into the overall risk management process, where issues concerning risk assessment and mitigation are also included in the monitoring of the SLA. But the SLA covers more than just the management of risk. Service providers will have obligations to provide availability of information, upgrades to hardware and software, and/or improvements in general customer service depending on what services are being provided. In short, the SLA can be considered an additional administrative control within the risk management process. The SLA should be enforced, but changes should be permitted as situations warrant. Communication is a vital part of ensuring that the SLA is never static and helps the healthcare organization and third party achieve a successful partnership.

To protect healthcare information for your organization, you may have to manage one or more SLAs. The SLA may be a portion of your overall risk management strategy. The following are some suggestions for properly managing the SLAs under your purview:

- Be proactive and review compliance regularly.
- Establish measurable objectives that meet business or clinical standards, comply with laws or regulatory requirements, and ensure that the service provider agrees to abide by.
- Monitor these objectives continuously.
- Communicate with the third party.
- Communicate to information governance within the healthcare organization.

Doing these activities can help you succeed in your duties. More importantly, active oversight will give the SLA the best chance of being efficient and effective. Too many SLAs are signed and shelved only to be reviewed after a data breach or after service levels have reached such low levels that the agreement is in jeopardy of being terminated for cause.

Interconnection Security Agreements

ISAs include the responsibilities and expectations that establish and maintain network interconnection. They specify technical and security requirements and controls the healthcare organization and third party are expected to implement to ensure information privacy and security. The ISA is intended to protect both organizations and their interconnected systems. This is related to the fact that an organization will not have control over a third party's firewalls, routers, or DLPs, for example. ISAs are a compensating administrative control to mitigate the risks.

The agreements are developed as early in the third-party negotiations as possible, preferably during system development. As business requirements change, the ISA can be modified to reflect these. The use of an ISA follows guidance from NIST SP 800-53 Rev. 4, *Security and Privacy Controls for Federal Information Systems and Organizations*, specifically control "CA-3 System Interconnections." For organizations establishing dedicated connections between information systems, the control asserts organizations can either develop ISAs or describe the interface characteristics between systems in the security plans for the respective systems.[32] Components of an ISA can include a description of the agreement's purpose and benefits, any security requirements, and a network diagram depicting the interconnection. The ISA is reviewed annually; as changes are made to the interconnections over the life of the contract, the ISA must be updated accordingly, not only at annual review.

Contracts (Standards and Practices)

When a formal, legally binding document is required, a contract may be used. Contracts include standards, practices, and clauses that exceed the level of formality and enforcement of an SLA. Contractual provisions are helpful for data security concerns. Every contract has variations, and an overall template is hard to illustrate, but some commonalities exist.

To begin with, the contract should hold the third party to relevant privacy and security standards that the healthcare organization complies with, including external regulations and internal policies and procedures. Additionally, contracts will consist of terms and conditions related to the following:

- **Compliance** The third party must adhere to relevant regulations. In the United States, this would start with HIPAA. The contract may be the business associate agreement (BAA), or the BAA may be part of the entire contract. The third party will also have to comply with relevant state laws. All compliance requirements must be covered specifically in the contract's compliance section. For organizations that extend globally, or those that transfer data across borders, the contract would include compliance requirements for laws of other countries, such as the EU GDPR. Beyond compliance with laws, compliance with standards should also be included.

For example, the third party must adhere to applicable Payment Card Industry Data Security Standard (PCI DSS) requirements or applicable NIST standards.

- **Confidentiality**   If the third party is required to handle sensitive healthcare information, the confidentiality provision must be present in the contract. The information is defined, permitted uses are explained, prohibited uses are described, and return or disposition provisions are outlined upon the termination of the contract.

- **Data loss prevention and response**   The third party will take on responsibilities for preventing data loss and will also need to know how to respond to potential or actual data loss by complying with the healthcare organization's incident response policies as well as any governing regulatory guidelines. The contract should allocate responsibilities and outline procedures accordingly.

- **Indemnification**   Some will argue the sections covering indemnification can be the most impactful in a contract. Indemnification, or the provisions for damages or compensation if things go wrong, becomes crucial in the event of a security breach or abuse of personal information. The contractual language should also include information regarding insurance to cover data loss events. Any regulatory obligations in the country where the patients reside will be provided. Also, the indemnification clause will include a duty to cooperate in investigations and resolution actions. In some cases, the healthcare organization will want to add provisions for controlling these investigations and any notification actions to patients or regulators, even if the vendor is responsible for some or all of the related costs.

- **Limits to liability**   In the event the third party causes a data loss or breach, the contract should limit liability (or hold harmless) for the healthcare organization. On the other hand, there can be limits imposed on the liability of the third party, because too high of a threshold or unlimited liability may far exceed the value of the contract. Not many third-party vendors would accept that much risk and would instead choose not to provide the service to the healthcare organization. It is a delicate balance. But the healthcare organization needs to be protected from undue litigation and data breach recovery costs resulting from a third party's failure to perform or to comply with applicable laws.

Chapter Review

Health information technology (HIT) involves the design, development, creation, use, and maintenance of information systems used within healthcare organizations. As the healthcare industry has evolved from paper documents and printed images to digital files and databases, the importance of HIT has increased. HIT helps providers and payers improve medical care and public health, lower costs, increase efficiency, reduce errors, and improve patient satisfaction, while also optimizing reimbursement for ambulatory and inpatient healthcare providers.

HIT consists of many types and formats of information systems along with technology peripherals such as scanners and printers. Some HIT may appear to be technically the same as regular office automation and business systems, but as an HCISPP, you must realize that HIT is not the same. HIT has important privacy and security concerns that must be addressed to ensure the secure use and transfer of healthcare information. The best information security practices used in other industries may not be appropriate for HIT. Understanding this and developing tailored approaches to delivering information privacy and security in healthcare is central to your success.

In this chapter, we introduced some of the HIT used. Major categories of HIT include electronic health records (EHRs), a central component of the HIT infrastructure. An EHR is a patient's official, digital health record and is often shared among multiple healthcare providers and agencies. Other types of HIT in the healthcare organization are the patient health record (PHR), or the patient portal that an individual may use to track his or her own record of care. The electronic record sources feed into a health information exchange (HIE), which is a group of healthcare providers who agree to share data to improve patient care for their defined population.

EHRs are a system of systems that connect to and depend on interoperability with networked medical devices. Medical devices are special-purpose computing systems that are regulated by the US Food and Drug Administration (FDA). Some examples are picture archiving and communication systems (PACS) and patient monitoring telemetry systems in the intensive care unit (ICU). The privacy and security impacts of these classes of HIT are numerous, and you must be aware of them and address them. The potential for increased patient safety risk and patient harm are significant if medical devices are not properly protected.

Added to privacy and security risks are interoperability issues between systems. Information blocking or other forms of system incompatibility bring about a specific problem in HIT that relates to data availability. This, too, is an area where you will play a role in designing, implementing, and monitoring systems that can communicate securely.

We also covered data lifecycle management (DLM) in terms of how to maintain confidentiality, integrity, and availability as data is created, stored, used, archived, and destroyed by the healthcare organization. At any of these phases, there are important tools, techniques, and practices to help you protect the data. The use of data leads to a discussion of the sharing of data with external, third-party organizations. It is important to note that some third parties, such as cloud service providers, that deal with data on behalf of the healthcare organization may provide services to other organizations in other industries. These cases emphasize the need for all third parties to interconnect with healthcare organizations using technical trust models. In addition to the technical configurations and concerns, administrative controls such as memorandums of understanding and interconnection security agreements are an imperative.

Implementation and enforcement of the information privacy and security concepts described in this chapter will help your healthcare organization realize the benefits of HIT. There is broad consensus that HIT improves patient care and research, enhances provider practices, and reduces cost over the long term.

Questions

1. You are provided a network vulnerability scan of the hospital network. There are numerous critical unpatched vulnerabilities on many of the devices. You work with the person who runs the centralized vulnerability patching team to develop a remediation approach that includes automated security patching of systems. Which of these steps would you take next?

   A. Contact system owners to advise them of the updates.

   B. Schedule the remediation patching after clinical hours.

   C. Exclude medical devices from the updates.

   D. Quarantine vulnerable systems per policy.

2. An organization that facilitates the electronic sharing of healthcare information between providers and payers is a description of

   A. Health information exchange (HIE)

   B. Health insurance exchange (HIE)

   C. Health information establishment (HIE)

   D. Health insurance establishment (HIE)

3. In using an electronic health record (EHR) with computerized provider order entry (CPOE), which is true?

   A. Nurses are permitted to change prescriptions when they see data entry errors.

   B. Insurers are able to suggest alternative medications or generic options in real-time.

   C. Patients with known allergies receive a contraindication alert prior to a prescription being submitted.

   D. Encryption enables providers to submit digital orders without any signature.

4. You receive an overnight package to your data center. The invoice describes an encrypted hard drive containing contents of a physician's office that is part of your healthcare network. There are directions for you to degauss the media and transfer it to the radiology department. Which phase in data lifecycle management would you consider the data?

   A. Archive

   B. Store

   C. Share

   D. Destroy

5. Which of these is an external threat to the privacy and security of HIT?

   A. Hacking of a medical device implanted inside a patient

   B. Health information exchanges between organizations

   C. Cloud hosting organization disclosing closure of potential vulnerability

   D. Laboratory specialist contracted to work in the clinic who copies patient data

6. Mainview Healthcare Systems has entered into merger discussions with Heart of Gold Healthcare. Each healthcare organization has an impressive HIT inventory, including EHRs, networked medical devices, and a significant presence for patients on the Internet through PHRs. You are the lead security engineer for Mainview. Which of these scenarios best depicts your main concerns at this point?

   A. The Heart of Gold EHR was implemented three years before your EHR. There is almost three times as much data to export into the disaster recovery storage systems.

   B. The EHRs are manufactured and supported by two competing companies. There may be a need for significant engineering to connect the systems securely.

   C. To connect the medical devices from Heart of Gold, multiple firewall rules must be implemented. These will expose Mainview to threats unlike any time before.

   D. Medical devices in Mainview are managed by a third-party biomedical firm with remote access to the network. Heart of Gold manages medical devices with internal staff and has expressed reluctance to allow any external, third-party access.

7. Which of the following appropriate medical device security approaches would explain why your organization provides input and follows the FDA MedWatch services?

   A. Medical devices are out of scope for the organization's information security incident response plan.

   B. Regulations mandate that medical device interoperability be maintained.

   C. Vulnerability management of medical devices is integrated into the organization's information security program.

   D. International sources contribute to security approaches and most manufacturers are global.

8. Which of the following security concerns would still be the responsibility of a healthcare organization that uses an EHR solution hosted by a cloud services provider that is proprietary to a customer of the cloud host organization?

   A. Patching

   B. Access

   C. Firewall

   D. Configuration

9. In an organization that mandates third-party connectivity by way of a virtual private network (VPN), which of the following would you expect?

   A. Medical billing contract employee receives monthly charges for patient care via secure e-mail

   B. Healthcare organization employees use Infrastructure-as-a-Service cloud hosting for storage

   C. Patients provided with unique credentials to establish a secure web portal for access

   D. Outsourced data science team use BYOD and special security application to login remotely

10. Which of the following is a set of documents that outlines expectations between two organizations to address items such as technical specifications and configuration responsibilities for interconnection?

    A. SLA

    B. MOU

    C. BAA

    D. ISA

Answers

1. **C.** This illustrates the concept that even the best practices for information privacy and security in other industries may not be best for healthcare. The first step when dealing with a scan of the entire healthcare network is to make sure you can separate medical devices from regular office automation or business systems. C is the best option of those given. Medical devices may require special handling, especially legacy systems, but medical devices are regulated by law and good manufacturing processes after their sale. You will need to identify those on the report and exclude them from the initial remediation. Then you will need to develop a plan to remediate the medical devices according to organizational policy, manufacturer guidance, and any patient safety concerns. The medical devices need to be as secure as possible, and the rest of the healthcare network must be as protected from the vulnerable medical devices as much as possible. None of that should put patient care at risk or disrupt the mission of the healthcare organization. A would be acceptable, but simply advising owners would not address the risk to medical devices by pushing a security patch automatically. The eventual patching may be done at night when the healthcare organization is closed or there is minimal patient care activity, but B would not prevent medical devices from being patched and possibly disrupted. D is partially correct in that the guidance for medical devices and all networked systems should be covered in organizational policy that must be followed, but quarantine or isolation is very likely going to cause disruption to medical devices and will negatively impact patient care.

2. A. More than just a play on words, it is important to distinguish the health information exchange from any other type of exchange. B is an actual exchange (or type of exchange) found in each US state in accordance with the Affordable Care Act. However, it does not support exchanging anything more than insurance information options for enrollees. Providers would not use a health insurance exchange to collect information about patients. C and D are not actual types of organizations.

3. C. With the computing capabilities to reconcile numerous databases and transactions, EHRs provide near-instantaneous drug–drug contraindication alerts that improve patient care and safety. A is incorrect because nurses (excluding advanced nursing professions such as nurse practitioners) would not have authority to alter a physician's prescription order. B is not typically a feature of EHRs, especially considering the variety of insurers that would require access. D is incorrect because encryption of the data would not remove the need for a signature (digital or otherwise).

4. D. Degaussing will destroy the data on the hard drive. In degaussing, the electronic media is sanitized so that no remnants of data could be re-created from the disk. A degaussed drive removes startup files along with all other data. We will never know why the radiology department wants a useless hard drive. All other answers are valid phases in data lifecycle management, but degaussing is a step taken when information is determined to be obsolete.

5. A. An implantable medical device hacked from an external source is the best example of an external threat to HIT. Along with the benefits of HIT, new information and privacy threats have emerged, some with internal sources and others external in origin. B is not a threat if the exchange has appropriate information security transfer controls in place. C is incorrect because, although cloud computing does introduce new threats, the disclosure and remediation of a vulnerability are normal operations. It is not the best example of a threat based on the actions the cloud hosting company appears to have taken. D is incorrect because it is an example of an internal threat to privacy and security through a third party. The contract employee is located within the organization and has access to the HIT network. Additionally, the fact that this party is copying data may be a required part of normal duties.

6. B. Interoperability is the major concerns at this point, and this answer suggests possible challenges. A is not an obstacle but may be more of a need for financial projections to increase storage capability if disaster recovery and business continuity requirements call for the data to be maintained. C is also a normal course of business, and although the risks of more interconnections are real, the process of managing firewall rules is a normal course of business. The management of medical devices by internal or external staff, onsite or remotely, as depicted in D is something the organizations will need to address. Of the choices, D is not as urgent as addressing interoperability challenges, which will directly impact patient care.

7. **C.** A successful approach to managing security for medical devices is to integrate them into the organization's overall information security program. This will include monitoring logs and responding to alerts, of which FDA MedWatch is a good source, as part of the incident response plan. A is incorrect because these devices are within scope of the security incident response plan according to MedWatch. B is incorrect because the use of MedWatch is voluntary and would not focus on interoperability issues. D is incorrect because international sources would not have a connection to the important content that would be covered in FDA MedWatch.

8. **B.** Access to the system and data will remain the responsibility of the healthcare organization, because the cloud service provider is probably not going to have the ability to determine authorized users and responsibilities. In most cloud computing environments, even in a Software as a Service (SaaS) relationship, the healthcare organization controls access. A is incorrect because as a hosted solution, the scenario assumes maintenance of the hardware and software is managed by the cloud services provider. C is also not likely the responsibility of the healthcare organization but would be part of the cloud provider's infrastructure. D may not be a security control, but it is also not the right answer based on the scenario, because the healthcare organization probably has no ability to configure the system or application other than to customize screens or administer users.

9. **D.** Of the options, this is the only one that is descriptive of a VPN connection with external access through a secure, dedicated connection. A describes a secure transfer to an external, third party but not via VPN. B is not a third party and does not describe a VPN connection, although the cloud-to-healthcare organization connection will be a secure connection. C involves patients, not third parties such as vendors, and the connection is web-enabled or certificate (PKI) based.

10. **D.** Interconnection security agreements (ISAs) outline the technical and configuration details that will establish and secure the interconnections. A, a service level agreement, will focus more on the satisfaction of terms and conditions for security and performance. B, the memorandum of understanding, is an important document but it addresses business and operational expectations. C, the business associate agreement, in the United States, will contain significant points of responsibilities and expectations between the healthcare organization and its third party, but not to the specificity of an ISA, which would the complement BAAs.

References

1. The ECRI Institute's "Top 10 Patient Concerns for 2019" can be downloaded by registering at https://www.ecri.org/landing-top-10-patient-safety-concerns-2019.

2. Browning, J. G., and S. Tuma. 2015. "If Your Heart Skips a Beat, It May Have Been Hacked: Cybersecurity Concerns with Implanted Medical Devices." *Southern Carolina Law Review*, 67, 637.

3. Kirk, J. 2012. "Pacemaker hack can deliver deadly 830-volt jolt." *Computerworld*, October 17, https://www.computerworld.com/article/2492453/pacemaker-hack-can-deliver-deadly-830-volt-jolt.html.

4. Newman, L. H. 2019. "A Model Hospital Where the Devices Get Hacked—on Purpose." *Wired*, August 6, https://www.wired.com/story/defcon-medical-device-village-hacking-hospital.

5. Beavers, J., and S. Pournouri. 2019. "Recent Cyber Attacks and Vulnerabilities in Medical Devices and Healthcare Institutions." In *Blockchain and Clinical Trial*, 249–267. Cham, Switzerland: Springer.

6. McLean, R. 2019. "A hacker gained access to 100 million Capital One credit card applications and accounts." *CNN Business,* July 30, https://www.cnn.com/2019/07/29/business/capital-one-data-breach/index.html.

7. Brewster, T. 2017. "Medical Devices Hit by Ransomware for the First Time in US Hospitals." *Forbes*, May 17, https://www.forbes.com/sites/thomasbrewster/2017/05/17/wannacry-ransomware-hit-real-medical-devices/#41f1d7a425cf.

8. Weiner, J. P., T. Kfuri, K. Chan, and J. B. Fowles. 2007. "'e-Iatrogenesis': The most critical unintended consequence of CPOE and other HIT." *Journal of the American Medical Informatics Association,* 14(3), 387–388.

9. The Joint Commission. 2019. "Sentinel Event." https://www.jointcommission.org/resources/patient-safety-topics/sentinel-event.

10. Scholl, M., et al. 2008. *An Introductory Resource Guide for Implementing the Health Insurance Portability and Accountability Act (HIPAA) Security Rule.* National Institute of Standards and Technology Special Publication 800-66 Rev. 1, https://nvlpubs.nist.gov/nistpubs/Legacy/SP/nistspecialpublication800-66r1.pdf.

11. Smallwood, R. F. 2018. *Information Governance for Healthcare Professionals: A Practical Approach.* Boca Raton, FL: Routledge/CRC Press.

12. Donaldson, S. E., S. G. Siegel, C. K. Williams, and A. Aslam. 2018. *Enterprise Cybersecurity Study Guide: How to Build a Successful Cyberdefense Program Against Advanced Threats.* Apress.

13. HealthIT.gov. 2019. "What is an electronic health record (EHR)?" https://www.healthit.gov/faq/what-electronic-health-record-ehr.

14. HealthIT.gov. 2019. "Guide to Privacy & Security of Electronic Health Information." https://www.healthit.gov/topic/health-it-resources/guide-privacy-security-electronic-health-information.

15. AHIMA. "Fundamentals of the Legal Health Record and Designated Record Set." *Journal of AHIMA* 82(2): expanded online version.

16. HealthIT.gov. 2016. "What is a personal health record?" https://www.healthit.gov/faq/what-personal-health-record-0.

17. Islam, S. R., D. Kwak, M. H. Kabir, M. Hossain, and K. S. Kwak. 2015. "The Internet of Things for Health Care: A Comprehensive Survey." *IEEE Access*, 3: 678–708.

18. US Food and Drug Administration (FDA). 2018. "Medical Device Overview." https://www.fda.gov/industry/regulated-products/medical-device-overview.

19. US Food and Drug Administration (FDA). 2020. "Cybersecurity." https://www.fda.gov/medical-devices/digital-health/cybersecurity.

20. US Federal Bureau of Investigation (FBI). 2015. "Internet of Things Poses Opportunities for Cyber Crime." Alert No. I-091015-PSA. https://www.ic3.gov/media/2015/150910.aspx.

21. US Food and Drug Administration (FDA). 2018. "Regulatory Controls." https://www.fda.gov/medical-devices/overview-device-regulation/regulatory-controls.

22. US Food and Drug Administration (FDA). 2020. "Classify Your Medical Device." https://www.fda.gov/medical-devices/overview-device-regulation/classify-your-medical-device.

23. Jansen, W., and T. Grance. 2011. *Guidelines on Security and Privacy in Public Cloud Computing*. NIST Special Publication 800-144. https://nvlpubs.nist.gov/nistpubs/Legacy/SP/nistspecialpublication800-144.pdf.

24. Ponemon Institute. 2016. "The Economic Risk of Confidential Data on Mobile Devices in the Workplace."

25. Grand View Research. 2016. "Health Information Exchange Market Analysis by Setup (Private, Public)…to 2024." https://www.grandviewresearch.com/industry-analysis/health-information-exchange-hie-market.

26. The Office of the National Coordinator for Health Information Technology (ONC). 2020. HealthIT.gov: "Guide to Privacy & Security of Electronic Health Information." https://www.healthit.gov/topic/health-it-resources/guide-privacy-security-electronic-health-information.

27. Candeias, V. 2018. World Economic Forum: "How to unleash the enormous power of global healthcare data." https://www.weforum.org/agenda/2018/12/global-healthcare-data-is-a-vast-untapped-resource-until-now.

28. Kent, J. 2018. Health IT Analytics: "Big Data to See Explosive Growth, Challenging Healthcare Organizations." https://healthitanalytics.com/news/big-data-to-see-explosive-growth-challenging-healthcare-organizations.

29. National Institute of Standards and Technology (NIST) 2015. *NIST Big Data Interoperability Framework: Volume 1, Definitions*. NIST Special Publication 1500-1. https://nvlpubs.nist.gov/nistpubs/SpecialPublications/NIST.SP.1500-1.pdf.

30. Isaak, J., and M. J. Hanna. 2018. "User Data Privacy: Facebook, Cambridge Analytica, and Privacy Protection." *Computer*, 51(8), 56–59.

31. Arghire, I. 2019. "InfoTrax Settles with FTC Over Data Breach." *SecurityWeek*. https://www.securityweek.com/infotrax-settles-ftc-over-data-breach.

32. Joint Task Force Transformation Initiative. 2015. *Security and Privacy Controls for Federal Information Systems and Organizations*. NIST Special Publication 800-53 Rev. 4, https://nvlpubs.nist.gov/nistpubs/SpecialPublications/NIST .SP.800-53r4.pdf.

Regulatory and Standards Environment

This chapter covers Domain 4, "Regulatory and Standards Environment," of the HCISPP certification. After you read and study this chapter, you should be able to:

- Recognize primary regulatory guidance in healthcare information protection
- Apply regulatory governance to healthcare information technology and practices
- Appreciate the types of sensitive personal information used in healthcare organizations
- Identify and compare US and international information protection laws and regulations
- Understand important information privacy and security compliance frameworks

The importance of understanding and applying the proper privacy and security controls on healthcare information is foundational to your success as a healthcare information security and privacy professional. The healthcare industry is highly regulated in the United States, as is the protection of personal data in most countries internationally. We must understand the regulatory environments that impact our healthcare organization. From the leading regulations come numerous frameworks and control standards. Understanding the regulatory environment has a very practical purpose. Even at an office or department level, policies and procedures should be informed by national regulatory guidance. As we study information governance, our starting point is an overview of the legal and regulatory environment. This chapter will prepare you to apply practical approaches to your local information protection policies and procedures based on relevant national, industry-specific, and international guidance.

Identify Regulatory Requirements

It is important to understand a few of the applicable regulations that govern healthcare. From a practical standpoint, you will need to know the local policies and procedures that govern your organization. From a daily perspective, you will refer to organizational guidance as you design, build, implement, and enforce privacy and security controls for information. However, you are also well served to be aware of the national and international laws that shape those policies and procedures at the local level. The local guidance must be aligned with prevailing national or international law. Within the United States there is additional oversight by state and local regulators (for instance, the state of New York has cybersecurity legislation that expands the definition of sensitive personal information). Those guidelines may in fact be even more relevant to your organization's day-to-day operations than national law. It is also important to know how state law *exempts* healthcare organizations. For example, California has passed the California Consumer Privacy Act of 2018 (CCPA), which is considered comparatively more stringent than many; however, if you work in a healthcare organization subject to CCPA and the Health Insurance Portability and Accountability Act (HIPAA), CCPA exempts organizations that comply with HIPAA. This knowledge can help you prevent redundancy or negative impacts to patient care in your organization. The relationship between state and national law in the United States is complex and important to understand. What follows is an overview of the pertinent higher-level regulations you need to know.

There are no shortage of local, state, and federal laws, rules, and public policies that are specific to healthcare. For instance, you should be the most familiar with HIPAA and its amendments—the Privacy Rule, the Security Rule, the Health Information Technology for Economic and Clinical Health (HITECH) Act, and the Omnibus HIPAA Final Rule. Along with numerous individual state medical privacy laws, healthcare organizations must also comply with regulations that apply across other industries, such as the Gramm-Leach-Bliley Act (GLBA) and the Red Flags Rule governed by the Federal Trade Commission (FTC) standards.

Internationally, much healthcare regulation is found in privacy and security directives that extend across all industries. Some have specific mentions and guidance for healthcare. In general, the international view of safeguarding an individual's identifying information is a human right, so every industry is held to a high but universal standard. Examples of these are the European Union's Data Protection Directive (DPD), which has been superseded by the General Data Protection Regulation (GDPR); Canada's Personal Information Protection and Electronic Documents Act (PIPEDA); and Australia's Privacy Amendment (Private Sector) Act of 2000.

Table 4-1 provides an overview of laws that impact privacy and security in industries including healthcare. You may want to be familiar with these even if you are not impacted by them on a daily basis. Each regulation covers similar protections and includes similar provisions.

EXAM TIP   Remember that the PCI-DSS standard differs from other industry-specific regulations and directives covered in Table 4-1. PCI-DSS is developed, updated, and enforced within the private sector; it's not authored or mandated by government entities.

Legal Issues Regarding Information Security and Privacy

The following sections cover some of the most important areas where legal issues pertain to the work of healthcare organizations. Legislatures and regulatory bodies alike have focused significantly on the potential issues of connected devices. With the increasing interconnection of healthcare organizations and countless IoT devices, medical devices,

Regulation	Intent	Jurisdiction
HIPAA, 1996	Ensures continuation of health insurance coverage and protection of individuals' health information privacy. Several amendments to the original law strengthened the focus and enforcement of confidentiality of patient information. Includes criminal and civil penalties for noncompliance.	Hospitals, health systems, doctor's offices, health insurers, health information exchanges, and healthcare clearinghouses as well as business associates, such as third-party external businesses that handle HIPAA-protected health information (PHI) on behalf of a covered entity or another business associate.
Sarbanes-Oxley Act (SOX), 2002	Prevents and punishes corporate fraud; includes civil and criminal penalties for security violations, systems of certification of internal audits, and provides job protection to whistleblowers.	US publicly traded companies (including healthcare organizations), their boards, and accounting firms.
Federal Information Security Management Act of 2002, (FISMA) and Federal Information Security Modernization Act (FISMA), 2014	Recognize information security as matters of national security and have attempted to keep pace with the dynamic and growing cybersecurity risks.	All information systems in the US government. Although it's not specific to healthcare, the security controls and security management requirements are fundamental and tailored to healthcare business and clinical requirements.
Gramm-Leach-Bliley Act (GLBA), 1999	Includes Safeguards Rule for privacy and security requirements; mandates protection of nonpublic personal information (NPI) such as Social Security numbers, credit and income histories, and credit and bank card information. Requires covered entities to create a written information security plan to secure NPI against unauthorized access, notify individuals of information sharing, and track user activity.	Federal banking agencies and other federal regulatory authorities, plus state insurance oversight agencies. Enforced by the US Consumer Protection Agency and Federal Trade Commission (FTC).
Family Educational Rights and Privacy Act (FERPA), 1974	Requires the use of reasonable methods to safeguard student records against unauthorized disclosure of personally identifiable information (PII) without the consent of a parent student aged 18 or older unless an exception to the law's general consent requirement applies. Contains provisions for record review and correction requests for parents and eligible students if there are claims of inaccuracy or misleading record entries.	Postsecondary institutions including universities, academies, colleges, seminaries, technical schools, and vocational schools.
Payment Card Industry Data Security Standard (PCI-DSS), 2004	Outlines 12 security and privacy requirements that are organized into the following control objectives to protect cardholder data: – Build and maintain a secure network and systems – Protect cardholder data – Maintain a vulnerability management program – Implement strong access control measures – Regularly monitor and test networks – Maintain an information security policy	Organizations that store, process, or transmit payment and cardholder data.

Table 4-1 Relevant US Privacy and Security Laws

and electronic health records (EHRs), the need for oversight and guidance grows. Better privacy and security measures are not going to happen automatically. Regulators will continue to play a lead role in encouraging businesses, system engineers, application developers, information protection professionals, and executives to work together to develop HIT that builds in security and privacy, versus bolting it on later. In short, many of the regulations you will encounter refer to a concept of security and privacy by design.

Following are some key methods by which security and privacy by design can be accomplished:

- Establish how consent and authorization will be received.
- Be clear with patients about information collection and sharing.
- Know where data will be stored and how the storage system will be protected.
- Connect and share data via secure data transfer methods.
- Enable limits to and enforce access and permissions to sensitive data.
- Log activity to support monitoring and alerting.
- Support required patching for vulnerabilities over time.

One thing to keep in mind as you read and contemplate the material that follows: Legal issues that pertain to information security and privacy for healthcare organizations have a common theme. The laws generally mandate that healthcare organizations implement information protection programs that attain fundamental control baselines for location, access, and use of information. The obligation is on the healthcare organization to comply. When an event occurs, the regulations require the healthcare organization to provide evidence that unauthorized access or data breach did not happen. In the absence of such evidence, the organization is compelled to make public notification of the event.

Medical Devices and Critical Infrastructure Issues

In short, medical devices are an extension of the clinical care provider and integral to patient care. There are legal implications in managing them from an information privacy and security standpoint. Using medical devices offers both benefits and risks. Regulations covering medical devices generally oblige medical device manufacturers to provide a reasonable assurance that the benefits the devices offer to patients outweigh the risks. From the healthcare organization perspective, medical device regulation typically focuses on safe and secure operation of the devices for the manufacturers' intended use.

The interconnectivity of medical devices has expanded over the past two or three decades to connect via the Internet, across healthcare systems, and to other medical devices. This has advanced medicine, improved healthcare, and increased quality. But these interconnections have also increased information risk to healthcare organizations. Much like regular office automation systems, medical devices face the likelihood of security breaches, which may impact the safe operation of a device and increase the risk to patient care and security.

That said, medical devices cannot be managed exactly like regular office systems. Actions such as updating vulnerability patches and applying any kind of additional software that is not part of the manufacturer's configuration can invalidate warranties or cause the device to malfunction. Most importantly, these updates may be the direct cause of patient harm, even if the updates are considered best-practice security measures. On the other hand, both manufacturers and healthcare providers have been warned by the US FDA that they have responsibilities to keep medical devices safe (to include privacy and security considerations). This creates an uneasy balance with significant government oversight.

With respect to the international concerns of medical device security, although the FDA does not have jurisdiction, it does have impact. The same concern for patient safety in the United States is a regulatory concern internationally. Medical device manufacturers that do business internationally base their requirements on the International Organization for Standardization (ISO) frameworks for securing systems. They also provide the same medical devices cleared for use in the United States through the FDA to their international customers. In this way, the FDA has an indirect reach across the globe.

Medical device manufacturers also self-regulate. An example of this is in the increasing use of a form called the Manufacturer Disclosure Statement for Medical Device Security (MDS²).[1] Medical device manufacturers complete this form and provide it to customers to document the device's significant security features. Because the form was developed in partnership with the Healthcare Information and Management Systems Society (HIMSS) and leading clinical engineering associations, the content is reflective of concerns the FDA has with medical device security. The effect is to ensure a baseline security measure so that medical devices can be networked safely. Of course, vulnerabilities that may be introduced by networking the medical devices must be addressed and mitigated; this just happens differently (sometimes) from addressing vulnerabilities for regular office automation systems.

When it comes to critical infrastructure, healthcare organizations certainly have a responsibility to manage the network according to standards such as National Institute of Standards and Technology (NIST) Special Publication (SP) 800-34 Rev. 1, *Contingency Planning Guide for Federal Information Systems,* which contains standards for disaster recovery, backup operations, and continuity of operations. Healthcare organizations also have much in common with other industries that have networks that are considered critical infrastructure. Healthcare infrastructure is included in landmark US government guidance starting with the February 2013 Executive Order (EO) 13636, "Improving Critical Infrastructure Cybersecurity," by President Barack Obama, and strengthened by the 2017 Executive Order issued by President Donald Trump, EO 13800, "Strengthening the Cybersecurity of Federal Networks and Critical Infrastructure." These EOs are intended to help cybersecurity professionals improve the US cyber posture and capabilities in the face of intensifying cybersecurity threats. Both are aimed at federal government systems but are relevant to private-sector healthcare organizations. Specific deliverables of the EOs are modernizing IT infrastructure and increased partnerships with public government and private sectors. Healthcare organizations in all sectors (and internationally) can benefit by abiding by the EOs' deliverables.

The work undertaken to implement EO 13636 and EO 13800 reflect the strong partnership between the federal government and industry partners to safeguard the security of critical infrastructure and reduce national cybersecurity risk. There is a distinction in healthcare-critical infrastructure and the other examples with respect to the impact of network disruption. In addition to the potential loss of revenue and cost of recovery, direct patient care may be at risk during unplanned network outages. This has the potential to open the healthcare organization to malpractice claims if there is patient harm. Information technology outages caused by cybersecurity incidents in healthcare are making headlines. What is viewed as a "bug" in other information security circles is a "a disruptive, potentially dangerous major malfunction of a life-critical enterprise medical device," in a healthcare context.[2] As we become more digital and less able to revert to manual processes, the chances of patient harm increase. In addition, if an unplanned outage causes an adverse event as defined by relevant healthcare accrediting agencies in the United States and internationally (the Joint Commission, for example), it must be reported to them.

Information Accountability

Information privacy and security laws are concerned with the roles and responsibilities of those who create, use, and dispose of healthcare information. HIPAA in the United States was enacted in 1996 to cover privacy and security issues, but also to solidify accountability for the use of medical information. HITECH concentrated even more on such concerns. To be clear, there really is no "ownership" of health information. However, patients do have legal, individual rights to access their health information and learn about disclosures of their health information. Patients are entitled to full disclosure regarding how their PHI is used and disclosed. If they want to restrict sharing of information, they can make that request. The healthcare provider does not have to honor every request, but the provider must evaluate and respond to each request. Patients also have the right to inspect and review the information, amend incorrect information, and receive a copy of health information about themselves held by the healthcare provider. The healthcare provider, in turn, has the right to use the patient information for defined reasons of treatment, payment, and operations without additional patient consent required.

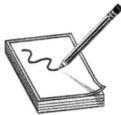

NOTE Although there have been several amendments to HIPAA over the years, the term "HIPAA" commonly refers to them all. In other words, it is acceptable to reference HIPAA requirements for patient notification of a data breach even though the requirement was implemented with the HITECH rule amendment in 2009.

In the United Kingdom and the European Union, the parameters for information accountability are similar to those in the United States. In the EU Data Protection Directive (DPD), accountability stems from the roles and responsibilities of those people, or *actors*, in the information chain of custody. Actors are data subjects who are, in essence, identified or identifiable natural persons whose personal data is processed. No one owns the information, but the EU DPD assigns roles to the actors in the information process that are similar to those in HIPAA. Table 4-2 defines these actors.

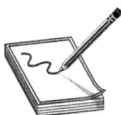

NOTE The EU replaced the DPD with the GDPR effective May 25, 2018. The DPD was considered outdated. Later in this chapter, we will explore the specific differences and updates in the change from DPD to GDPR. The main reason to include DPD information is for use as testable material in certification exams.

Term	Definition
Data subject	The person to whom the data pertains.
Data controller	An entity (or entities) that determines the purposes for why and how any personal data is, or will be, processed. This entity can be a person, an organization, or a group of people who are not collectively an organization. The data controllers must ensure that information use complies with the EU DPD.
Data processor	The person or entity that manages the data for a data controller but is not employed by the data controller. In the European Union, these entities are not directly subject to the DPD in their role as data processor.

Table 4-2   Definitions for Information Accountability from EU DPD

Cloud Computing

Across multiple industries, cloud computing has gained acceptance and momentum. Cloud computing is a collection of software, platforms, and infrastructure provided as a service to consumers via the Internet from remote locations (outside the consumer's organization). The cloud service provider hosts all the equipment on its premises and is responsible for power and availability. The consumer just logs on and uses the resources. Cloud services are offered by a variety of vendors, but some that may be the most familiar to you are Google, Amazon, and Microsoft. Cloud computing presents unique risks to healthcare. These risks are magnified in that many cloud computing vendors are unfamiliar with the special requirements of healthcare. One such unique requirement is the need for all healthcare organizations to conduct a third-party risk assessment of vendors that handle PHI on their behalf. Because other industries may not require these assessments, or a legal requirement for assessments, vendors can be reluctant to comply with these requirements or reluctant to comply with mitigating any findings.

Another concern with cloud computing is the location of the PHI. For example, PHI that is hosted in cloud locations outside the United States is a potential issue, where cloud providers are not subject to HIPAA, or training of workforce members is insufficient for protection of PHI. There are also concerns when data hosted in a non-US jurisdiction could be subject to discovery and disclosure requirements of the host nation's jurisdiction. Where those access requirements potentially violate HIPAA, US healthcare organizations have to understand the impact from a regulatory and reputational perspective. For this reason, many healthcare organizations require that servers hosting PHI be located within the United States. For Canada, the transfer of data across borders is not prohibited by PIPEDA, but more and more government agencies are requiring that restriction in their business contracts. The location of data (even if not stored across borders) raises concerns about requirements for audits and e-discovery. In many cloud computing environments, resources are so co-mingled that the level of auditing and e-discovery that supports forensics and accounting of disclosures is nearly impossible. Cloud computing vendors may be able to accommodate privacy and security provisions, but when they exceed their other non-healthcare customers' needs, costs increase, and value to the healthcare customer may decrease.

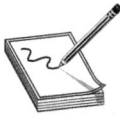

NOTE With the September 23, 2013, effective date of the HIPAA Omnibus Final Rule, cloud vendors that support healthcare are mandated to sign business associate agreements (BAAs). Some larger vendors with multiple clients (many not in healthcare) were not willing to sign these agreements. In fairness, many saw it as an added, redundant requirement to their already rigid compliance processes such as the Federal Information Security Management Act (FISMA), Statement on Standards for Attestation Engagements no. 16 (SASE 16), and others. However, US government agencies suggest that if a cloud service provider is unwilling to sign a BAA, it should not be chosen to store healthcare data. With HIPAA updated to include strong clarification language, requirements for signing a BAA for cloud computing vendors with US healthcare customers is in reality non-negotiable.

Data Breach Regulations

Many nations, including the European Union, have been considering formal government mandates for data breach notification for individuals, or data subjects. Those efforts continue, and in reality, specific organizations already do some notification to data subjects and data controllers. These, of course, span all industries that handle personal information.

In the United States, HIPAA mandates that the healthcare industry investigate potential and actual data breaches that may exceed other industries' standards for sensitive personal information. For instance, the US government has determined a measurement threshold to determine whether there is a data breach of PHI. The standard measures whether there was a risk of disclosure of the information. Previous to the HIPAA Omnibus Rule in 2013, the risk threshold was risk of harm to the individual. There is clearly a shift in emphasis today, and a risk assessment must be done to address the following:[3]

- The nature and extent of the PHI involved, including the types of identifiers and the likelihood of re-identification
- The unauthorized person who used the PHI or to whom the disclosure was made
- Whether the PHI was actually acquired or viewed
- The extent to which the risk to the PHI has been mitigated

After these conditions have been evaluated, the healthcare organization must report the breach unless the risk of unauthorized access or disclosure is assessed as low. If the breach involves more than 500 individual records and the probability of compromise is not rated low, the organization must notify the US Department of Health and Human Services (HHS) of the loss, theft, or certain other impermissible uses or disclosures of unsecured PHI. Additionally, in this scenario, the organization must alert the media if the breach affects more than 500 residents of a single state. Of course, in this scenario, the organization must notify the affected individuals as well, as they would in most other data breaches. This risk assessment and formal process for notification differs from privacy laws governing data breach of things such as credit card information or Social Security numbers. The differences are applicable to US healthcare organizations that respond to data breaches of both PHI and financial information.

When it comes to protecting healthcare information, nothing influences the perception of success or failure like a data breach. It may be unfair to use data breaches as an outcome measure of program effectiveness, because some believe breaches are not a matter of "if," but "when." As of spring 2020, Thales eSecurity reports that 77 percent of healthcare organizations have been breached at some point, and 48 percent have been breached in the past year.[4] Organizational reputation is certainly affected by a data breach. Data breaches may also cause patients to lose trust in the organization, which would result in patient care implications. In addition, a breach may cause an organization to lose revenue if patients choose to switch to a competitor as a result. All these impacts may occur with a data breach, in addition to the most publicized impact of data breaches in healthcare, which are fines and penalties from regulators.

These impacts are not unique to the United States; internationally, aggressive scrutiny on protection of healthcare information and increasing government fines for data breaches of sensitive information are making the headlines. Organizations that have data breaches lose more than just patient data, and Figure 4-1 helps illustrate this by presenting some of the data from surveys from organizations such as Ponemon Institute for IBM, which conducts annual independent assessments of organizations relative to data breaches and their impact.[5] There is no shortage of these data points, and they are often shocking. There are numerous considerations above and beyond the negative impact a data breach can have from a regulatory perspective. Data breaches can also have detrimental effects to the organization in terms of reputational harm, financial costs, medical and financial identity theft, and patient embarrassment.

Figure 4-1
A small sample of results from the 2019 Cost of a Data Breach Report

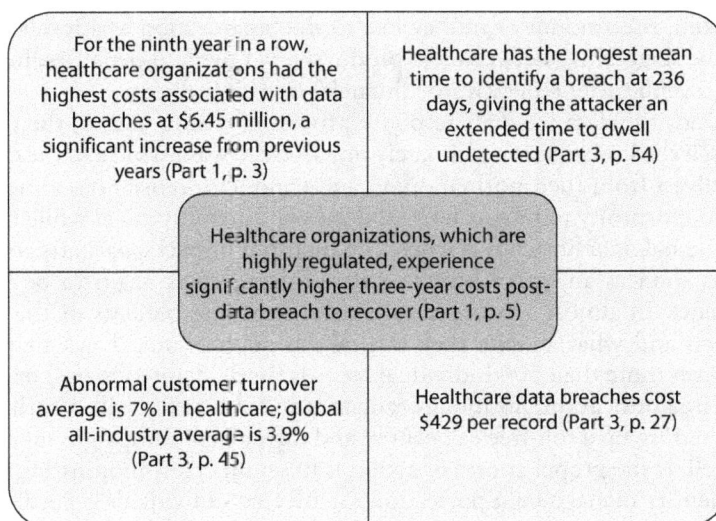

For the ninth year in a row, healthcare organizations had the highest costs associated with data breaches at $6.45 million, a significant increase from previous years (Part 1, p. 3)

Healthcare has the longest mean time to identify a breach at 236 days, giving the attacker an extended time to dwell undetected (Part 3, p. 54)

Healthcare organizations, which are highly regulated, experience significantly higher three-year costs post-data breach to recover (Part 1, p. 5)

Abnormal customer turnover average is 7% in healthcare; global all-industry average is 3.9% (Part 3, p. 45)

Healthcare data breaches cost $429 per record (Part 3, p. 27)

Organization Reputation

Nobody wants to be the subject of headlines like these: "Hospital Loses 200,000 Medical Records," or "Healthcare Organization Fined $5 Million for Data Breach." Such headlines have a negative impact on the organization's reputation. Many organizations invest heavily to cultivate and promote the assets of public perception, brand image, and reputation, which have a high intrinsic value for an organization. Something like a data breach can have immediate and lasting effects on an organization's reputation, which may have taken years to earn.

Depending on its size of the organization and the industry served, an organization's reputation has been valued as high as 70 to 80 percent of the its market value.[6] Although not specific to healthcare organizations, adverse public events such as a data breach may reduce that value significantly and in real financial losses. In an industry such as healthcare, where trust is so important, reputation value leads to positive perceptions by patients and other stakeholders, such as regulators. To help soften the blow of a data breach and mitigate the negative effects it has on reputation, the organization can take several actions: It can do what is necessary to investigate and understand why the data breach happened. Applying forensics to determine the root cause will help the organization plan for mitigation and will help prevent another similar data breach later on. Also, how closely and openly the organization works with law enforcement, complies with regulatory inquiry, and communicates to the media propels the organization in the right direction from a public perception perspective. Finally, organizations fare much better after a breach if they provide support mechanisms such as call centers for customer inquiry, identity protection, credit monitoring, and tips on other actions affected individuals can take.

Financial Impact

The easiest way to measure the impact of a data breach in healthcare is by looking at the financial impact. In fact, reputation can also be measurable in dollars and financial loss. All told, the amount of money lost to the organization as a result of losing information can be staggering. Between lost productivity, fines and penalties, investigation costs, and lost revenue after a breach, the financial impact is direct.

Once the data incident response process goes into action, the costs begin to mount. Even if the investigation ultimately reveals there was no breach, the cost of having employees divert from their normal duties and conduct forensics has a measurable impact. The lost opportunity to pursue normal duties or other initiatives while investigating potential and actual data breaches is where the financial impact also starts to become evident.

As soon as an actual breach is determined, costs begin to be incurred in notifying patients. In almost any breach scenario, notifying patients of the circumstances of the breach and what actions they can take is appropriate, if not mandated. If the breach involves more than 500 individual records (in the United States) or regulations otherwise require notification, notifying regulators and the media will contribute to cost. Advertising, setting up a toll-free call center, and direct-mail campaigns take significant financing as well. If the proper course of action is to set up credit monitoring or if some other form of identity management protection for affected individuals is needed, more financial cost is incurred.

Once the event is mitigated and notification actions have been taken, the organization may face the possibility of fines and penalties from regulators. These dollar amounts tend to get the biggest headlines. However, although the mean US fine under HIPAA/HITECH was a substantial $2.6 million in 2018, fines and penalties are only a portion of the average annualized costs of cybercrime against healthcare organizations, which was about $12.47 million in 2017.[7,8]

Another component of financial cost is the resulting loss of future revenue. For publicly traded companies, stock prices can be affected after a breach occurs. For nonprofit healthcare organizations, the risk of having a bond rating lowered is a possibility. The impact of a lower bond rating makes it more expensive to invest in capital improvements and can make an otherwise solvent healthcare organization a better target for acquisition or merger. These are somewhat extreme outcomes, but they are very real possibilities if information protection is not a focus of the healthcare organization and data breach is a periodic occurrence rather than a rare one.

Data breaches can have another financial impact on healthcare organizations: increased patient turnover. Every organization experiences patient turnover—that is normal—but the hope is that the net turnover results in a positive, or increase, in overall patients that visit the healthcare organization. Studies in 2017 showed that healthcare organizations that have suffered a data breach actually experienced turnover at a rate of 4 percent more than they expected.[9]

Medical and Financial Identity Theft

The information contained in a medical record can be worth quite a bit more than the amount accessed via a stolen credit card file or stolen bank account information. This is due, in large part, to two factors:

- Medical records tend to include financial data as well as health information.
- Elements in the medical record can be sold separately for maximum gain.

In either scenario, stolen health information is usually used to gain inappropriate access to medical services and prescription medication. An emergency department, where patient care is delivered rapidly, can be a likely source of the illegal medication or service procurement. A "patient" visits the ER with an injury (perhaps even self-inflicted) and offers a fake ID created from stolen data. In an effort to care for the patient first, a medical professional makes a diagnosis and prescribes treatment such as medication. In an ER, it is common for at least a small amount of medication to be provided to a patient even when insurance or identity has not been verified. But even if a prescription is filled later at a retail pharmacy requiring proof of identity, the fraudulent ID may fool the dispensary. The person whose identity was stolen may not be aware that any of this has happened until his insurance company provides an accounting of the benefits paid, which may result in increased premiums. Although the effect on insurance is germane mainly to the United States, the effect of medical identity theft on an international audience with a single payer-system, where insurance fraud is nonexistent, is nonetheless impactful. Where resources are limited, such fraud can make treatment or resources unavailable to those who truly need it.

Healthcare organizations, especially those in the United States, handle sensitive financial information such as bank card information, credit card numbers, home addresses, and birthdates. Even if the criminal does not care about the healthcare data, access to viable financial data makes a healthcare organization a profitable target.

To date, in a few cases, patients have been able to win lawsuits based on the loss of their PHI or PII as a result of a healthcare organization's data breach. It is difficult to prove harm that is directly attributable to the data loss by the healthcare organization. That can change quickly, however; if a healthcare organization is judged to be willfully negligent in the data breach, class action lawsuits may be won more frequently by patients as time goes on. In growing numbers, however, the general public expresses complacency about the loss of their financial data. Far too often, individuals whose PII has been stolen or compromised view cancelling their accounts and cards and setting up credit monitoring as the remedy to an inevitable reality of having the convenience of digital banking and retail. The costs incurred to banks and credit card companies for account re-creation and card issuance are passed back to organizations (healthcare organizations, for example) that lose the data in the first place. This is a good reason for companies to increase efforts to protect the information.

Patient Embarrassment

According to Ponemon Institute, an oft-cited source on this subject, when healthcare providers are asked what they believe to be the greatest fear patients have with respect to the potential unauthorized disclosure of their health data, they respond that public exposure or embarrassment rank above both medical identity theft and financial identity theft.[10] It is significant to note that unauthorized disclosure of PHI can be more emotionally damaging to an individual than financial information being lost or stolen. Figure 4-2 puts these responses into perspective.

Figure 4-2
Healthcare providers' 2016 responses to what risks patients face when their data is lost or stolen

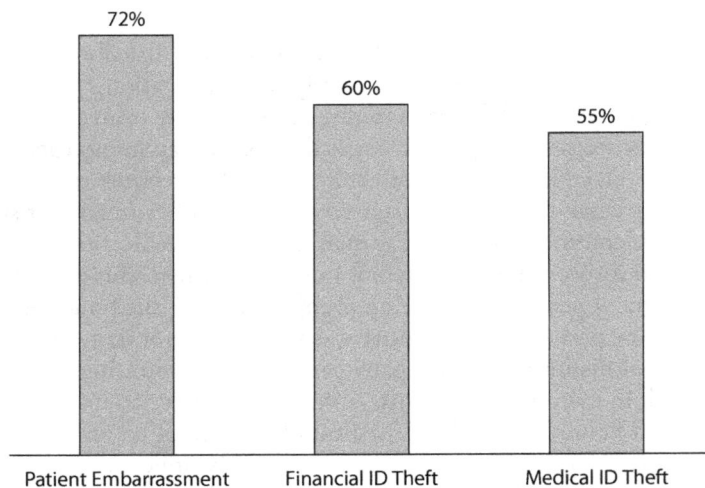

Patients may have valid personal reasons for wanting information to be protected from employers, friends, family, and the community at large. Once medical history and status information is disclosed in an unauthorized manner, it cannot be retrieved, reversed, or forgotten. Unlike financial information, one cannot "cancel" a medical record or change the number and make the old information useless. No monitoring service exists to determine whether any of the sensitive information has been disclosed further, whether employment or personal reputational decisions are made because of it, or whether other actions have been taken based on the information. So there is no way to prove a level of harm; if there were, maybe affected individuals could better execute class-action lawsuits on the basis of embarrassment alone.

Evidence suggests that patients may actually withhold relevant medical information in fear that the healthcare organization will improperly safeguard their sensitive information, or in fear of the organization sharing it.[11] When it comes to sensitive health data, the impact of withholding information, delaying care, or not seeking care is worrisome enough when it affects a single individual. Unfortunately, however, it is often the case that the delay or failure to seek care is more of a public health issue to the immediate family and/or to the community at large. Conditions such as PTSD and other behavioral health issues can result in patients harming themselves and others around them. Domestic violence and mass shootings top the list of tragic outcomes of failures to seek out or comply with treatment. Patients who seek care for mental health or substance abuse issues often withhold relevant parts of their medical history from providers, which can actually sabotage the care plan.[12]

And some diseases, such as sexually transmitted diseases (STDs) and HIV/AIDS for example, can be spread if a patient delays care out of fear of exposure.

Healthcare Information Protection Is a Patient Care Issue

The idea that patient embarrassment is a factor in data breach impact helps to illustrate the convergence of responsibility for biomedical engineers, clinical system administrators, health information managers, and health information technology professionals in the practice of healthcare information security and privacy. To those who have come into information protection from a clinical background, patient care and patient safety have always been at the core of risk management (including information risk management), but the digitizing of patient information with its ease of access to huge amounts of data in a short period of time has shed new focus on the patient safety and patient care impacts of a data breach.

Protected Personal and Health Information

With the proliferation of technology and the increasing awareness that PII and PHI are stored online or electronically in some way, shape, or form, there is growing pressure to protect such information. Almost weekly, global media reports of databases being compromised, files being lost, and attacks being made against businesses and systems that store PII. This has spurred concerns over the proper collection, use, retention, and destruction of information of a personal or confidential nature. Public concern has prompted the creation of regulations intended to foster the responsible use and stewardship of personal information. In the context of this discussion, privacy is one of the primary areas in which business, in almost all industries, is forced to deal with regulations and regulatory compliance.

Personally Identifiable Information

Personally identifiable information data, also known as personal information or sensitive personal information, is personal information that relates to and identifies a particular person. For legal purposes, the effective definitions of personal information vary depending on the government jurisdiction and the purposes for which the term is being used. PII is, however, commonly addressed in international guidance, US privacy laws, and information security.

Any information that is unique to a single person or any combination of information elements that together identify a single person is considered PII. International privacy laws tend to have more expansive or differing definitions for the term "personal data" than the United States does, and this difference impacts regulatory scope. Australia's 1988 Privacy Act, for example, defines personal information as any information or opinion (true or not) from which the person's identity is reasonably ascertainable, and it potentially covers some personal information not covered by US regulations, such as a person's religion, union membership, or political party. In the US, NIST SP 800-122 defines PII as "any information about an individual maintained by an agency, including (1) any information that can be used to distinguish or trace an individual's identity, such as name, social security number, date and place of birth, mother's maiden name, or biometric records; and (2) any other information that is linked or linkable to an individual, such as medical, educational, financial, and employment information."[13] The components of the definitions are found in 18 identifying elements, listed next, that are also defined in SP 800-122:[14]

- Name, such as full name, maiden name, mother's maiden name, or alias
- Personal identification number, such as Social Security number (SSN), passport number, driver's license number, taxpayer identification number, patient identification number, and financial account or credit card number
- Address information, such as street address or e-mail address
- Asset information, such as Internet Protocol (IP) or Media Access Control (MAC) address or other host-specific persistent static identifier that consistently links to a particular person or a small, well-defined group of people
- Telephone numbers, including mobile, business, and personal numbers
- Personal characteristics, including photographic images (especially of the face or other distinguishing characteristics), X-rays, fingerprints, or other biometric image or template data (such as retina scan, voice signature, or facial geometry)
- Information identifying personally owned property, such as vehicle registration number or title number and related information

- Information about an individual that is linked or linkable to one of the previous items (such as date or place of birth, race, religion, weight, activities, geographical indicators, employment information, medical information, education information, or financial information)

Any one of these elements by itself may not be considered PII. Note, for example, that a user's IP address is not classed as PII on its own, but it is classified as a linked PII when the IP address is assigned to a networked technology for one person or a small enough number of people that identification is very possible. In the European Union, by way of contrast, the IP address of an Internet subscriber is likely to be categorized as personal data.[15]

EXAM TIP Be on the lookout for PII questions referencing web page "cookies," a small, persistent piece of data transferred from a web site to a user's web browser and stored on the individual's computer during the web session. Cookies are typically considered PII. There is a growing awareness and concern about the persistent nature and identifying properties of cookies.

Another caveat of note is that some examples of personal data are not always considered PII. The context of the data element is also a factor in determining PII. For example, while an SSN is automatically considered PII because the number corresponds to one and only one person, without any need of additional PII data, a home address by itself may not identify one person, especially if the street address is a high-rise building that does not include an apartment number, and is not automatically considered PII. In any case, the context of typical PII data elements helps you be aware of your information protection requirements.

Protected Health Information

Protected health information (PHI) can also be called personal health information, depending on the regulatory source. You can consider the terminology synonymous for individually identifiable information containing elements of health data. PHI is a subset of PII. Under various laws, PHI is a separate classification of sensitive, personal information with legal implications specific to healthcare organizations. When PII is combined with patient health data elements, it becomes legally protected PHI. There's one important caveat to note: The regulation of PHI depends on whether or not the organization using the information is covered by the protection law. This is not an issue in most international countries, as privacy law is not industry-specific. In the United States, it is possible for an organization to handle PHI but not be subject to HIPAA. For instance, a public K–12 school may have health information on a student, but the organization is not a healthcare organization. However, under FERPA, that school would be subject to a law that requires safeguarding of sensitive data, though it is not directly subject to HIPAA. This is complex. Dealing with PHI requires you to be versed in relevant laws as they impact your organization's information privacy and security policies and procedures.

> **CAUTION** It is possible to have PHI without any of the traditional PII elements included. For example, even without an SSN in the record, multiple health data elements, such as diagnosis, age, gender, and date of treatment can collectively be considered identifying information unique to one person. In such cases, the data elements are considered PHI and are subject to HIPAA.

Another component of PHI is the existence of some type of health information related to the PII. The PHI relates to health information of an individual that is being collected, used, transferred, stored, or disposed of by an organization subject to HIPAA. The category of information applies to information that is kept as well as transmitted in all forms, such as electronic, paper, or speech. Some examples of PHI elements are X-ray image information, diagnosis codes, dates of treatment, images, genetic information, or DNA. According to HIPAA, these are the general categories of healthcare information:

- The past, present, or future physical or mental health or condition
- The provision of healthcare to the individual
- The past, present, or future payment for the provision of healthcare to the individual

As you know, HIPAA defines two types of organizations: the covered entity and the business associate. As a refresher, Figure 4-3 shows an easy-to-understand illustration of different types of covered entities and business associates. These organizations, in the United States specifically, would handle PHI routinely and be subject to HIPAA.

The significance of PHI related to information privacy and security concerns continues to grow. The value of PHI to criminals coupled with the reported ease of committing cybercrimes erodes the trust of the general public. Globally, regulators have increased

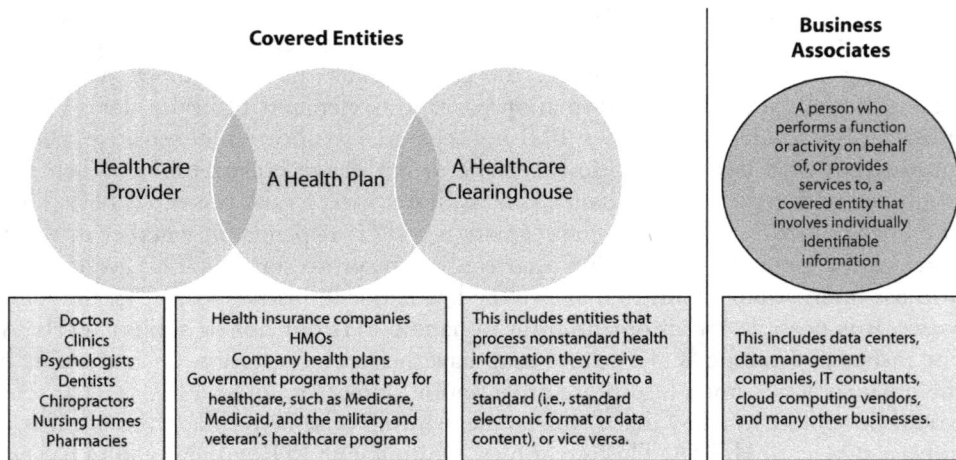

Covered Entities

Business Associates

Healthcare Provider	A Health Plan	A Healthcare Clearinghouse

A person who performs a function or activity on behalf of, or provides services to, a covered entity that involves individually identifiable information

| Doctors Clinics Psychologists Dentists Chiropractors Nursing Homes Pharmacies | Health insurance companies HMOs Company health plans Government programs that pay for healthcare, such as Medicare, Medicaid, and the military and veteran's healthcare programs | This includes entities that process nonstandard health information they receive from another entity into a standard (i.e., standard electronic format or data content), or vice versa. | This includes data centers, data management companies, IT consultants, cloud computing vendors, and many other businesses. |

Figure 4-3 Covered entities and business associates

guidance, oversight, and enforcement to address privacy protections. Their tools are sanctions, fines, and penalties, and all of these have increased in frequency and severity. The 2018 implementation of GDPR is a relevant example of the regulatory perspective. The potential fines for a GDPR violation (albeit, not necessarily by a healthcare organization), depending on the severity of the infraction and the size of the organization, can be as much as €10 million to €20 million, or 2 percent to 4 percent of the firm's worldwide annual revenue from the preceding financial year, whichever amount is higher.[16] The intent is to prompt organizations to invest in every effort to provide due diligence and due care in handling sensitive information. The first step in proper adherence to regulatory guidance is to know the regulations applicable to your industry and jurisdiction. Then you can take steps to align that guidance with organizational policy and procedures.

Jurisdiction Implications

Those who work in healthcare organizations that have third-party business associates in different US states or countries, or that provide patient care across the globe, may need to consider cross-border jurisdictional issues. We mentioned one specific case that raises jurisdiction implications: You must consider trans-border issues when transferring or storing data using a cloud provider that has physical servers outside the United States. Of course, this can also be an issue for Canadian and EU providers. In these cases, you certainly want to ensure that your local policies and procedures outline how to gain the necessary consent and approvals for sharing PHI and PII. When one jurisdiction requires stricter controls than those that apply to your organization's jurisdiction, you will need to assess how to comply. An example of how this process has been addressed between the European Union and foreign organizations wanting to share information is the Privacy Shield Agreement, discussed in more detail later in this chapter.

Agreements and treaties such as Privacy Shield can help bridge jurisdictional issues. As US cloud providers take on EU business partners, US companies may not fully understand the reach of the EU laws such as GDPR. The European Union places additional limitations on the use of an individual's consent to permit data processing, for example, internationally. As far back as 2013, efforts were made to strengthen the international applicability of the EU DPD, which was replaced by GDPR, in business relationships outside of the European Union. US cloud providers need to adjust their standards in some cases to satisfy those of EU organizations. Of course, this is not specific to healthcare, but it does include EU healthcare organizations. The European Union is the most important bilateral trade area for the United States. Having a way to permit these business arrangements and adequately protect information is profoundly significant.

Another jurisdictional implication would be within various breach notification rules. Imagine an international organization getting a contract to help develop a healthcare web site in the United States. If the web site collected healthcare information and was hacked because of a failure to maintain proper OS vulnerability patch management, the liability may be shifted to the third-party business associate. While the actual notification of individuals may not be the responsibility of the international firm, the costs and fines certainly would be. These same liabilities and costs may not be levied in their home country.

An area where jurisdictional impacts are possible is in offshore third-party support of organizations subject to HIPAA. Such impacts of jurisdiction have not been tested by the US government by HHS yet, but you can expect that they will. Offshore third-party contracts for support and services are increasingly popular because of the cost-efficiencies of outsourcing for labor in countries outside the United States. Following are some of the types of offshore business associates that you may find in your organization:

- Data centers
- Medical transcription services
- Radiology readings
- IT customer support
- Application and system development
- Billing and clinical decision support

The HIPAA Omnibus Rule holds business associates and subcontractors directly liable for compliance with HIPAA. If there are data breaches, theoretically, the offshore business associates would be fined or would have penalties levied against them. It is not clear whether or not the authority of HHS would be recognized or honored by the offshore organization. The offshore organization could be penalized by the healthcare organization for a contractual violation in that the third party failed to meet the terms and conditions of an agreement. That does not relate to HHS enforcement authority, however. In the absence of an ability to enforce HIPAA sanctions against offshore entities, HHS may instead apply pressure to and increased scrutiny of the healthcare organization that entered into the contract. You will need to make sure your organizational policies and third-party risk management procedures include this jurisdictional complexity.

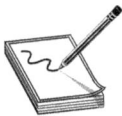

NOTE Many offshore third-party organizations operate a US-based location as well as international office locations. They may still be considered offshore if the actual work is done outside the country of the healthcare organization. In the United States, the jurisdictional impacts are different in these cases, as HIPAA scope and authority cover the US-based location and extend to international locations. Even if the data breach occurred as a result of events at a non-US location, HHS can address and evaluate the offshore company directly.

Data Subjects

A *data subject* is the individual about whom any organization or government entity collects, stores, shares, and analyzes data. In a healthcare context, the data subject is the person or patient who is the subject of a medical record or healthcare transaction. A common consideration of information security and privacy regulations is that healthcare organizations must know and adhere to applicable laws. The organizations also must be open and transparent about their information handling practices, and data subjects must be notified of these practices. Data subjects generally have important rights that healthcare organizations will have to accommodate in compliance with the law and aligned with healthcare delivery and payment. One right is the requirement for data subjects to provide consent to the healthcare organization before any data collection and processing can happen. Another important right is the data subject's legal ability to access any data that is collected about them.

EXAM TIP If there is an exam question with a scenario of a person requesting deletion of their record, pay attention to the patient's location. Don't forget that in the European Union, the right to be forgotten differentiates the privacy framework. For example, under HIPAA in the United States, a healthcare provider does not have to erase a healthcare record from its databases just because a patient requests to be forgotten.

Data Owners

Similar in definition to data subjects, a *data owner* is an important role that has clearly defined roles and responsibilities in information security and privacy regulations. Other regulations may use synonymous terms for data owner, such as information owner or data steward. Data owners are not usually the data subject, however.

Data owner responsibilities are founded in regulatory guidance, and organizational policy will outline the manner by which the data owner may use, collect, share, and store data that they own. All data, but especially data with a sensitivity level, must be assigned to an owner. The data owners will have legal rights to the information and complete control over it. The data owner can authorize or deny access to that information. Their role in the context of privacy is central. The data owner is the person or group of individuals in an organization responsible and accountable for the data. This person could be as senior as the CEO or president of the company, especially in terms of ultimate accountability for protecting the data. Normally, the daily responsibility is delegated to another senior person more directly involved in implementing information security and privacy controls. It is important to note that there are legal and regulatory consequences for the data owner if they commit negligent acts resulting in misuse or disclosure of sensitive data in an unauthorized way.

EXAM TIP If asked about roles and responsibilities in the exam, you'll want to remember that the data owner establishes the required security controls for access and use of data in collaboration with system owners. In a healthcare environment, this may describe the relationship between departments such as Health Information Management and the system administrators for the organization's EHRs.

A primary responsibility of data owners is to provide information protection at a standard that meets legal obligations and regulatory requirements. The measurement of these responsibilities can be generalized by the concepts of due care and due diligence.

Due care is defined as the amount of attention that an ordinary and reasonable person would be expected to provide to avoid negative consequences. Information protection due care would include employing security protection of networked assets using firewalls and intrusion detection devices, at a minimum. The complementary term, *due diligence*, relates to ensuring that information protection policies and procedures are in place and that all practical steps are taken. Under the concept of due diligence, you would advocate a sufficient vulnerability management process. That process would include using risk assessment of vulnerabilities as well as timely application of patches.

Note that due care and due diligence are not synonymous, but they are often used together because of their importance and relationship. Neither force compliance as a goal, but both focus on reasonable and practical approaches based on risk. This is important to remember, because the concepts change legal obligation and regulatory requirements from a checklist activity with pass or fail outcomes. Due care and due diligence, when demonstrated correctly, permit healthcare organizations to manage liabilities under the law, yet provide patient care and operations. The point is that healthcare organizations face advanced persistent threats daily that will eventually succeed given enough time and effort. Due care and due diligence set a standard high enough to be effective, but not so high that the goal is cost-prohibitive or excessively impedes the mission of the organizations.

Data Steward

In the various functional areas of a business such as finance, human resources, sales, and IT, the organization will assign people the responsibility of creating and executing policies for the management of data and metadata. These individuals play an important role in the data governance process as subject matter experts on the categorization of the data, data definitions for its use, and implementing the data governance policies in their area of responsibility. They manage the data quality requirements to ensure fitness of data that is within their business area. Fitness of data includes concerns such as the ability to use the data for its intended purpose in a format that is readable. Data stewards establish internal and external data access requirements for data in their functional area.

Data Controller

An entity (or entities) determines the purposes for why and how any personal data is, or will be, processed. The entity can be a person, an organization, or a group of people who are not collectively an organization. The data controllers must ensure that information use complies with prevailing legal and regulatory guidance. The GDPR defines a data controller as the natural or legal person, public authority, agency, or other body that, alone or jointly with others, determines the purposes and means of the processing of personal data.[17] The controller is responsible for adhering to the principles relating to processing personal data. To that end, the controller has to be able to demonstrate compliance with the principles of lawfulness, fairness, transparency, data minimization, accuracy, storage limitation and integrity, and confidentiality of personal data. The responsibility for ensuring that data subjects are able to rectify, remove, or block information that is reported as incorrect rests with the data controllers. These entities also negotiate privacy protections for personal data from data processors via secure contractual terms and assurances called data processing agreements.

Data Custodians

In an organization, the data governance process should include a role for the *data custodian*. The data custodian role differs from the data steward. Data custodians implement the data delivery process in partnership with the data steward. However, the data custodian is much more concerned with the technologies used in data management and the tools that assist data users with the secure use of the data. Compared to the data steward, the data custodian is more concerned with protection of data as it is transferred and stored instead of the contents of the data. There may be one or more people assigned as data custodians.

Data Processor

The person who processes the data on behalf of the data controller but is not an employee of the controller (such as a third-party business associate) is considered a *data processor*. In the European Union, these entities were not directly subject to the EU DPD in their role as data processor. However, in the enactment of GDPR, data processors are subject to EU law. You should think of this change much like the changes in HIPAA through the Omnibus Final Rule in 2013 that clarified how business associates were directly subject to HIPAA rules.

The value in data is often in the sharing or exchange of the information between authorized entities. The party responsible for transferring, transmitting, or otherwise sharing data on behalf of a data owner is a data processor. Data processors have a distinct role in the protection of data. In a healthcare setting, the data exchange can be important in the safe and proper conduct of patient care, appropriate treatment, managing billing, and other organizational operations. In banking, the data supports business and individual investments as well as credit worthiness. The regulatory focus in GDPR and HIPAA, as examples, reflects the importance of data processing responsibilities.

A data processor is not synonymous with a data controller. The key difference is that a data processor does not have legal responsibility and accountability for the data as does a data controller. The processor performs data manipulation on behalf of the data controller. A data controller is an entity that determines the purposes, conditions, and the means of processing the personal data. Figure 4-4 depicts the relationship between data processors and data controllers.

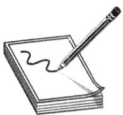

NOTE In some instances, people in organizations play both roles as data processor and data controller. For instance, a human resources firm would have data about their own employees and would be a data controller in this sense. However, if the firm provides outsourced human resource actions for other clients, the human resources firm would be a data processor for the client data, while the individual clients remain the data controllers.

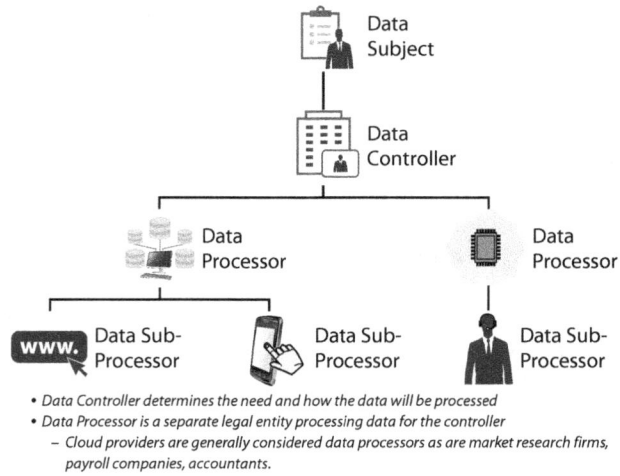

Figure 4-4
Relationship between data processors and data controllers

- Data Controller determines the need and how the data will be processed
- Data Processor is a separate legal entity processing data for the controller
  - Cloud providers are generally considered data processors as are market research firms, payroll companies, accountants.

Research

It is often beneficial to use patient information in clinical research. Unlike in public health reporting, researchers try to conduct clinical research after obtaining patient consent for the use of the information for that specific purpose. This is not always possible, however. In those cases where obtaining consent is impractical or impossible, researchers in the United States can use an internal institutional review board (IRB) or a privacy board to obtain a waiver to any required patient consent. The IRB was mandated by government through the passing of the National Research Act in 1974. Oversight for IRBs is currently under the purview of the Office for Human Research Protections (OHRP) at the federal government level. An IRB is a group of knowledgeable research peers led by one or two board administrators from the organization sponsoring the research. The IRB or privacy board will have documented protocols and controls to safeguard the PHI. This incorporates assurances that the use or disclosure of patient information adds only a minimum of risk to privacy for the individual. The IRB would require researchers to demonstrate the following:

- A plan that includes alternate measures to safeguard PHI
- A plan to destroy patient information when it's no longer needed (to include any bona fide need to keep the information for research or legal reasons)
- Written statements to prohibit reuse or disclosure of patient information unless permitted by law or the IRB or privacy board
- No research without a waiver
- No research without access to and use of the patient information

The IRB is an important safeguard to behavioral and medical studies. It is a foundational process for adhering to ethical conduct in research that an investigator will use.

Each IRB has a defined review process with specific requirements. The following should be the guiding principles of any IRB:[18]

- **Respect for people**   People should be treated as autonomous agents (individuals), and those with diminished autonomy must be protected.

- **Beneficence**   The well-being of study participants should be protected by adhering to "do no harm" and maximizing benefits while minimizing potential damages.

- **Justice**   Participants should have equal opportunity to be selected, because even if there is benefit, there is probably a burden some people will need to bear.

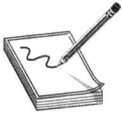

NOTE   In the United States, the IRB is governed by 45 Code of Federal Regulations (CFR) part 46 (HHS regulations for the protection of human subjects) and 21 CFR parts 50 and 56 (FDA regulations on the protection of human subjects). Closely related to IRBs is the provision under HIPAA, specifically the Privacy Rule, which has a provision for a privacy board. Both the IRB and the privacy board are permitted to allow PHI disclosure without additional patient consent for research. You can find this provision at 45 CFR parts 160 and 164, specifically, section 164.508. Privacy boards differ from IRBs, though. Privacy boards have no other authority within human subject research or FDA-sponsored research like the IRB does.

For clinical research, several of the alternative steps that are taken to remove patient information from the data or at least limit it to the least amount required are important to know. We will cover security and privacy controls in more depth in Chapter 5, but here we introduce them as a component of conduct research securely and protecting patient privacy:

- **De-identification of patient information**   This consists of removing any PII or PHI from the data set so that you can be reasonably certain no one can identify someone based on the remaining information. There are two ways to do this. The first way is to use a person trained in rendering the standard categories of identifiable data anonymous through mathematical manipulation so that the risk of re-identifying the information is low. The second way is simply to remove completely these same categories of identifiable data.

- **Limited data sets**   This establishes that some of the patient information can be excluded, and what remains is the minimum number and types of identifiers needed, if any. You would usually have a data use agreement in place for using a limited data set that would also determine who has a need to know the information and for what purposes.

- **Accounting of disclosures**   Researchers must keep and be able to provide a record of all information disclosed, by whom, and to whom outside of the research organization (for example, another research organization doing similar trials) during the life of the research.

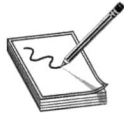

NOTE Under HIPAA, researchers must be able to account for disclosures for up to six years prior to the request of the individual and must include particular data elements required by the law.

Noteworthy clinical research done by a third party is through a contract research organization (CRO). This organization provides support to healthcare organizations conducting specialized types of biopharmaceutical development, preclinical research, clinical trials management, and drug safety. For the most part, these advanced research types are used by leading pharmaceutical, biotechnology, and medical device industries. CROs also support academic medical centers, the government, and international organizations. The ability to partner with CROs enables the development and evaluation of all the various trials safely and effectively, but they do not need to have internal staff from the healthcare organization dedicated to the research. For medical devices, the CRO gathers clinical data to support a regulatory before-market submission, drive product adoption, support product reimbursement, or monitor after-market product use. CROs bring expertise and streamlined processes at a much more cost-effective level than what the healthcare organization could do alone.

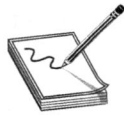

NOTE Increased disclosure of patient information is authorized for the purposes of clinical research under HIPAA. Where a scenario of information exchange includes clinical research, controls that would be required under HIPAA may be absent. Be aware of the impact of clinical research on any data use scenario.

The Belmont Report (Protection of Human Subjects)

The seminal research done on the importance of ethics in research was the Belmont Report in 1974. The report included an examination by researchers on the ethical principles and guidelines for the protection of human research subjects. The genesis of the report was the exploitation of 399 African American men in the Tuskegee Syphilis study, who were told they were receiving treatment. Researchers instead provided a placebo and monitored the long-term effects of the syphilis infection. Three major principles come from the Belmont Report. You will recognize these, as they became the guiding principles of all IRBs. The first is beneficence. Researchers should minimize potential harm to a subject and balance the risks against the potential for the betterment of the community.[19] Respect for persons is the second principle. Researchers must treat study subjects as autonomous, as each individual has the opportunity to make their own decisions, including to consent to participation. The third principle from the Belmont Report is justice. Research done on prisoners and other misfortunate populations has benefited more privileged society. Researchers need to apply a measure of equality and apply the risks or burdens fairly on populations that may benefit from the outcomes.

Recognize Regulations and Controls of Various Countries

Protecting healthcare information is a global concern. In the United States, specific laws are in place to govern the handling of healthcare information. Internationally, laws address healthcare information specifically, though typically within the context of protecting all personal information. Privacy regulations and controls cover individually identifiable information, and health information is included in this. You may not encounter many international laws and regulations, but your awareness will improve your understanding of commonalities and context, and will dispel confusion about various approaches. A major point in this discussion is that information security and privacy is a concern across the globe. The issues transcend borders and industries. In some cases, an information security issue may begin in one country or industry before it impacts healthcare in another. Consider a malware attack launched from a foreign nation against critical infrastructure in the United States. As a healthcare information security and privacy professional, it is imperative that you have a broad understanding of regulations and controls governing international entities.

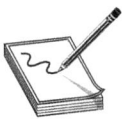

NOTE Particularly in the United States, regulations are enacted following a rule-making process that consists of engaging relevant stakeholders to develop a proposal, the open proposed legislation in draft for public comment, and then publication as a final rule.

Treaties

Healthcare organizations operate in environments where laws, regulations, and compliance requirements must be met. Healthcare professionals must understand the laws and regulations of the country and industry they are working in. An organization's governance and risk management processes must consider these requirements from an implementation perspective and a risk perspective. Laws focus on situations specific to the country subject to the law. There may be differences in similar laws between countries.

A process is needed to make sure laws and regulations with differences can be made agreeable to both parties. An example of how that mutual agreement is established is through the concept of "safe harbor" provisions. A safe harbor is typically a set of "good faith" conditions, which if met, may temporarily or indefinitely protect an organization from the penalties of a new law or regulation. You should know about several international examples of treaties, particularly EU–US Safe Harbor and Privacy Shield.

EU–US Safe Harbor

The EU–US Safe Harbor framework was declared invalid in 2015 and was replaced with the Privacy Shield agreement, covered in the next section. However, the framework is still illustrative for understanding treaties meant to ensure adequacy of the protection of personal data transferred to other countries. More importantly, the newer privacy guidance and treaties directing EU data transfer and sharing is built from this earlier agreement. A Safe Harbor Agreement indicates that from the EU perspective, data transfer could happen only if there is a determination of third-party "adequacy." In other words, the entity that is collecting the data has adequate privacy processes and safeguards in place. The European Union does not automatically grant that assurance of adequacy for non-EU member nations, as the United States and Canada does. To facilitate data transfer, to enable international trade, and to bridge any privacy differences, the European Union and United States, through the Department of Commerce, developed a Safe Harbor framework that satisfies the EU adequacy requirement.[20] Figure 4-5 provides an overview of the Safe Harbor gap assessment process. Again, the underlying approach and evaluations remain, with newer privacy guidance of data transfer and sharing.

To be certain, the United States and the European Union have different approaches to privacy and security. However, both have a commitment to protecting private information. The Safe Harbor process did not infer that the United States lacked privacy and security controls. The United States uses an industry perspective, versus an individual rights approach. There are specific laws governing each industry (HIPAA for healthcare, for example). The governing approach is a combination of these laws and a measure of

EU Safe Harbor Gap Assessment

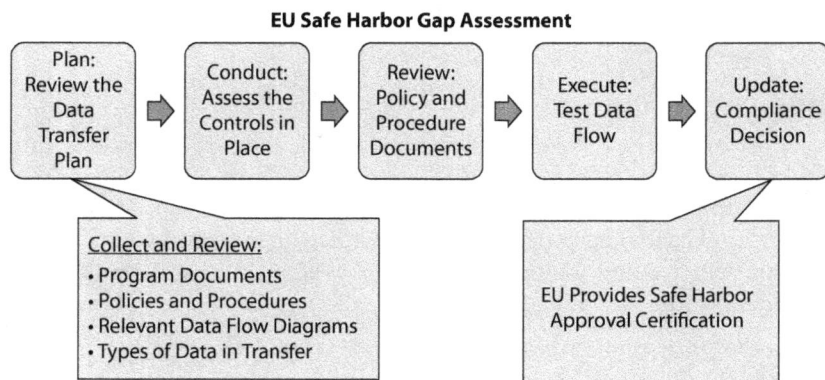

Figure 4-5 Process to address the privacy gap between US and EU data transfer

voluntary self-regulation. The European Union, however, considers privacy a human right, and protections are directed and monitored by the national governments (across health and all industries). Therefore, there is significant control over data collection with comprehensive legislation in the European Union. Independent government data protection agencies are prevalent, and data controllers must register their databases with those agencies. In some cases, the government must provide prior approval before personal data processing may begin.

Keep in mind that the Safe Harbor framework applied to more industries than healthcare. But for healthcare organizations that need to transfer data between the United States and the member nations of the European Union, Safe Harbor was (and still is) something to appreciate. Not understanding international laws and treaties may lead to disruption of patient care or prosecution under European law. Under newer privacy guidance, that statement is still true.

EXAM TIP Don't be confused. "Safe Harbor" is a term that can still be confused by those who work in the US healthcare industry, because specific actions that are taken "in good faith" are usually exempted in most US laws, called *Safe Harbor provisions*. HIPAA, governing healthcare, provides several Safe Harbor provisions such as using full-disk encryption to render protected health data unreadable. In the event a laptop is lost or stolen with PHI but is protected by full-disk encryption, the data loss is generally not reportable. The US use of Safe Harbor in legal terms in dealing with state and federal regulators remains relevant and unaffected by EU changes.

Many healthcare organizations have integrated EU–US Safe Harbor policies into their existing policies. Those practices remain practical and effective. Additionally, healthcare vendors that conduct business internationally should have signed up for EU Safe Harbor provisions and should continue those practices. Annually, organizations conducted a self-certification and submitted a letter to the EU to appear in the list of Safe Harbor participants.

To become EU Safe Harbor certified, a US organization was required to comply with the following seven principles, which should look familiar with respect to the privacy principles used in the other guidance, although they are not identical:[21]

- **Notice** The organization must let the individual know why it is collecting the information and how it will be used.
- **Choice** The individual must have the opportunity to opt out of the information collection, and the organization must inform the individual of the resulting alternatives to not providing the information.
- **Onward transfer** Safe Harbor–certified organizations can transfer information to third parties only if those organizations also agree to follow adequate information protection principles.
- **Access** Individuals must be able to access their information. When it is inaccurate, they must have remedies available to them to correct or delete it.

- **Security**   There must be reasonable controls in place to protect personal information from loss and unauthorized disclosure.

- **Data integrity**   Organizations must limit information collection only to that which is relevant to its use. The information must be protected so that it remains reliable for that use.

- **Enforcement**   Organizations must have procedures to enforce these principles. For instance, sanctions must be convincing enough to encourage compliance.

Privacy Shield

The Safe Harbor treaties and agreements had a long history. They were started in 1998 under the provisions of the EU DPD standards. The European Union used Safe Harbor to assure its citizens that adequate privacy controls were in place to protect their personal information when it was transferred to other countries. One of the primary countries that used and maintained Safe Harbor provisions was the United States. The adequacy of US privacy controls was deemed adequate in 2000. At that time, the European Union also granted authority for US companies to self-certify, with oversight for certification and compliance through the US Department of Commerce.

In 2015, the European Union determined that a new and stricter privacy framework and controls for transatlantic data flows were needed because there were too many US infractions to the DPD, including infractions by the US government. After the Safe Harbor agreement was invalidated, the European Union and United States developed a new framework for transatlantic data flows, and the EU–US Privacy Shield was launched in December 2016. Its purpose is to protect the privacy of personal information of EU citizens who share information with US commercial organizations. One note—the Privacy Shield is specific to the United States. The agreement intends to make data transfer easier while assuring data subjects' adequate privacy protection they expect from the EU member nations.

Other data transfer arrangements have been approved by the European Union for other countries. For some countries with privacy laws and guidance in place—Andorra, Argentina, Canada (only commercial organizations), Faroe Islands, Guernsey, Israel, Isle of Man, Jersey, New Zealand, Switzerland, Uruguay, and Japan—the European Union has determined that no additional treaties or agreements are needed. For countries that are not explicitly approved, adequacy for data protection in non-EU nations is achieved by the use of standard contract clauses in individual agreements with EU data controllers, called model clauses, to meet EU requirements.

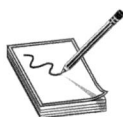

NOTE   The EU–US Privacy Shield satisfies adequacy only for data transfer for US organizations.

Another component of compliance for non-EU companies is the use of binding corporate rules that adhere to EU requirements. Binding corporate rules are like a code of conduct for a company and its information protection practices. In sum, the Privacy Shield is an example of the privacy protection agreements implemented by the European

Union to determine adequacy before data transfer is approved. However, the scope of Privacy Shield being limited to US companies is important in comparison with the other methods for data transfer treaties and agreements from the European Union.

Laws and Regulations

In the United States, data privacy is handled as a functional concern or regulated within an industry. Healthcare, retail, government, and telecommunications, for example, are affected by privacy and security laws and regulations that govern those industries only. To demonstrate practical impact, consider the category of PII, which is any information that can be used for the purpose of identifying, locating, or contacting a specific individual, either combined with other easily accessible sources or by itself. Government regulations require adequate safeguarding of PII, and commercial organizations may be subject to those regulations, but they must also answer to contractual requirements. Depending on the industry, laws may be written to cover PII, individually identifiable information, PHI, or sensitive personal information. Not all of these terms are interchangeable. Applicable terms and definitions are included in many US privacy regulations, including the Fair Credit Reporting Act (FCRA), Gramm-Leach-Bliley Act (GLBA), Privacy Act, Children's Online Privacy Protection Act (COPPA), and Family Educational Rights and Privacy Act (FERPA).

Working in the healthcare industry, you can expect to interact with laws and regulations directly through external entities or indirectly through compliance with internal policies and procedures. Remember that internal policies and procedures should have a connection with prevailing laws and regulations in addition to any moral or ethical obligations that pertain to the organization.

There are two major categories of law—criminal law and civil law:

- Criminal law prohibits and punishes bad conduct using fines, imprisonment, or both. Criminal law punishes the offender but usually does not compensate a victim.

- Civil law refers to rules for disputes between private parties. In civil cases, one party sues or brings an action to a court of law against another for financial compensation for some wrong.

Torts are a related concept to civil law, where financial redress or remedy is provided through a judgement by court. The implementation of torts developed almost entirely from common law practices. Common law consists of judgments based on earlier judicial outcomes. Common law does not involve interpretation of statutes, regulations, treaties, or codified law.

Another category of law is statutory law. This source comes from written (and published) statutes, most of which are written and voted into law by a government entity. In the United States, this entity is the Congress, the legislative branch of the federal government. Statutory law can also be enacted by placing a proposed new law on a ballot so that private citizens can vote for or against it. Although you don't need to be a legal scholar, becoming familiar with the purposes and sources of laws and regulations will give you context and help you develop policies and procedures for your organization.

EU Data Protection Directive

The EU DPD (officially, Act 95/46/EC) regulates the processing of personal data within member states of the European Union. The DPD is an important component of privacy and human rights law. The prevailing principle of the DPD is that the first consideration is not to collect personal data at all. But when that is not possible, certain conditions must be met. This is consistent with the idea of limiting collection of personal data included in other frameworks, such as the Organization for Economic Cooperation and Development (OECD). The conditions that must be met for necessary collection fall into three categories:[22]

- **Transparency**   The data subject has the right to be informed when her personal data is being processed. The controller must provide his name and address, the purpose of processing, the recipients of the data, and all other information required to ensure the processing is fair.

- **Legitimate purpose**   Personal data can be processed only for specified explicit and legitimate purposes and may not be processed further in a way incompatible with those purposes.

- **Proportionality**   Personal data may be processed only insofar as it is accurate, relevant, and not excessive in relation to the purposes for which it is collected and/ or further processed.

  - **Accurate**   The data must be up-to-date, and every reasonable step must be taken to ensure that data that is inaccurate or incomplete is erased or rectified.

  - **Relevant**   The data shouldn't be kept in a form that permits identification of data subjects for longer than is necessary for the purposes for which the data was collected or for which it is further processed. Member states shall devise appropriate safeguards for personal data stored for longer periods for historical, statistical, or scientific use.

  - **Not excessive**   Only the minimum amount of identifying data that is needed should be collected.

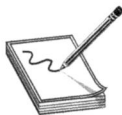

NOTE   When it comes to healthcare, some exceptions are allowed. EU member states should adhere to the principle of limiting collection except where the data is needed for preventive medicine, medical diagnosis, or the provision of care or treatment. Additionally, the data must be handled by a healthcare entity that is subject to national laws, rules, or obligations for professional confidentiality (privacy) or the equivalent level of obligation of confidentiality.

This provision impacts data transmitted to the United States. As mentioned, this transfer is initially prohibited, because the European Union considers the United States lacking in the national or equivalent level of obligation to ensure individually identifiable information is kept confidential. This is why the Safe Harbor provisions are so important. Between adhering to HIPAA and certifying through the Department of Commerce, the US healthcare entities can also satisfy the EU DPD requirement to demonstrate adequacy of safeguarding personal information. If you work for a US healthcare business and your work includes data transfer between the United States and the European Union, you will want to make sure your compliance with the HIPAA final privacy and security rules is complemented by certification under Safe Harbor.

General Data Protection Regulation

GDPR was created to reform the EU DPD because of the recognition that online and digital capabilities require an evolution of privacy rights. The interconnections and increased volume of data transfer in our global economic environment required an update to principles that were almost 20 years old in the EU DPD. While many principles remain, you should be aware of the significant and relevant changes, including the following changes to daily healthcare operations:

- A single market is constructed to enforce a single set of rules on data protection. Even though each EU nation has national authority for data protection, the single market ensures that GDPR is valid across the European Union to reduce administrative complexity, cost, and burden for compliance.

- GDPR increases the rights of individuals to provide more control. The intent is to provide visible assurance that the collection and use of personal data is limited to the minimum necessary.

- Requirements for data portability are clearly defined to transfer personal data more easily from one service provider to another.

- The "right to be forgotten" is explicitly recognized. The EU DPD had provisions to destroy information when it was no longer needed, but GDPR empowers citizens to demand the destruction when applicable.

- The GDPR clarified and strengthened data breach notification requirements for organizations outside of the European Union.

- The GDPR increased fines and penalties. Between 2 percent and 4 percent of a business organization's annual revenue is at risk for data protection infractions.

- The GDPR provided more effective enforcement of the rules in that police involvement and criminal prosecution are tied to violations of privacy rules.

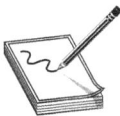

NOTE GDPR features the concept of "privacy by design" or "privacy by default." The law obliges companies to build-in data privacy in all phases of the information management lifecycle.

Depending on where you work, you may be affected by GDPR. If you use personal data that was subject to EU DPD, you will be subject to GDPR. The implementation of GDPR gives your organization an opportunity, regardless, to look inward at your governance, risk, and compliance programs. GDPR is a precursor to how other countries will continue to update and enhance their own privacy and security frameworks.

EXAM TIP For the exam, commit the following concept to memory and remember where it comes from: the GDPR's Article 17, The Right to Erasure, is commonly called "the right to be forgotten." This causes organizations to evaluate previous record retention requirements against the right to be forgotten considerations introduced by Article 17.

HIPAA/HITECH

HIPAA and all of its amendments—the Privacy Rule, the Security Rule, HITECH, and the recent Omnibus HIPAA Final Rule—are a voluminous set of regulations established over a long period of time. The privacy of healthcare data was covered at the US state level before HIPAA. However, the reality was a highly variable set of state-level standards with very little patient benefit. HIPAA was established as a national series of regulations to govern all US organizations that provide certain services using PHI. HIPAA also addresses the issues of health insurance portability and patient privacy rights. The administrative simplification provisions of HIPAA called for the establishment of standards and requirements for transmitting certain health information to improve the efficiency and effectiveness of the healthcare system while protecting patient privacy.

Another feature of HIPAA evolution has been the manner by which the regulations have kept pace with the digitization of healthcare information. The power for the federal government to enforce compliance through fines and penalties has always been a component of HIPAA, but there has been an upward progression of severity and strength in the publication of HIPAA amendments. It was determined that because of failures of regulated entities to comply, an enforcement rule was needed. The HIPAA Enforcement Rule in 2006 codified the power for the HHS to investigate complaints against covered entities for failing to comply with the Privacy Rule or for violating the Security Rule when the outcome is a preventable data breach of PHI. Enforcement was further strengthened by HITECH in 2009, which was enacted as part of the American Recovery and Reinvestment Act (ARRA) to promote the adoption and meaningful use of healthcare information technology and addresses the privacy and security concerns associated with the electronic transmission of health information, in part through several provisions that strengthen the civil and criminal enforcement of the HIPAA rules.

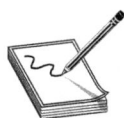

NOTE HIPAA was introduced to the US Congress as a bill by the name the Kennedy-Kassebaum Act, after Senators Ted Kennedy and Nancy Kassebaum, the act's two leading sponsors.

Table 4-3 shows a summary of all the HIPPA amendments.

HIPAA Privacy Rule In 1996, HHS enacted the Privacy Rule. Also known as "The Standards for Privacy of Individually Identifiable Health Information," the rule was the first standard for the protection of certain health information applicable across all US states. The definition of PHI was established in the rule, and this was the first source of the identifying data elements that make up PHI. The following identifiers

Amendment	Summary
HIPAA Privacy Rule, 1996	Implements the requirements of HIPAA. Addresses the use and disclosure of PHI by organizations subject to the Privacy Rule—covered entities—as well as standards covering individuals' rights to understand and control how their health information is used.
HIPAA Security Rule, 2005	Establishes national standards to protect ePHI that is created, received, used, or maintained by a covered entity. The Security Rule requires appropriate administrative, physical, and technical safeguards to ensure the confidentiality, integrity, and security of ePHI.
HITECH Act, 2009	Provides designated funding to modernize the healthcare system by promoting and expanding the adoption of HIT. HITECH supports the rapid adoption of HIT by hospitals and clinicians through Medicare and Medicaid incentive payments to physicians and hospitals for meaningful use of EHRs. It also authorizes grant programs and contracts that support HIT adoption by providing technical assistance to healthcare providers, especially in rural and underserved communities; training a HIT workforce; and developing standards for certification of EHR privacy and security.
HIPAA Omnibus Final Rule, 2013	Clarifies earlier provisions to the law and implements several new requirements. It provides a clear definition of a business associate and strengthens how these agents are subject to HIPAA—whether they sign a business associate agreement or not. Includes requirements for determining when a data breach has occurred. The previous standard was to determine "risk of harm" to the affected person. The new standard is "risk of disclosure," which is designed to be more objective.

Table 4-3 Summary of HIPAA Amendments

of the individual or of relatives, employers, or household members of the individual, are removed:[23]

- Names
- All geographic subdivisions smaller than a state, including street address, city, county, precinct, postal code, and their equivalent geocodes, except for the initial three digits of the postal code if, according to the current publicly available data from the Bureau of the Census:
  - The geographic unit formed by combining all postal codes with the same three initial digits contains more than 20,000 people; and
  - The initial three digits of a postal code for all such geographic units containing 20,000 or fewer people is changed to 000
- All elements of dates (except year) for dates that are directly related to an individual, including birth date, admission date, discharge date, death date, and all ages over 89 and all elements of dates (including year) indicative of such age, except that such ages and elements may be aggregated into a single category of age 90 or older
- Telephone numbers

- Vehicle identifiers and serial numbers, including license plate numbers
- Fax numbers
- Device identifiers and serial numbers
- E-mail addresses
- Web universal resource locators (URLs)
- Social Security numbers
- IP addresses
- Medical record numbers
- Biometric identifiers, including finger and voice prints
- Health plan beneficiary numbers
- Full-face photographs and any comparable images
- Account numbers
- Any other unique identifying number, characteristic, or code
- Certificate/license numbers

The Privacy Rule also outlines which types of organizations, or covered entities, are subject to the rule, such as health plans, healthcare clearinghouses, and healthcare delivery organizations such as hospitals. These organizations are expected to adhere to standards for appropriate use and disclosure of PHI. The rule provides for individuals' privacy rights too. For the first time, people providing their information to covered entities were given specific rights to understand and control how their health information is used. For example, the Privacy Rule established an individual's rights to examine and obtain a copy of personal health records, and to request corrections.

Another main component of The Privacy Rule was guidelines for de-identification of PHI. Remember that there are two methods for de-identification of sensitive information, which were provided within the Privacy Rule: The first is expert determination that sufficient methods have been used to result in very little risk that the information could be re-identified. The second method is to remove all of the types of identifying elements so that the organization has no knowledge of any residual identifying information. The Office for Civil Rights (OCR), a government agency that reports to HHS, is designated as responsible for implementing and enforcing the Privacy Rule.

CAUTION The Privacy Rule predates the digitization of healthcare and EHRs. The main focus of the Privacy Rule is PHI in written and oral formats. It is not sufficient for electronic PHI.

HIPAA Security Rule In recognition of the evolution of healthcare information technology (HIT), the HIPAA Security Rule was published in 2005. The rule supported the transition of healthcare data collection, storage, use, and transfer from paper processes to increasingly more electronic information systems to pay claims, answer eligibility questions, provide health information, and conduct a host of other administrative and clinically based functions.

With the increase in mobile applications, electronic information systems, and data access from anywhere at anytime, the risks of unauthorized data access and loss of confidentiality is significant. There is little debate about the benefits HIT has brought to patient care and healthcare organization capabilities. EHRs, networked medical devices, and data analytics are standard, if no longer state-of-the-art. Patients have unparalleled access to their claims and care management through self-service applications. In this environment, to maintain adequate privacy and security protections, the Security Rule was implemented to outline administrative, technical, and physical security controls to guide covered entities to protect the privacy of individuals' health information while allowing them to adopt new technologies to improve the quality and efficiency of patient care.

The Security Rule recognized a new format for PHI. As data evolved from paper, film, or audio storage to digital, the designation "electronic PHI," or ePHI, was established. Covered entities must attend to the same concerns of confidentiality, integrity, and availability with ePHI, just as they are required to do for PHI under the Privacy Rule. The Security Rule introduced standards for protecting ePHI according to security controls categorized as administrative, physical, and technical administrative safeguards. It is important to recognize specific types of solutions that fall into several categories.

Administrative safeguards are policies and procedures governing activities such as

- Establishing security training requirements, including sanction policies for personnel who violate policy and procedures

- Outlining security roles and responsibilities, including designation of a security official responsible for implementing the security program

- Authorizing access to ePHI based on role or need-to-know similar to the Privacy Rule standard of limiting uses and disclosures of PHI to the "minimum necessary"

- Periodic evaluation of how well the security policies and procedures meet the requirements of the Security Rule

Physical safeguards are physical measures that protect electronic information systems and related buildings and equipment, from natural and environmental hazards, and unauthorized physical access. The following are some examples of physical controls:

- Facility access and control systems of badges, ID cards, or biometric scanners to limit physical access to authorized personnel only

- Workstation and device security that ensures proper use and access to hardware and software, maintained by limiting systems in plain view or provide tamper-proof locations

- Protect electronic media during transfer, removal, disposal, and reuse

Technical safeguards are technology, information systems, or software applications that are used to ensure reasonable and appropriate levels of protection for ePHI. There are many examples that provide access, audit, integrity, and transmission security. The following are some examples:

- Data encryption for information at rest (storage) or in transit
- Hardware solutions such as firewalls, network intrusion detection systems, and data loss prevention systems
- Auditing tools that use system and security log files, such as a security incident and event management system (SIEM)
- Various forensic analysis applications as well as vulnerability scanning software, antimalware, and antivirus applications
- Authentication and access control systems, including passwords and multifactor authentication systems

An important addition implemented by the provisions in the Security Rule is a requirement for healthcare organizations to perform risk analysis as part of their security management processes. The risk analysis and management provisions of the Security Rule are necessary to determine which security measures are reasonable and appropriate for a healthcare organization. Remember that each organization will differ in their evaluation of risk. The results of the risk analysis will impact the implementation of the security controls listed in the Security Rule.

As outlined in the Security Rule, a general overview of the requirements includes, but is not limited to, the following activities:

- Assess events or threats for likelihood and impact.
- Address risks identified with appropriate security measures.
- Document security measure and the reasons for the choices.
- Maintain continuous, reasonable, and appropriate security protections.

Risk analysis is not an event. It should be a continuous process. A healthcare organization should continually review the reasonableness and appropriateness of security controls, track access to ePHI, and detect response to security incidents. As opportunities to improve security controls are identified, the healthcare organization should evaluate and implement to stay ahead of the dynamic risks.

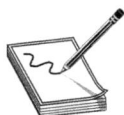

NOTE NIST published *An Introductory Resource Guide for Implementing the Health Insurance Portability and Accountability Act (HIPAA) Security Rule* (SP 800-66 Rev. 1) in October 2008 to assist covered entities in understanding and properly using HIPAA. It is not meant to supplement, replace, or supersede the HIPAA Security Rule itself, but it is a guide for program implementation and to other information sources.

HITECH Act   The next amendment to HIPAA was the HITECH Act. This law was enacted as part of the American Recovery and Reinvestment Act of 2009. The overall intent of HITECH was to promote the adoption and meaningful use of HIT. HITECH strengthened the HIPAA enforcement regulations and actions. For example, HITECH introduced a tiered responsibility and penalty structure that included significant increase of the minimum penalty amount for each violation. The maximum penalty for each identical infraction was raised from $50,000 to as much as $1.5 million. Prior to HITECH, there was a perception that healthcare organizations were not fully implementing information protection standards. The total number of complaints and total enforcement actions from OCR rose steadily through 2009. Increasing minimum and maximum fines for civil infractions in conjunction with the authority for criminal charges that may include jail time was deemed necessary.

The HITECH Act clarified the legal obligations of business associates, making them directly liable for compliance with certain requirements of the HIPAA Rules. OCR was granted authority to take enforcement action against business associates directly for certain violations, including the following:[24]

- Noncompliance with OCR requests for program documentation or failure to cooperate in an official investigation to determine compliance
- Retaliation against anyone filing a complaint under HIPAA provisions
- Failure to comply with the requirements of the Security Rule
- Not following breach notification rules in support of a covered entity or another business associate
- Impermissible uses and disclosures of PHI
- Failure to disclose a copy of electronic PHI (ePHI) to the covered entity, the individual, or the individual's designee (whichever is specified in the business associate agreement)
- Failure to make reasonable efforts to limit PHI to the minimum necessary to accomplish the intended purpose of the use, disclosure, or request
- Failure, in certain circumstances, to provide an accounting of disclosures
- Failure to extend business associate agreements to subcontractors that create or receive PHI on their behalf and failure to implement the standards
- Failure to take reasonable steps to address a material breach or violation of the subcontractor's business associate agreement

HITECH had many clarifications and changes, making it a significant amendment to the previous rules that were published. Strengthening civil and criminal penalties, redefining breach notification guidelines, and clarifying business associate accountability are just a few very important examples. As HITECH was tied to ARRA Meaningful Use provisions that offered financial incentives for implementing EHRs, it follows that privacy and security provisions were highly relevant. Regulators had to ensure that increased digitization of healthcare information through expanded use of EHRs had appropriate focus on protecting the data as well. HIPAA was extremely important when it emerged in 1996, and the increased use of technology via computers and electronic storage devices made HITECH a necessity to help protect individuals whose records might be divulged or altered through unauthorized access and malicious hacking.

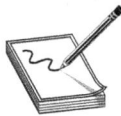

NOTE HITECH provides clarification of "unsecured PHI" to mean "unencrypted PHI," but it does not require encryption.

HIPAA Omnibus Final Rule The HIPAA Omnibus Final Rule is not necessarily a new rule, but a finalization of the interim provisions that were part of earlier rules, particularly the HITECH Act and another related information protection law, the Genetic Information Nondiscrimination Act (GINA). The HIPAA Omnibus Rule went into effect on September 23, 2013. Here is a summary of the most relevant provisions of the HIPAA Omnibus Rule:

- Extends the direct obligation of business associates under HITECH to authorize OCR to audit business associates for compliance
- Changes the threshold for determining a data breach from risk of harm to an individual to a more objective standard—risk of unauthorized disclosure
- Modifies the HIPAA Privacy Rule as required by GINA to prohibit most health plans from using or disclosing genetic information for underwriting purposes

Before the HIPAA Omnibus Final Rule, there was some disagreement about the definition of "business associate." The practical implication of the disagreement was that US healthcare organizations were reluctant to enter into supplier relationships with entities that did not consider themselves business associates and would not enter into business associate agreements. For example, many cloud service providers fit into this category. This slowed adoption of many cloud-enabled technologies and potential improvements for healthcare organizations. With the HIPAA Omnibus Final Rule, the definition of business associate was modified to include any entity that "creates, receives, maintains, or transmits" PHI to include providers of cloud computing platforms. In fact, the law stipulates that performing the actions with PHI and acting as a business associate obligates an entity under the law with or without a formal contract such as a business associate agreement. This modification resulted in many cloud providers accepting obligations as a business associate subject to HIPAA.

Stark Law

The Physician Self-Referral Law, commonly referred to as the Stark Law, is related to healthcare information security and privacy in that it helps to govern patient transfer and referrals. The Stark Law is primarily a civil law and a safeguard against fraud. Unethical practitioners may attempt to defraud the government by referring a patient to a family member or financial partner, whereby the referring physician receives some financial reward. The foundation for Stark Law is found in the AMA Code of Medical Ethics Opinion on "Conflicts of Interest." It is both illegal and unethical to practice referrals that would involve information sharing based on family or financial relationships.

Anti-Kickback Enforcement Act

While failing to comply with the Stark Law is not a criminal offense, failing to comply with the Anti-Kickback Enforcement Act is. Physicians, administrators, and facility owners alike should be familiar with this federal law, which prohibits the exchange, or offer to exchange, of anything of value in an effort to induce or reward a referral of federal healthcare program business. Violating the Anti-Kickback Statute exploits the healthcare system, drives up program costs, and hinders fair competition in the industry. Kickbacks may also compromise the medical decision-making processes of physicians and hospitals in the form of patient steering.

Criminal penalties can include jail time as well as steep fines. Civil fines can also be expensive if the offense is not considered a criminal act. If a provider is found guilty of accepting a kickback, they can be excluded from receiving reimbursement under government programs such as Medicaid and Medicare. Thirty-six US states have anti-kickback statutes in addition to the federal law.

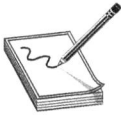

NOTE In October 2019, HHS proposed changes to modernize and clarify the regulations that interpret the Stark Law and the federal Anti-Kickback Statute. The change to the law allows hospitals to give free cybersecurity software to local providers they frequently work with, as part of an effort to facilitate more coordinated patient care.

The Privacy Act of 1974 (United States)

A foundational privacy regulation that was passed in 1974 and is still in effect today, the Privacy Act applies to the US government with regard to how personal information is collected, used, and stored. The Privacy Act protects the creation, use, and maintenance of records that contain personal identifiers such as a name, Social Security number, or other identifying numbers or symbols. Federal agencies are required to give the public notice of the systems that exist to use and store the personal information. They post this notice in the US Federal Register, which is a repository posted to the Internet. Individuals can inquire about and be provided access to information maintained about them. They can also seek corrections if they think there is an error in their record.

Many nongovernment organizations have used the Privacy Act and subsequent rules and laws as a basis for their own regulations. Like HIPAA, the Privacy Act requires agencies to use administrative, technical, and physical safeguards to protect personal information contained in systems of records. A collection of related records that are organized together based on uniquely identifying information, such as a patient's name, is part of a system of records covered in this law. Another example of the lineage connecting the Privacy Act to later regulation is the Fair Credit Reporting Act (FCRA) enforced by the Federal Trade Commission to promote the accuracy, integrity, fairness, and privacy of consumer information.

The Privacy Act (Canada)

The Canadian Privacy Act relates to a person's right to access and correct personal information that the government of Canada holds about them. It applies to all of the personal information that the government collects, uses, and discloses, including personal information about federal employees, though it does not apply to political parties and political representatives. It offers protections for personal information, which it defines as any recorded information "about an identifiable individual." The act also gives individuals the right to access personal information held by the federal government. All provinces and territories have laws governing their public sectors.

The act also applies to the government's collection, use, and disclosure of personal information in the course of providing services such as the following:[25]

- Old-age security pensions
- Employment insurance
- Border security
- Federal policing and public safety
- Tax collection and refunds.

Much like other privacy and security regulations, the Canadian Privacy Act defines a number of data elements that are considered personal information. You will notice many similarities to the US Privacy Act, but there are interesting differences. For example, the Canadian Privacy Act covers personal opinions or views, which are protected with a few exceptions. A specific exception is also made for identifying information of current and former government individuals relevant to their service as an employer or a supplier of contractual services. Discretionary financial benefits such as granting of licenses or permits to an individual may not be covered. The Privacy Act does not apply to individuals who have been dead for more than 20 years.

The types of data elements that are subject to the Privacy Act in Canada include the following:[26]

- Race, national or ethnic origin, color, religion, age, or marital status
- Education, medical, criminal, or employment history of an individual or information about financial transactions
- Any assigned identifying numbers or symbols
- Address, fingerprints, or blood type
- Private or confidential correspondence sent to a government institution
- The views or opinions of another individual about the individual
- The views or opinions of another individual about a proposal for a grant, an award, or a prize to be made to the individual by an institution
- The name of the individual where it appears with other related personal information and where the disclosure of the name itself would reveal information about the individual

Personal Information Protection and Electronic Documents Act (Canada)

The Canadian approach to regulation provides stricter controls for the collection, use, and storage of personal information, compared to other countries, such as the United States. In Canada, the federal Privacy Commissioner and various provincial privacy commissions have authority to oversee and investigate privacy matters. PIPEDA applies to private-sector organizations across Canada that collect, use, or disclose personal information in the course of commercial, for-profit activities. PIPEDA also mandates that such use must only be for purposes that a reasonable person would deem appropriate given the circumstances. Federally regulated organizations that conduct business in Canada are subject to PIPEDA. Similar legislation is in place for companies operating in the provinces of British Columbia, Alberta, and Quebec. Federal and provincial privacy commissioners may jointly investigate privacy complaints and/or data breaches. PIPEDA contains 10 Fair Information Principles:

- **Accountability**   An organization is responsible for personal information under its control as well as information transferred to a third party. Each organization must appoint someone to be accountable for compliance with these fair information principles. The organization must develop and implement relevant policies and procedures.

- **Identifying purposes**   The purpose for collecting personal information must be documented. Customers must be told why their personal information is needed before or at the time of collection, and their consent must be obtained if a new purpose or uses emerge.

- **Consent**   An essential component of the principles, knowledge, and consent of the individual are required for the collection, use, or disclosure of personal information, except where inappropriate. The form of consent can vary depending on the sensitivity of the information, and individuals can withdraw consent at any time with notice.

- **Limiting collection**   To prevent organizations from collecting information by misleading or deceiving individuals, information can be collected only for a legitimate and identified purpose through fair and lawful means.

- **Limiting use, disclosure, and retention**   Organizational use or disclosure of personal information must be limited to the identified purposes for which it was collected. Personal information should be stored only for as long as it is needed to serve those purposes, and then it must be destroyed, erased, or anonymized.

- **Accuracy**   Before information is shared, the organization must ensure that it is as accurate, complete, and up-to-date as possible when using it to make a decision about an individual.

- **Safeguards**   Personal information must be protected at a level appropriate to the information's sensitivity. All personal information must be protected against loss, theft, or any unauthorized access, disclosure, copying, use or modification regardless of how it is stored.

- **Openness** An organization must have clear and easily understood personal information management practices that are made available on request. Informed decisions and consent are possible only when an individual can understand what they are acknowledging and signing.

- **Individual access** An individual has the right to access information that an organization collects and holds on them. The individual also has the right to challenge the accuracy and completeness of the information and have it amended as appropriate.

- **Challenging compliance** An individual must be able to challenge an organization's compliance with the fair information principles. Their challenge should be addressed to the person accountable for the organization's compliance with PIPEDA.

There are laws at the province level that impact the applicability of PIPEDA. The provincial government can exempt an organization, a class of organizations, an activity, or a class of activities from the application of PIPEDA with respect to the collection, use, or disclosure of personal information that occurs within a province that has passed legislation deemed to be substantially similar to the PIPEDA. This does not mean the local laws are less strict; the exemption is possible only when the provincial laws are substantially similar. They must provide privacy protection that is consistent with and equivalent to that found under PIPEDA, incorporate the 10 Fair Information Principles, and provide for an independent and effective oversight and redress mechanism with powers to investigate and restrict the collection, use, and disclosure of personal information to purposes that are appropriate or legitimate. PIPEDA has national jurisdiction, and the national law continues to apply to information protection in connection with operations involving the Canadian government or in data use scenarios that extend outside of the province.

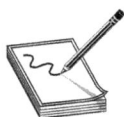

NOTE PIPEDA has been given adequacy designation, which enables EU-to-Canada data transfers. The designation is reviewed periodically.[27]

Separate statutes govern control of PHI by provincial government organizations and by anyone with access to that information, such as doctors and nurses. Across all Canadian provinces, as in the United States, there is no prohibition against sharing personal data across the border, and PIPEDA does not specifically forbid the transfer. However, the common practice in Canada is not to share personal data outside of Canada. Canadian officials have jurisdictional concerns with trans-border data flows, much like their American counterparts. In particular, the US Patriot Act, enacted after September 11, 2011, as a response to acts of terrorism, presents issues. Data pertaining to Canadian citizens that crosses the border and resides in a US company for storage or other use falls under US regulatory jurisdiction. In this case, the US Patriot Act may allow US government access to the personal information of Canadian individuals without their knowledge, which is a violation of Canada's PIPEDA. Therefore, contracts negotiated with Canadian healthcare organizations will likely mandate that such data remain within Canadian jurisdiction.

Understand Compliance Frameworks

Compliance frameworks are important, because organizations can use them to help organize their approach to stay within the guidelines of regulatory and legal requirements. There are numerous examples of compliance frameworks at a national or industry level. We will concentrate on frameworks that guide information security and privacy. Where applicable, we will examine those frameworks that are prevalent in healthcare settings too. No matter what type or size of healthcare organization you work in, from a one-person physician practice to an entire integrated healthcare delivery system, you will encounter and use various compliance frameworks.

Privacy Frameworks

With the advent of digitization of healthcare information and sharing of data across the world via the Internet in a matter of seconds, the focus on the confidentiality of PII has never been more important. Privacy frameworks foster privacy engineering practices that support privacy by design concepts to support healthcare organizations' privacy programs. According to NIST, there are several key areas where privacy frameworks provide benefit to customers and organizations:[28]

- To instill trust that the organization will make ethical decisions about product and service design as well as use sensitive information use with a balanced approach, with optimized beneficial use of information and minimal adverse consequences to individuals and society

- To meet current compliance obligations and build products and services as much as possible in anticipation of future privacy obligations in the dynamic technology environment

- To support and simplify communication about privacy practices with individuals, business partners, assessors, and regulators

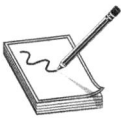

NOTE Just before publication of this material, NIST presented the document *NIST Privacy Framework: A Tool for Improving Privacy through Enterprise Risk Management,* Version 1.0. During 2020, the draft document will go through the process of obtaining comments from stakeholders before being published as a guidance document. It is worth reviewing at https://www.nist.gov/system/files/documents/2020/01/16/NIST%20Privacy%20Framework_V1.0.pdf.

The use of privacy frameworks helps to support the variety of privacy requirements that exists across organizations. The leading privacy frameworks are flexible so that privacy requirements are met while the organization can stay current with technology trends. A privacy framework is not merely a checklist. Risks and benefits must be calculated while addressing the principles or standards presented in the frameworks. Organizations must make informed decisions about privacy practices and communicate that to their customers.

Caldicott Guardian Program (United Kingdom)

The "Caldicott Committee's Report on the Review of Patient-Identifiable Information," or the Caldicott Report, led by Dame Fiona Caldicott, emerged in 1997 from a review of how information was handled by organizations in the UK's National Health Service (NHS). The Caldicott Report provided recommendations to the NHS on principles that would help guide safe use of patient identifiable data (PID). There are the seven Caldicott principles:[29]

- Justify the purposes for using confidential information.
- Use it only when absolutely necessary.
- Use the minimum that is required.
- Access should be on a strict need-to-know basis.
- Everyone must understand his or her responsibilities.
- Understand and comply with the law.
- Providers must be able to share information securely because they have an almost equivalent duty to do both.

Because privacy of patient information was a central tenant of the proper practice of medicine, the report established the need for a senior person to be made responsible for safeguarding the information-sharing processes. With the digital evolution of health-care information sharing, the need for these "Caldicott guardians" has not changed. In fact, the complexity of information sharing has expanded the scope of responsibilities. The Caldicott guardians are central to understand the risks and benefits for information exchange and to develop robust practice protocols to protect both patients and practices. Here is an overview of the responsibilities of a Caldicott guardian:

- **Strategy and governance**   The guardian should report to the organization's governance board and management group on information privacy issues and act as "conscience" of the organization while facilitating appropriate information sharing processes.

- **Confidentiality and data protection expertise**   The guardian should be a subject matter expert on confidentiality and data protection and should collaborate with individuals within the organization and seek process improvement solutions from external sources.

- **Internal information processing**   The guardian should use tools and resources such as the Information Governance Toolkit to provide oversight for currency and accuracy of organizational policies and procedures for information privacy.

- **Information sharing**   The guardian should oversee the arrangements and information-sharing procedure involving sensitive patient information, including disclosure for research purposes and to law enforcement.

The call to action is for NHS organizations and those organizations with whom they share data to appoint a Caldicott guardian to guide information collection and use according to the seven principles.

Organisation for Economic Cooperation and Development Privacy Principles

The Organisation for Economic Cooperation and Development (OECD), headquartered in Paris, has developed policy around the general principles all 29 member countries should follow with the aim of fostering international trade. The United States is a member of the OECD and is one of the largest funders of its $200 million annual budget.[30]

The OECD framework categorizes fair information practices for collecting, storing, and using PII. It aims to help individuals participate in the use of their own information. The principles assign responsibility for protecting information to the entities that collect and maintain it. As you familiarize yourself with US and international data protection laws, you will find the following principles well integrated and perhaps even repetitive; the list is taken from the 2013 document "The OECD Privacy Framework":[31]

- **Collection limitation principle**   There should be limits to the collection of personal data, and any such data should be obtained by lawful and fair means and, where appropriate, with the knowledge or consent of the data subject.

- **Data quality principle**   Personal data should be relevant to the purposes for which it is to be used and, to the extent necessary for those purposes, should be accurate, complete, and kept up to date.

- **Purpose specification principle**   The purposes for which personal data is collected should be specified no later than at the time of data collection, and the subsequent use should be limited to the fulfilment of those purposes or any occasions that are not incompatible with those purposes and as specified on each occasion of change of purpose.

- **Use limitation principle**   Personal data should not be disclosed, made available, or otherwise used for purposes other than those specified except in the following cases:
  - With the consent of the data subject
  - By the authority of law

- **Security safeguards principle**   Personal data should be protected by reasonable security safeguards against such risks as loss or unauthorized access, destruction, use, modification, or disclosure of data.

- **Openness principle**   There should be a general policy of openness about developments, practices, and policies with respect to personal data. Means should be readily available for establishing the existence and nature of personal data and the main purposes of its use, as well as the identity and jurisdiction of the data controller.

- **Individual participation principle**   An individual should have the right to do the following:
  - Obtain from, or otherwise, obtain confirmation of whether the data controller has data relating to him
  - Have communicated to him data relating to him, within the following parameters:
    - Within a reasonable time
    - At a charge, if any, that is not excessive
    - In a reasonable manner
    - In a form that is readily intelligible to him
  - Be given reasons if a request made by an individual to access their information is denied and be able to challenge such denial
  - Challenge data relating to him and, if the challenge is successful, have the data erased, rectified, completely amended, or annotated in the case where the patient and provider are not in agreement
- **Accountability principle**   A data controller should be accountable for complying with measures that give effect to the principles stated earlier.

EXAM TIP   Privacy frameworks (and security frameworks, as you will see later in this chapter) have significant overlap, which is to be expected. You can assume that principles or standards are defined similarly across frameworks, including transparency, openness, purpose limitation, and so on. However, if the exam specifies a framework, you will need to know the version of the term or definition used within that specific framework.

Fair Information Practice Principles   The Fair Information Practice Principles (FIPPs) are commonly adopted from sources such as the US Privacy Act and have been used in publications from entities such as the US Federal Trade Commission (FTC) and the Department of Homeland Security (DHS). They are voluntary guidelines but are often used to develop privacy law, such as OECD privacy principles and the EU DPD. Although the FIPPs are not law, government entities can intercede and consumers have ways to address complaints. For organizations that conduct business over the Internet and collect, use, and store digital information, the FIPPs are considered a baseline requirement. The adherence process relies on organizations to self-assess and make corrections where needed. The principles are categorized as follows:[32]

- **The Collection Limitation Principle**   Collectors of personal information should restrict the amount and types of sensitive data to only what is required. Collection should follow regulatory constraints and the individual subject should be given the opportunity to provide informed consent when possible.

- **The Data Quality Principle**   Data that is collected and maintained should remain relevant to why it was obtained and used. While it is in the possession of the information collector, the data should remain accurate, complete, and up-to-date.

- **The Purpose Specification Principle**   The reason for collecting and using the data should be made known when it is collected. If the reasons change over time, additional notice should be made and consent should be obtained.

- **The Use Limitation Principle**   The uses of the information should stay true to the purpose that was originally disclosed. Changes are permitted only when consent is updated or under some law enforcement scenarios.

- **The Security Safeguards Principle**   Confidentiality, integrity, and availability of data should be ensured through reasonable security control implementation.

- **The Openness Principle**   Information collectors should be forthcoming about their privacy practices and they should make those policies and procedures easily available. Individuals should be able to identify and determine the existence of their data in possession and use by those information collectors.

- **The Individual Participation Principle**   This principle relates to a person's right to know that an information collector has data and, when possible, obtain that data in a readable format, at a reasonable cost, in a timely manner. This principle also applies to an individual's right to challenge a denial for access to their data as well as a right to challenge perceived errors through change or deletion request.

- **The Accountability Principle**   An entity that controls the sensitive information should be accountable to follow these principles.

Asia-Pacific Economic Cooperation Cross-Border Privacy Rules

Asia-Pacific Economic Cooperation (APEC) is a regional economic forum established in 1989 to leverage the growing interdependence of the Asia-Pacific region. APEC's 21 members, including Russia, Japan, Australia, the Republic of Korea, and China, aim to create greater prosperity for the people of the region by promoting balanced, inclusive, sustainable, innovative, and secure growth and by accelerating regional economic integration. The APEC Cross-Border Privacy Rules (CBPR) were developed to build trust in cross-border flow of personal information.[33] Industry and civil authorities have collaborated to develop a framework aligned with prevailing requirements. Over the years, additional countries have joined APEC and aligned with the CBPR, including Canada, Mexico, and the United States. An independent APEC CBPR accountability agent—an entity authorized by the APEC—assesses participating businesses for ongoing compliance. The agent's assessments are enforceable by law. The GDPR is being discussed for certification within the APEC CBPR system. Currently, CBPR permits an assessment and endorsement program similar to the EU–US Privacy Shield. Both provide a means for self-assessment, compliance review, adoption of the principles, dispute resolution, and enforcement by an authority. The authority would be a data protection authority, in the United States it is the FTC. The CBPR differs from the GDPR in that the CBPR does not replace or supersede the member countries' laws.

Generally Accepted Privacy Principles

The Generally Accepted Privacy Principles (GAPP) are rooted in the principles found in the OECD and leading international guidance. They also attempt to regulate the collection and use of PII in adherence with FIPP and prevailing law. Major proponents of GAPP include Canadian privacy practitioners. That is likely related to the fact that the principles were developed by the American Institute of Certified Public Accountants (AICPA) and the Canadian Institute of Chartered Accountants (CICA).

Generally accepted privacy principles are founded on a main privacy objective. The organization must collect, use, retain, disclose, and dispose of personal information following the entity's privacy notice and with criteria set forth in GAPP.

Following are the ten generally accepted privacy principles:[34]

- **Management**   The organization defines, documents, communicates, and assigns accountability for its privacy policies and procedures.

- **Notice**   The organization provides notice about its privacy policies and procedures and identifies the purposes for which personal information is collected, used, retained, and disclosed.

- **Choice and consent**   The organization describes the choices available to individuals and obtains implicit or explicit consent with respect to the collection, use, and disclosure of personal information.

- **Collection**   The organization may collect personal information only for the purposes identified in the notice.

- **Use, retention, and disposal**   The organization limits the use of personal information to the purposes identified in the notice and for which the individual has provided implicit or explicit consent. The entity retains personal information for only as long as necessary for the stated purposes, or as required by laws or regulations, and then disposes of such information appropriately.

- **Access**   The organization provides individuals with access to their personal information for review and update.

- **Disclosure to third parties**   The organization discloses personal information to third parties only for the purposes identified in the notice and with the individual's implicit or explicit consent.

- **Security for privacy**   The organization protects personal information against unauthorized access (both physical and logical).

- **Quality**   The organization maintains accurate, complete, and relevant personal information for the purposes identified in the notice.

- **Monitoring and enforcement**   The organization monitors compliance with its privacy policies and procedures and has procedures to address privacy-related complaints and disputes.

Security Frameworks

Organizations should use an information security framework to guide their information protection programs, and there are many to choose from. It is as important that you understand the components of the security framework as it is to know how to apply the framework to your organization. To choose and tailor your options, you'll need to be aware of regulatory requirements, organizational size, geographic location, investment constraints, and current capabilities of the security program. As important as the framework you choose is its implementation. The frameworks featured here can assist you and your organization in complying with and, in most cases, exceeding the various international, national, local, and industry-specific information security regulations.

Health Industry Cybersecurity Practices

In 2015, the US Congress passed the Cybersecurity Act of 2015 (CSA), a landmark legislation that promotes public and private information sharing across industry entities. One of the relevant components of the legislation for healthcare information security is in Section 405(d), "Aligning Health Care Industry Security Approaches." In 2017, HHS convened the CSA 405(d) Task Group, leveraging the healthcare and public health sectors to advance critical infrastructure security and resilience in the public–private partnership. This task group comprises a diverse group of more than 100 members representing many areas and roles, including cybersecurity, privacy, healthcare practitioners, HIT, and other subject matter experts.[35] A primary outcome of this group is a cybersecurity framework publication entitled "Health Industry Cybersecurity Practices: Managing Threats and Protecting Patients."

The HICP has a broad mission concerned with generating more cybersecurity awareness in the healthcare industry. The group is also a clearinghouse and source of advocacy for proven security practices developed and recommended by experts in various healthcare organizations and government agencies. Focused on sharing threat and risk-reduction intelligence, the HICP sees problems faced by one organization as potentially affecting all organizations. At the center of the mission is the requirement to protect patient safety and improve patient care through information protection. The group takes a very practical approach, with most of its effort focused on the most likely and impactful threats, including e-mail phishing attacks; ransomware attacks; loss or theft of equipment or data; insider, accidental, or data loss; and attacks against connected medical devices that may affect patient safety.

The initial publication was extensive and will grow over time with revisions and additions. While it is not itself a security framework, the documents or deliverables from the directives in Section 405(d) should be known by US healthcare information privacy and security professionals. The recommendations of the group are helpful in assisting practitioners remain aligned with the NIST Cybersecurity Framework and the privacy and security provisions of HIPAA.

The work of the group that authored the first version is an example of public–private partnerships formed to study the prevailing frameworks. By analyzing the most prevalent threats facing US healthcare organizations and practical approaches, the group formulated a controls implementation approach suitable for healthcare organizations.

International Organization for Standardization

The International Organization for Standardization (ISO) is an international standard-setting body that consists of qualified subject matter experts from more than 150 countries that attempt to integrate national standards such as those from the American National Standards Institute (ANSI), ISO Technical Committee (TC) 215 Health Informatics, the BSI Group from the United Kingdom, and the Standards Council of Canada, to name a few.

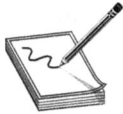

NOTE We are mentioning ISO standards here because you should familiarize yourself with their existence and their relationship to other regulations. These standards are copyrighted and not distributed for free. However, draft ISO standards are available during review periods, and some versions of standards can be found online through various sharing agreements.[36]

As a tool for daily use, the concepts and principles found in the ISO guidance are sufficiently available in other sources as well. However, they are important to acknowledge and, when available, reinforce the processes and procedures required for safeguarding individually identifiable information. We will discuss a few relevant standards related to managing risk, provide a brief description, and summarize their relevance.

The following are governance standards for information privacy and security:

ISO/IEC 27001, Information security management This standard helps organizations implement security as a system rather than using numerous controls to solve seemingly isolated issues. The standard includes handling of electronic information as well as paper-based information. From the management perspective, this standard's main contribution is to formalize the concept of risk assessments and organize information security as a quality improvement activity. The standard includes the plan–do–check–act (PDCA) concept as well as the principle of continually assessing the organization, rather than doing so episodically.

ISO/IEC 27799, Health informatics – Information security management in health using ISO/IEC 27002 This standard defines information security management in health, which uses ISO/IEC 27002 and augments its requirements with healthcare-specific considerations for information security management.

ISO/IEC 29100, Information technology – Security techniques – Privacy framework This standard defines requirements for properly safeguarding PII used by a data collector. The standard introduces terminology, outlines roles and responsibilities, and describes the following 11 privacy principles:[37]

- Consent and choice
- Purpose legitimacy and specification
- Collection limitation
- Data minimization
- Use, retention, and disclosure limitation

- Accuracy and quality
- Openness, transparency, and notice
- Individual participation and access
- Accountability
- Information security
- Privacy compliance

Another salient point about this standard is that it defines identifiability and related terms. *Identifiability* is the extent to which information serves to identify an individual. Of course, there are varying degrees of identifiability: from full anonymity (not identifiable) to full "verinymity" (positively identified). This is related to the concept of *linkability*, which is the extent to which you can link various data elements together to identify someone. *Unlinkability* means that even after complex combinations and attempts, you cannot determine identity by linking the information. The other concept the standard introduces is *observability*. This is the extent to which you can identify or link an identity to a system by virtue of an individual's use of the system. It includes a consideration of factors such as time, location, and data contents.

ISO/IEC 29101: Privacy Reference Architecture   A tactical guide, this standard contains best practices collected from the industry for processing PII. The guidance delivers consistent, technical implementation of privacy requirements. By using the guide, you can build a privacy reference architecture with the necessary privacy safeguarding measures built into the system functionally and systematically across the entire enterprise. The goal is to include all relevant systems and integrate with already existing safeguarding controls.

ISO/IEC 29190: Privacy Capability Assessment Model   This standard gives an organization the tools to determine its level of maturity in its processes for collecting, using, disclosing, retaining, and disposing of personal information. The level of maturity is assessed based on whether the organization has evidence of processes related to information governance, risk assessments, third-party management, and relevant policy, among other areas of concern.

National Institute of Standards and Technology

NIST, through a collaboration of industry stakeholders and government experts, published the initial version of the Cybersecurity Framework (CSF) in 2014. The initial CSF was a response to Executive Order (EO) 13636, "Improving Critical Infrastructure Cybersecurity" (February 2013). Version 1.0 envisioned future iterations of the CSF and provided guidance for accomplishing the evolution. The NIST CSF was updated in 2017 and has become one of the most widely adopted cybersecurity approaches. It is popular because the organization of the framework is understandable, uses a common language to address and manage cybersecurity risk, applies cost-effective considerations based on business and organizational needs, and aligns with applicable regulatory requirements.[38]

The NIST CSF is a US source, but it references globally recognized standards for cybersecurity. The reason the framework is so popular is because of its relevancy and practicality across organizations with critical infrastructure, including organizations with computing and networking technology that are significantly important to industrial control, energy, military, commerce, banking, telecommunications, healthcare, and retail. The CSF is a valuable tool and benchmark that you can use to evaluate, design, implement, and improve how your organization protects personal information and sensitive data collected, stored, used, and shared. It is also a template for continuous cybersecurity improvement when used in the information security management program.

Many organizations, public and private, have adopted the NIST CSF. Healthcare organizations of various missions and sizes find the framework compatible with patient care and safety. The CSF is also popular because it brings together the requirements into a common set of terminologies and measures. This helps regulators and healthcare leaders implement, monitor, and report fairly with less administrative burden. The framework also guides cybersecurity programs that are based on control effectiveness and structured on risk reduction to be scalable and relevant across various types and missions of organizations.

The CSF is the cornerstone of owners and operators of information security measures and controls in industries with critical infrastructure, such as healthcare, to help identify, assess, and manage cyber risks. Using the CSF starts with defining the organization's cybersecurity profile. The profile is one part of the overall framework and is the compilation or tailoring of standards, guidelines, and practices, based on business needs, cost effectiveness, and cybersecurity risk. Profiles can be used to identify opportunities for improving cybersecurity postures by comparing the organization's "as is" state with a target "to be" state. Building from the CSF, there are two additional parts to build: the Framework Core and the Implementation Tiers. The Framework Core is a set of cybersecurity activities, outcomes, and informative references that are common across sectors and critical infrastructure. Elements of the Framework Core provide detailed guidance for developing individual organizational profiles.[39] Figure 4-6 shows and defines the categories of the Framework Core. The tiers are assessed as a function of the organization's responses to cybersecurity approaches, characterized across a continuum of implementation. Do not think of the tiers as organizational maturity levels; they are a mechanism for organizations to manage and assess their tailored approach to reducing risks and effective operation of controls.

Common Criteria

The Common Criteria (CC) is particularly applicable within risk management frameworks because it has standards and controls built in. These controls are used by independently licensed testing and evaluation laboratories to assess the effectiveness of various hardware and software tools. The output or list of evaluated products can be used by healthcare information privacy and security personnel to select, purchase, and implement "approved" products. The approval that the CC list offers enables users to be more confident in what they use. They can be assured that testing was conducted in a rigorous, standard, and repeatable manner. The products will provide adequate security so long as users choose and implement products rated for a level of protection ability sufficient for the organizational threat environment. That said, authorities behind the CC make it clear that their approval is not a guarantee.

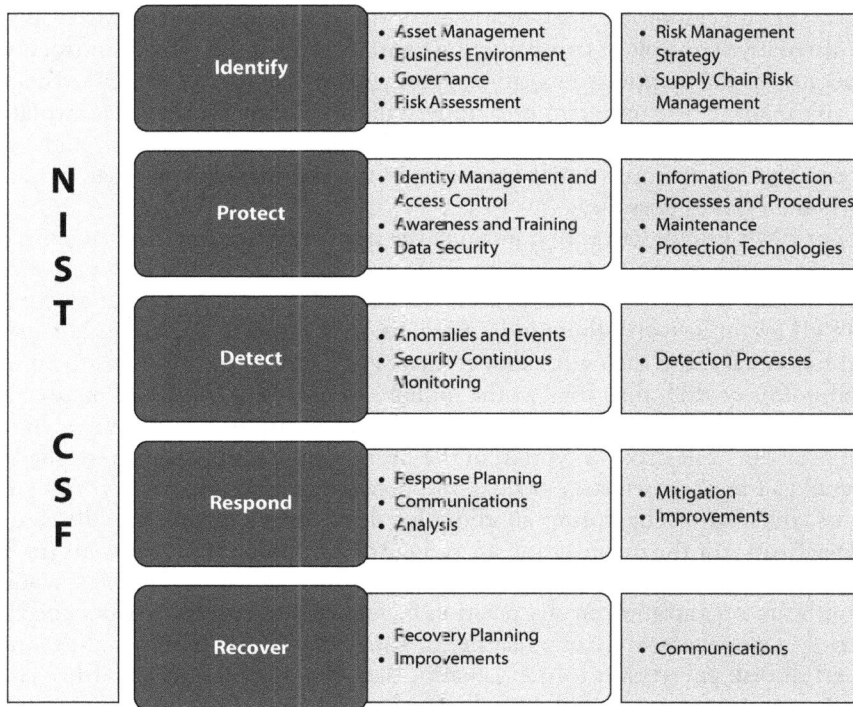

Figure 4-6 NIST CSF core elements

The CC international standard, ISO/IEC 15408, is honored by many countries, including the United States, the United Kingdom, Canada, Australia, Japan, Germany, France, Spain, and Italy, to name a few. Product evaluations through the CC program are recognized by all the countries that have signed the agreement, called the Common Criteria Recognition Arrangement (CCRA). Most often, CC considerations are part of government system implementations and critical infrastructure. The output of the CC traditionally has been the evaluation assurance level (EAL). This is a numerical value (EAL 1–7) that corresponds to the level of security requirements a product has been tested against. In recent years, the group has begun to move away from having EALs in favor of a more flexible assurance criteria based on the product profile. For day-to-day purposes, this philosophy is of little impact. What remains important is the idea of applying a risk management framework around products and applications. From there, an evaluation or accreditation is provided.

Factor Analysis of Information Risk

One of the drawbacks of using risk management frameworks is they are not typically good at giving the results much context. Of course, subjective input based on organizational mission, culture, risk tolerance, and cost are identified as variables to prioritize the categories of vulnerabilities. Also, nearly every risk management framework calls for the use of alternative controls or compensating controls when a prescribed control is not feasible because of the mentioned variables. Another way to integrate this tailored approach into a risk management program is to understand the factor analysis of information risk (FAIR), which is a categorization of the factors that contribute to risk and how they affect one another. In short, FAIR concentrates the risk manager on what is more probable versus all that is possible.

To put FAIR into practice, first imagine the information assets in an organization. In the United States, a mobile device with PHI stored on it is considered a vulnerability. If it is lost or stolen, which often happens, it can be used in a data breach. A device without stored PHI might be worth thousands of dollars, so controls to prevent its loss or damage should not equal more than a fraction of that value. However, if PHI is stored on it, its value after loss or theft may total in the millions of dollars. This would increase the feasibility of investing more heavily in securing the device from vulnerabilities. In fact, the cost of providing full-disk encryption of the device probably amounts to negligible costs compared to the likely scenario of fines and penalties after a breach. According to some accounts, the cost of encrypting an endpoint device is about $200, while a breach of that device can cost the organization an average of $3.9 million per incident (in 2019).[40] Of course, in addition to monetary fines and penalties, device loss or theft would place the healthcare organization in the position of loss of reputation, patients delaying care or seeking it elsewhere, and costs relating to patient notification and credit monitoring. Adding full-disk encryption to the scenario, that same mobile device, if lost, is almost assuredly not considered a data breach. In this scenario, a risk management decision around whether to implement a bring-your-own-device (BYOD) program to the healthcare organization in the United States is supported by integrating the FAIR probability thought process.

Health Information Trust Alliance

Developed in collaboration with healthcare and information security professionals, the Health Information Trust Alliance (HITRUST) Common Security Framework (CSF) is a security framework for protecting health information tailored for the US healthcare industry. The CSF includes and integrates federal and state regulations, standards, and frameworks such as HIPAA, NIST, ISO, and COBIT to provide a healthcare organization with a broad and adaptable tool for assessing risk.

Because, to date, no specific risk management framework or tool has been prescribed for healthcare organizations, there is a tremendous amount of variation in risk management programs. That means some organizations do not have a formal process, some do but it is inadequate, and some do too much just to be safe. Few organizations reportedly manage risk management correctly. The results of studies such as the HIMSS annual privacy and security surveys and the judgments after data breaches reveal this. It is not the healthcare organizations' fault entirely. In an effort to allow for flexibility in the guidance to accommodate organization size, mission, complexity, and capabilities, the guidance ends up open to interpretation. For instance, HIPAA calls for controls for protecting information that are "reasonable and appropriate." Depending on the healthcare organization, the decision-makers involved, and the level of information risk tolerance, these are terms with overly broad definitions, which can result in vulnerabilities that are not addressed, wasted resources, and ineffectiveness.

This is where a framework like HITRUST CSF has proven beneficial. The CSF is a product of collaboration among healthcare and IT professionals. The approach is to be more prescriptive because the diverse set of existing requirements from NIST, HIPAA, and so on, are integrated into an efficient set of standards that make sense to healthcare. Prescriptive does not mean inflexible, however. The CSF accommodates the diversity of information systems found in healthcare organizations. Built into the CSF is a concept of approved alternate controls to meet risk mitigation or compensation strategy against an identified vulnerability when the prescribed control is infeasible. As the CSF grows in use and popularity, it will be more of a trusted benchmark for compliance, rather than the current state of healthcare testing itself to be "reasonable and appropriate," with each organization for itself.

Chapter Review

Understanding the dynamic regulatory environment in healthcare can be overwhelming. The protection of information is rooted in national privacy and security laws. Those laws typically match international governing directives, although most countries do not have healthcare-specific laws like those in the United States. Where US law and international laws differ and healthcare information must be shared, agreements such as Safe Harbor, and more recently Privacy Shield, have been enacted to help bridge the differences. You will rely primarily on local laws and industry-specific guidelines to inform internal policies and procedures to govern the use of PHI. However, you must be familiar with prevailing national and international guidance, most of which we covered in this chapter.

In this chapter, we introduced some of the primary regulatory guidance that directs healthcare information protection. You must be familiar with guidance in leading regulations to avoid legal problems and improve your organization's policies and procedures. There are regulations with national and international impact, such as PIPEDA and the EU DPD, which has been replaced with the GDPR. These are examples of regulations that outline safeguards for privacy and security across all entities that collect, store, and transfer sensitive personal information. You also studied pertinent regulation applicable to the healthcare industry specifically. The HIPAA Privacy and Security Rules, HITECH, and the Omnibus Final Rule are examples of significant legislation you will want to understand as you work in the US healthcare industry. Knowing the laws and directives that govern information protection includes awareness of the regulatory agencies that are responsible for creating and enforcing the guidance. You may desire to take advantage of opportunities to participate in rulemaking with these organizations, such as HHS with HIPAA.

Understanding regulation and standards that have jurisdiction or applicability will also determine some important components of data collection and use as well as implementation of technology in healthcare organizations. It is important to know the types of sensitive personal information that you will handle and use in your work as a healthcare information security and privacy practitioner. In this chapter we introduced the categories of personally identifiable information (PII) and protected health information (PHI) and the data elements of which each consists. There are regulatory authority issues that emerge when dealing with these categories of information. As we applied technology advancements such as cloud computing and medical device management, we explored the concerns relevant to trans-border data flows and regulatory jurisdiction. Related to the regulatory authority, we also covered the roles and responsibilities that some regulations, such as EU DPD and GDPR, have established with specific obligations. To be specific, roles such as data collector and data steward carry codified expectations in those regulations.

The chapter also emphasized the value of compliance frameworks. Frameworks are useful to help organize, implement, and enforce standards and controls within an organization. Another important aspect of the frameworks we examined is the way they assist with providing a common language and set of expectations across multiple organizations with varying missions, sizes, investment levels in information protection, and other variables that differentiate organizations. In short, frameworks enable tailored approaches to information security and privacy that make sense for a single organization and simultaneously foster a public standard of information protection. In this way, important healthcare practices such as interconnection of technologies such as EHRs, and information sharing between HIEs, for example, are made possible while ensuring the protection of patient information. Some of the leading frameworks you must recognize and use are OECD for privacy practices and NIST CSF for information.

We have introduced the complex and consequential components of the regulatory environment that surrounds information protection in general and the healthcare industry specifically. You will be expected to have a solid understanding of these areas. However, legal interpretation or jurisdictional concerns are areas in which you will rely on partnerships with attorneys and legislative liaison personnel in your organization, where these exist.

The key takeaway from this chapter is that healthcare information protection occurs in a complex and dynamic environment. Your roles and responsibilities are steeped in laws, standards, and frameworks in a highly regulated industry. As you continue through the rest of the book, you will see that the material in this chapter is foundational to protecting healthcare information.

Questions

1. A data incident reporting policy would identify that breaches of at least what number of individual records must be promptly reported to the US Department of Health and Human Services?

   A. All breaches

   B. More than 500

   C. More than 5000

   D. A number based on hospital average daily census

2. Which amendment of HIPAA first made business associates directly subject to the law?

   A. HIPAA Security Rule

   B. Omnibus Final Rule

   C. Business associate agreement

   D. HITECH Act

3. Of the following, which would be found within the Organization for Economic Cooperation and Development (OECD) privacy principles?

   A. Collection limitation

   B. De-identification

   C. Onward transfer

   D. Choice and consent

4. The Cybersecurity Act of 2015 led to the establishment of several groups, including the 405(d) task force, with objectives that include which of the following?

   A. Public and private information sharing across industry entities

   B. Development of a cybersecurity framework for healthcare

   C. Recommendations for government sanctions against medical device manufacturers

   D. Nomination of a US National CISO for healthcare

5. According to PIPEDA, informed decisions and consent are possible only when an individual can understand what he or she is acknowledging and signing. This is an element of which principle?

   A. Openness

   B. Identifying purpose

   C. Consent

   D. Accounting of disclosures

6. To bridge any privacy differences between the European Union and United States, the _____ was developed using the EU DPD.

   A. Fair information principles

   B. Privacy Rule

   C. Generally acceptable privacy principles

   D. Safe Harbor

7. The international standard that requires that data collection meet the conditions of transparency, legitimate purpose, and proportionality is the _____.

    A. EU DPD

    B. ISO/IEC 29100, Information technology – Security techniques – Privacy framework

    D. Health Insurance Portability and Accountability Act

    E. Generally acceptable privacy principles

8. ISO/IEC 27001: Information Security Management outlines the concept and implementation of risk _____.

    A. assessment

    B. tolerance

    C. measurement

    D. perspective

9. A healthcare organization in France receives a request by an individual French citizen to delete the information the organization has about them. A patient visit was recorded for an emergency department outpatient event because of a drug overdose when the individual was a minor, seven years ago. How should the organization handle the request?

    A. Amend the record with the request for deletion

    B. Deny the request because the event may be relevant to law enforcement

    C. Data mask the reason for the visit and provide a copy to the individual

    D. Explain why it will take a week to identify the data and delete the record

10. One of the categories of the Framework Core in the NIST CSF that would include measurement of security control maturity for threat intelligence and security incident alerting is:

    A. Identify

    B. Protect

    C. Detect

    D. Respond

Answers

1. **B.** This is a straightforward question that is fundamental to understanding and reporting healthcare data breaches. HHS has determined that 500 records delineate the requirement for prompt notification. After 500 records, various additional actions must happen, including notifying patients and the local media in some cases. Of course, more than 5000 records would also meet this requirement, but the phrase "at least" makes option B the correct answer and matches the HIPAA law. All breaches are eventually reported in aggregate.

Because this data incident reporting procedure is not established by any internal considerations, a measure such as average daily census is not applicable. But, knowing this fundamental number (500) helps you take the proper internal steps to respond to data breaches and mitigate any data loss.

2. **D.** The first amendment of HIPAA, the HITECH Act, made it clear that not only are covered entities subject to the HIPAA regulations, but third-party suppliers, called business associates, are also directly subject to the laws. Subsequent updates to HIPAA have clarified and strengthened this. B, Omnibus Final Rule, does include direct obligation for business associates, but it was not the first to do so. A is incorrect because the HIPAA Security Rule applied to covered entities. C, business associate agreement, is a special type of contract that outlines the obligations of the third party under HIPAA, but it is not the actual law.

3. **A.** A is the best choice because collection limitation is the one option provided that is included in the OECD Privacy Principles. Knowing and differentiating between the frameworks and international principles is difficult, because they are similar. However, in some organizations and countries, you are required to be able to distinguish the principle and the source. That said, B, de-identification is a process of taking PHI and either removing all the identifiers or creating an algorithm to change the identifiers to make them unconnected to a person. C, onward transfer, is a concept covered under Safe Harbor, and D, choice, and consent, is a principle under GAPP. If your responsibilities do not include memorizing the principles and their sources, you should concentrate on knowing the definitions of the principles themselves.

4. **A.** A strategic objective of the Cybersecurity Act of 2015 was to foster greater public and private information sharing across industry entities such as healthcare organizations, government agencies, academic institutions, and other healthcare and security-focused organizations. B is not accurate because the group was not specifically tasked with creating a framework and, in fact, concentrated on recommendations for adopting current frameworks. C is incorrect because the security of medical devices was a concern with the task groups, but punishment or sanctions against medical device manufacturers was not a focus. D is incorrect because the groups were not charged with creating any national-level positions, including a CISO for healthcare.

5. **A.** The definition of the principle of openness includes the concept of consent and understanding. A data collector must provide openness in their policies and practices so individuals can make proper choices. B is a valid principle but relates to the data collector assuring that information is gathered and used for a specific purpose. When that purpose ends, the data is no longer maintained and is destroyed in a secure fashion. Consent, C, is only partially current because it is a part of the question but does not satisfy the element of making sure the individual can understand to what he or she is consenting. D is incorrect primarily because it is not a principle under PIPEDA. However, knowing that accounting of disclosures is a retrospective view of the use of information, it would support the principle of openness and possibly continued consent and understanding, but not prior to information collection, as openness does.

6. D. The correct answer is Safe Harbor, which is the method to address any perceived gap in the privacy practices of the United States from the EU perspective. A, the fair information principles, in this context, are related to the OECD framework that represents widely accepted concepts concerning protecting privacy. B, the Privacy Rule, is an amendment to US HIPAA law and is not applicable to the European Union. Though generally acceptable privacy principles, C, are internationally recognized, they are more prevalent in United States and Canadian data exchange.

7. A. As we introduce the EU DPD in this chapter, the guiding conditions of transparency, legitimate purpose, and proportionality foreshadow the finer details covered later in the book. Of course, the DPD starts with a caution to collect personal information only if you must. B, the ISO Privacy Framework, does not include these components, and C, the Health Insurance Portability and Accountability Act, is not international. Finally, the generally acceptable privacy principles, D, have similar concepts, but because the EU DPD specifically frames itself around these conditions, the EU DPD is correct.

8. A. ISO 27001 is the central source from the ISO family of standards that introduces and formalizes the process of risk assessment in organizations. B is incorrect because tolerance is a way to mitigate or deal with risk, so it is a response to issues found in the risk assessment. C, measurement, and D, perspective, are at best synonymous terms for assessment or mitigation (of risk) but are not used by ISO/IEC 27001.

9. D. Key to this question is the location of the healthcare record. GDPR includes a "right to be forgotten," which has exceptions, but none of the options given would satisfy a reason to deny the request by the individual, an EU citizen, to have their information deleted. Although the one-week timeframe for processing may seem long, a valid explanation is implied by the scenario. The right to be forgotten is satisfied in this option as long as the action is taken in a timely manner. A, amending the record with the request for deletion, would not satisfy the requirement for a right to be forgotten; in fact, the action would be in direct opposition of the requirement. B is incorrect because law enforcement is not actually requiring the information and after seven years it is unlikely this information would be useful to law enforcement. C, masking the reason for the visit, does not fulfill the right of the individual to have all of the information removed from the healthcare organization data stores.

10. C. According to the NIST CSF, Anomalies and Events and Security Continuous Monitoring are components of the Detect core framework element. Gathering and using threat intelligence as well as the security alerting for anomalies fits within this category. The other answers are valid core framework elements and have measurable control specifications, but the specific actions presented by the question are measured elsewhere.

References

1. From the 2019 National Electric Manufacturing Association standard, *Manufacturer Disclosure Statement for Medical Device Security,* ANSI/NEMA HN 1-2019, which can be downloaded or purchased from https://www.nema .org/Standards/Pages/Manufacturer-Disclosure-Statement-for-Medical-Device-Security.aspx.

2. Silver, J. D. 2011. "Computer outage at UPMC called 'rare': Systemwide disruption potentially dangerous, expert warns." *Pittsburgh Post-Gazette,* December 24, http://old.post-gazette.com/pg/11358/1199140-53-0 .stm?cmpid=news.xml#ixzz2sNyCu9SQ.

3. US Department of Health and Human Services. 2013. "Modifications to the HIPAA Privacy, Security, Enforcement, and Breach Notification Rules Under the Health Information Technology for Economic and Clinical Health Act and the Genetic Information Nondiscrimination Act; Other Modifications to the HIPAA Rules." 45 CFR Parts 160 and 164. p. 78. https://www.govinfo.gov/ content/pkg/FR-2013-01-25/pdf/2013-01073.pdf.

4. From the Thales eSecurity website at https://dtr-healthcare.thalesesecurity.com/. The *2018 Data Threat Report – Healthcare Edition,* can be downloaded from the same site.

5. From the 2019 IBM Security and Ponemon Institute, *2019 Cost of a Data Breach Study: Global Overview.* Register to download the report at https://www.ibm .com/security/data-breach.

6. Reese, F. 2019. "Ranking the reputation of the 100 most visible companies in America." *Stacker,* June 19, https://thestacker.com/stories/3211/ranking-reputation-100-most-visible-companies-america.

7. *HIPAA Journal.* 2019. "Summary of 2018 HIPAA Fines and Settlements," https://www.hipaajournal.com/summary-2018-hipaa-fines-and-settlements.

8. From 2017 Accenture Security study, "Cost of Cyber Crime Study: Insights on the Security Investments that Make a Difference in Healthcare." https://www .accenture.com/_acnmedia/pdf-81/accenture-health-cost-of-cyber-crime-study.pdf.

9. Ponemon Institute and Accenture Security. 2017. "2017 Cost of Cyber Crime Study: Insights on the Security Investments that Make a Difference." https:// cdn2.hubspot.net/hubfs/85462/2018/2018_VUENUE/2018_BLACK%20HAT/ Accenture-2017CostCybercrime-US-FINAL.pdf?t=1521831469946.

10. Ponemon Institute. 2016. *Sixth Annual Benchmark Study on Privacy & Security of Healthcare Data.* https://www.ponemon.org/local/upload/file/Sixth%20 Annual%20Patient%20Privacy%20%26%20Data%20Security%20Report%20 FINAL%206.pdf.

11. Cobb, S. 2016. "Healthcare data breaches lead patients to withhold information from doctors." welivesecurity, Feb 18, https://www.welivesecurity.com/2016/02/18/security-privacy-patients-withholding.

12. From Hu, L., S. Sparenborg, and B. Tai. 2011. "Privacy protection for patients with substance use problems." *Substance Abuse and Rehabilitation*, 2: 227–233. Download at https://www.dovepress.com/privacy-protection-for-patients-with-substance-use-problems-peer-reviewed-article-SAR.

13. US Government Accountability Office. 2008. "Privacy: Alternatives Exist for Enhancing Protection of Personally Identifiable Information," GAO-08-536. http://www.gao.gov/new.items/d08536.pdf.

14. National Institute of Standards and Technology. 2010. *Guide to Protecting the Confidentiality of Personally Identifiable Information (PII)*, Special Publication 800-122. https://nvlpubs.nist.gov/nistpubs/Legacy/SP/nistspecialpublication800-122.pdf.

15. Regulation (EU) 2016/679 of the European Parliament and of the Council of 27 April 2016 on the protection of natural persons with regard to the processing of personal data and on the free movement of such data, and repealing Directive 95/46/EC (General Data Protection Regulation). https://eur-lex.europa.eu/legal-content/EN/TXT/HTML/?uri=CELEX:32016R0679&from=EN.

16. Wolford, B. 2020. "What are the GDPR fines?" GDPR.eu, https://gdpr.eu/fines.

17. Information Commissioner's Office (ICO). 2020. "What are 'controllers' and 'processors'?" ICO, https://ico.org.uk/for-organisations/guide-to-data-protection/guide-to-the-general-data-protection-regulation-gdpr/controllers-and-processors/what-are-controllers-and-processors/.

18. Office for Human Research Protections. 2018. "Protection of Human Subjects." Title 45, Subtitle A, Subchapter A, Part 46, Code of Federal Regulations. HHS.gov. p. US 45 CFR 46.101. e-CFR, https://www.ecfr.gov/cgi-bin/retrieveECFR?gp=&SID=83cd09e1c0f5c6937cd9d7513160fc3f&pitd=20180719&n=pt45.1.46&r=PART&ty=HTML.

19. Department of Health, Education, and Welfare. 1979. "The Belmont Report: Ethical Principles and Guidelines for the Protection of Human Subjects of Research." https://www.hhs.gov/ohrp/regulations-and-policy/belmont-report/read-the-belmont-report/index.html.

20. US Department of Commerce. 2000. "Safe Harbor Privacy Principles." https://2016.export.gov/safeharbor/eu/eg_main_018475.asp.

21. US Department of Commerce. "Safe Harbor Privacy Principles."

22. Directive 95/46/EC of the European Parliament and of the Council of 24 October 1995 on the protection of individuals with regard to the processing of personal data and on the free movement of such data. http://eur-lex.europa.eu/LexUriServ/LexUriServ.do?uri=CELEX:31995L0046:en:HTML.

23. US Depart of Health and Human Services. 2012. "Guidance Regarding Methods for De-identification of Protected Health Information in Accordance with the Health Insurance Portability and Accountability Act (HIPAA) Privacy Rule." https://www.hhs.gov/sites/default/files/ocr/privacy/hipaa/understanding/coveredentities/De-identification/hhs_deid_guidance.pdf.

24. Office for Civil Rights. 2020. "Direct Liability of Business Associates." HHS .gov. https://www.hhs.gov/hipaa/for-professionals/privacy/guidance/business-associates/factsheet/index.html.

25. Office of the Privacy Commissioner of Canada. 2019. "The Privacy Act in brief." https://www.priv.gc.ca/en/privacy-topics/privacy-laws-in-canada/the-privacy-act/pa_brief.

26. Office of the Privacy Commissioner of Canada. "The Privacy Act in brief."

27. Commission Decision of 20 December 2001 pursuant to Directive 95/46/EC of the European Parliament and of the Council on the adequate protection of personal data provided by the Canadian Personal Information Protection and Electronic Documents Act (notified under document number C(2001) 4539) (2002/2/EC). https://eur-lex.europa.eu/legal-content/EN/TXT/?uri=CELEX:02002D0002-20161217.

28. National Institute of Standards and Technology. 2020. *NIST Privacy Framework: A Tool for Improving Privacy Through Enterprise Risk Management.* https://www.nist.gov/system/files/documents/2020/01/16/NIST%20Privacy%20Framework_V1.0.pdf.

29. UK National Health Service (NHS), Department of Health. 2013. "What are the Caldicott Principles?" Information Governance Toolkit, https://www.igt.hscic.gov.uk/Caldicott2Principles.aspx.

30. The Organisation for Economic Co-operation and Development (OECD). 2019. "Member Countries' Budget Contributions for 2019." http://www.oecd.org/about/budget/member-countries-budget-contributions.htm.

31. The Organisation for Economic Co-operation and Development (OECD). 2013. "The OECD Privacy Framework." http://www.oecd.org/sti/ieconomy/oecd_privacy_framework.pdf.

32. International Association of Privacy Professionals (IAPP). 2020. "Resource Center: Fair Information Practice Principles." https://iapp.org/resources/article/fair-information-practices/

33. Asia-Pacific Economic Cooperation. 2019. "What is the Cross-Border Privacy Rules System?" https://www.apec.org/About-Us/About-APEC/Fact-Sheets/What-is-the-Cross-Border-Privacy-Rules-System.

34. American Institute of Certified Public Accountants, Inc. (AICPA) & Canadian Institute of Chartered Accountants (CICA). 2011. "AICPA/CICA Privacy Maturity Model." https://iapp.org/media/pdf/resource_center/aicpa_cica_privacy_maturity_model_final-2011.pdf.

35. US Department of Health and Human Services. 2018. "Health Industry Cybersecurity Practices: Managing Threats and Protecting Patients." https://www.phe.gov/Preparedness/planning/405d/Pages/hic-practices.aspx.

36. An example of relevant ISO standards that are made publicly available found at the ISO website at http://standards.iso.org/ittf/PubliclyAvailableStandards/index.html.

37. ISO/IEC 29100 is available for download at https://standards.iso.org/ittf/PubliclyAvailableStandards/c045123_ISO_IEC_29100_2011.zip

38. National Institute of Standards and Technology. 2018. *Framework for Improving Critical Infrastructure Cybersecurity.* https://nvlpubs.nist.gov/nistpubs/CSWP/NIST.CSWP.04162018.pdf.

39. National Institute of Standards and Technology. 2019. "Cybersecurity Framework." https://www.nist.gov/cyberframework/frequently-asked-questions/framework-basics#components.

40. HIPAA Journal. 2019. "2019 Cost of a Data Breach Study Reveals Increase in U.S. Healthcare Data Breach Costs," July 24, https://www.hipaajournal.com/2019-cost-of-a-data-breach-study-healthcare-data-breach-costs.

CHAPTER 5

Privacy and Security in Healthcare

This chapter covers Domain 5, "Privacy and Security in Healthcare," of the HCISPP certification. After you read and study this chapter, you should be able to:

- Identify key information security objectives and attributes
- Understand common information security definitions and concepts
- Know fundamental privacy terms and principles used in information protection
- Comprehend the interdependence of privacy and security in healthcare organizations
- Categorize sensitive health information according to US and international guidelines
- Define privacy and security terms as they apply to healthcare
- Distinguish methods for reducing or mitigating the sensitivity of healthcare information

The importance of understanding and applying proper privacy and security controls on healthcare information is foundational to your success as a healthcare information privacy and security professional. The healthcare industry is highly regulated in the United States as is the protection of personal data in most other countries. As we move from our discussion of the regulatory environments that impact our healthcare organizations, we will examine specific information security and privacy definitions and concepts that regulations and ultimately our policies and procedures are built upon. In this chapter, you will learn to understand security objectives and attributes, including the principles of confidentiality, integrity, and availability. You'll also learn about accountability, which is often a major part of the discussion of security as it relates to healthcare organizations. You will also learn general security definitions as they apply to healthcare.

As with most healthcare organizations, your organization likely faces a multitude of challenges, not the least of which is the need to apply a reasonable standard of due care and due diligence to safeguard the confidentiality, integrity, and availability of patient healthcare information. Whether the intent is to improve patient care, to protect the sensitive information we need to serve our customers, or to ensure compliance with regulatory requirements, the challenges are significant.

This chapter addresses security- and privacy-related topics together. This is in part because it also includes an overview of the relationship between information security and privacy. *Privacy* involves controlling access to personal information and the control a person can have over information discovery and sharing. *Security* is administrative, technical, and physical mechanism that protects information from unauthorized access, alteration, and loss. In short, privacy is about *what* we protect, and security is about *how* we protect it.[1]

> **EXAM TIP** You will be tested on your basic understanding of security and privacy concepts and principles, the relationship between security and privacy, and the types of information requiring protection in the healthcare industry.

Privacy and security are important to everyone involved in healthcare, including health facility employees, patients, family members, and care givers. It also applies to anyone who works for organizations that play cursory roles in patient care—for example, workers at a clearinghouse for healthcare information who never work directly providing patient healthcare. These workers also have obligations to ensure that the privacy and security of patient data are maintained in accordance with their employers' policies and applicable regulations.

Guiding Principles of Information Security: Confidentiality, Integrity, and Availability

Data security has three guiding principles: confidentiality, integrity, and availability (CIA).[2] In general, it does not matter where you work, where you live, or what organizations you support; these principles remain the same. In addition to understanding CIA, you need to understand the importance of accountability, another central concept akin to CIA.

The CIA model is driven by the implementation of a combination of technical, administrative, and physical information protection controls. You should understand the relationship between CIA components in general and within your organization. Depending on a variety of concerns, including your role in the organization, the organization's mission and size, applicable regulatory authorities, and sensitivity of information, one component may be emphasized over the others. For example, as a system administrator, providing integrity and availability may be more appropriate to your job description than providing confidentiality.

The prevailing illustration used for the CIA triad is an equilateral triangle that indicates the "weight" of each component as being equal to the others. The reality of these relationships, however, depends on situational factors. This is an important concept, because the emphasis placed on these three factors represents the assessment and balance

Figure 5-1
The CIA is often depicted as a triangle that implies the relationship of the three components.

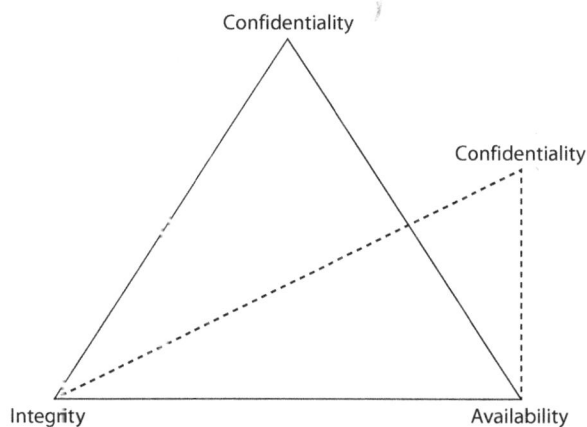

of choices for security and privacy tools within your organization. So, for example, in your organization, confidentiality may be considered more of a priority than the other two factors, which means you'll have increased focus on access controls and encryption. Or if data availability takes precedence, you may invest more in technical solutions for disaster recovery.

Figure 5-1 shows a comparison of the CIA triad in two scenarios. In the solid line triangle, each component is weighted equally. The triangle comprising dotted lines depicts an emphasis on confidentiality in implementing security and privacy controls.

Confidentiality

Confidentiality relates to protecting sensitive proprietary information or personally identifiable information (PII) from unauthorized disclosure. The objective is to control access to a limited amount of data so that only those with proper authorization are allowed to access it. Security controls are implemented to protect confidentiality and avoid unauthorized disclosure In healthcare, a breach in confidentiality could include an employee calling a media outlet to "anonymously" inform them that a public figure has been admitted to a rehabilitation facility. A similar example of a confidentiality breach, though beyond the scope of healthcare, also occurs when a fan magazine publishes photos of famous people enjoying personal time at a beach or other locale.

Although confidentiality is an important aspect in protecting information in any organization, healthcare information, in particular, warrants a higher level of protection and enforcement—consider, for example, an unauthorized disclosure that an individual has HIV, a psychiatric disorder, or another health concern.

Healthcare data confidentiality requirements are recognized internationally. For example, in the United States, the National Institute of Standards and Technology (NIST) has issued directives regarding CIA for healthcare information, and within the scope of confidentiality it states the following in a 2008 publication:

> The confidentiality impact level is the effect of unauthorized disclosure of health care delivery services on the ability of responsible agencies to provide and support the delivery of health care to its beneficiaries will have only a limited adverse effect on agency operations, assets, or individuals. Special Factors Affecting Confidentiality Impact Determination: Some information associated with health care involves confidential patient information subject to the Privacy Act and to HIPAA [Health Insurance Portability and Accountability Act]. The Privacy Act Information provisional impact levels are documented in the Personal Identity and Authentication information type. Other information (e.g., information proprietary to hospitals, pharmaceutical companies, insurers, and care givers) must be protected under rules governing proprietary information and procurement management. In some cases, unauthorized disclosure of this information such as privacy-protected medical records can have serious consequences for agency operations. In such cases, the confidentiality impact level may be moderate.[3]

In Canada, the Canadian Privacy Act, Section 63, states the following:

> Subject to this Act, the Privacy Commissioner and every person acting on behalf or under the direction of the Commissioner shall not disclose any information that comes to their knowledge in the performance of their duties and functions under this Act.[4]

In healthcare, confidentiality is not only important to protect individuals from medical and financial identity theft, but research shows that a breach of confidentiality can impact patient care. In some cases, where breaches are all too common, some patients are worried their private information will fall into the wrong hands.[5] As mentioned in Chapter 4, providers understand that patients who fear their information might be disclosed in an unauthorized manner may delay seeking care or withhold information.

Specific circumstances require additional confidentiality considerations. For example, patient care information related to HIV, behavioral health, substance abuse, and children's health often have even more restrictive confidentiality requirements than other types of information.

Whether in the United States under HIPAA or in the European Union under the General Data Protection Regulation (GDPR), confidentiality requirements often continue even after an employee's role has changed or after an employee leaves a position or an organization. Most healthcare regulatory requirements clearly state that even when an individual no longer has access to the information, he or she is still required to keep the information confidential. For example, in the European Union, the Data Protection Directive, Article 28, Section 7, states the following:

> Member States shall provide that the members and staff of the supervisory authority, even after their employment has ended, are to be subject to a duty of professional secrecy with regard to confidential information to which they have access.[6]

By law, data collectors are responsible, in the United States and in most other nations, for maintaining the confidentiality of the information forever, even if the patient discloses the information. Of course, the patient can give consent for specific disclosures, but generally, regulations do not permit the healthcare organization to disclose the information outside of legal allowances. Further, the organization must protect the information from disclosure until it can legally and properly destroy it.

Integrity

Integrity is a security pursuit that is intended to protect information from unauthorized editing, alteration, or amendment. Imagine a scenario in which malicious code (such as a software virus) is introduced via a malware software application into a medical device. If, for example, that medical device is responsible for dosing medications to a patient, and the virus causes all decimal points to move to the right one space, the resulting dosage change can be significant, and potentially life-threatening, to the patient (for example, a dose of 0.5 ml may have a disastrous effect if only 0.05 ml is indicated). The integrity of healthcare data is important for patient safety and for many other reasons.

Data integrity is achieved by protecting the accuracy, quality, and completeness of the information. Integrity of information is maintained by assuring that any changes made to data are authorized and correct or not made at all. Security controls for integrity follow the data flow through the lifecycle of the information. When you examine the process of data collection and use in a healthcare setting, the data often changes format, and various data elements are combined, parsed out, or even aggregated. Throughout this process, however, the integrity of the data must remain intact. A patient name or date of birth, for instance, must remain the same even if it is collected as Jane Doe, December 14, 1970, at admissions and then changed to Doe, Jane, 12/14/70, after it gets transcribed into the billing system. Although this is an exceedingly simplified example, maintaining data integrity across data flow is one reason for the existence of standards such as the US Centers for Disease Control and Prevention (CDC) guideline ICD-10 for coding patient encounters, and Health Level (HL7), a set of international standards for transmitting health information across organizations and systems. Using standard data sets and transaction codes helps to assure data integrity.

To accomplish integrity, several methods are used, including error checking and validation procedures. The following list includes some generic data integrity approaches that apply, some sample technical methods, and the security improvements that are addressed. The list is adapted from data integrity guidance from the NIST SP 1800-11 (Draft), *Data Integrity: Recovering from Ransomware and Other Destructive Events*:[7]

- **Corruption testing**   This procedure includes the use of extract-transform-load (ETL) data testing applications, reliable backups, and TCP/IP checksum testing to examine unauthorized changes. The process includes logging and auditing for a retrospective review of data. The testing uses file hashing and encryption algorithms to identify cybersecurity events and data alteration.

- **Secure storage**   This process includes encrypted backups and immutable (unchangeable) storage solutions with write-once, read-many (WORM) properties. Technical processes, such as redundant storage—namely RAID— are storage configuration solutions that satisfy secure storage and data integrity protection.

- **Logging**   A significant component of data integrity is to collect and enable the review of access to data and user activity. In this case, logging is used in alerting and analysis to discover any unusual or unauthorized activity and in legal discovery and e-forensics. It can be generated from individual systems. Several analysis tools can be used, such as security incident and event monitoring (SIEM) applications and network data capture systems.

- **Backup capability**   Data integrity is preserved through procedures that enable data to be replicated and recovered periodically. Related to secure storage, backup tools support full, incremental, and differential schedules for backup. Another approach to backups is mirroring, which is similar to a full backup except that an exact copy of the data is stored separately, matching the source. Other backup procedures store files in one encrypted storage repository.

In healthcare, information integrity has a strong association with patient care and patient safety. While unauthorized disclosure (confidentiality) may lead to an unauthorized individual having access to healthcare data, and while the unavailability of data may hinder care, the fact remains that if the data we have on a patient is not accurate, it can in fact lead to death. For example, an unconscious patient who has an allergy to a specific medication undergoing treatment cannot advise staff about his allergy. In such a case, the availability of accurate data can save his life.

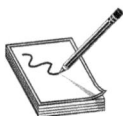

NOTE   Security controls for integrity also apply to technology and processes that assure nonrepudiation. This means that the controls in place assure the authentication of a data user or sender without the possibility of another actor impersonating the user.

Availability

Information is valuable only if it is accessible and timely. The data can be accurate and kept private, but if it is not available when it is needed, this third part of the CIA triad has failed. Availability of data is generally described as proper access at the time the information is needed. In healthcare, we can certainly understand the failure of protecting PII and ensuring that patient records are accurate. But experiencing network downtime with no contingency operations plan in place would mean the information is not available at the point of care. If the provider does not have the ability to access the information he or she needs, patient care is affected and patient safety risks increase.

Paper-based health records and procedure manual processes can exacerbate the availability issue, because they may not be as easily accessed or enacted as digitally stored information. Not having availability of information can result in improper diagnosis, inefficient or redundant tests, and in some cases adverse drug-to-drug interactions. A major assurance of availability from an information security and privacy perspective is reached through implementation of business continuity and disaster recovery procedures. These focus areas require the use of administrative, technical, and physical controls to oversee high-availability system architectures, reliable backups, secondary operating locations, and practiced recovery procedures.

Availability also relates to having only the necessary information available. Having too much information available or having unorganized raw data can pose a security issue. Privacy and security frameworks such as the DPD, GDPR, and HIPAA, for instance, address the issue of having relevant information versus having more information than is needed. Consider an example: A provider who requires a relevant prior MRI image when treating an orthopedic injury must certainly have the most recent MRI on the affected body part to compare against the latest image. However, that provider would be overwhelmed by having to search through all the images on record for unrelated care of that patient. If nothing else, the search would be time consuming and wasteful.

In addition, by limiting availability, we can prevent unauthorized disclosures or data breaches simply by not sharing unused or extra data in the transaction. For illustration, consider an example from the past. There was a time in the United States when credit card numbers were printed in their entirety on receipts. This was useful for identification purposes and convenient for the payer when proving a purchase or seeking a refund. But eventually the practice ceased, because proof of purchase could be determined in more discrete ways, such as using only the last four to six digits on the card with the other digits masked. The practice of including the entire credit card number introduced too much risk of data loss and identity theft. This is a good example of the security impact of unnecessarily disclosing too much information.

Accountability

While generally not considered part of the CIA principles, accountability is often included as a high-level security principle. Within the healthcare environment, compliance standards often treat accountability as a basic principle. Accountability in information security and privacy refers to the determination of who is responsible for proper and improper information access and use. For example, a clinician treating a patient who enters data, thereby editing the patient record, is accountable for the actions they take to enter the information. The clinician should be responsible for ensuring that the information is accurate when it is entered. Accountability intersects with the CIA principles. The individual with access should ensure the integrity of the data entered, while leveraging availability of the system, and ensuring confidentiality that the information is available only to those with proper authorization.

An organization must also demonstrate accountability for the information it collects and uses. Data use actions must be logged and audited to various degrees to prove that measures of accountability are in place. Accountability incorporates tracking actions and identification of responsible parties in retrospect after cybersecurity incidents and data breach recovery. Auditing information disclosure reports enables us to view and remediate any disclosures that may have been unauthorized, or at least to prove to government regulators that disclosures are tracked as required. Nonrepudiation also applies to account-ability. By providing protections such as digital signatures and encryption algorithms, an organization can ensure that the sender of an electronic message cannot deny sending it and that the receiver cannot deny receiving it. In this way, nonrepudiation assists organiza-tions by providing ways to prove accountability.

Understanding Security Concepts

The concepts that shape information security can seem abstract and complex. To help you understand the approaches and practices of information security, this section describes some basic approaches and methods to security that you should be familiar with. These concepts are central to information security practices and compliance, and many pro-gressive security processes are based on them.

You should be familiar with three basic aspects of security that will help you better understand the information that follows in this and other chapters: security controls, defense-in-depth, and security categorization. Understanding these important concepts may also improve your ability to do a good job in supporting and providing security and privacy in your organization.

Security Controls   Security controls include management controls (often administra-tive, such as policies or procedures), operational controls (the processes we follow to do things), and technical controls (hardware and software implementations to assist in securing computer-based resources). The organization's cost considerations and interre-lationships between security controls have a great deal of influence on the ability of the organization to deliver on its mission.

Defense-in-Depth   Defense-in-depth consists of implementation of various defen-sive controls working together for your systems or applications to protect the overall security of organizational assets. In the IT world, examples of defense-in-depth include the integrated use of antivirus and antimalware software, firewalls, encryption, intru-sion detection and prevention systems, and biometric authentication. An example of defense-in-depth in your home is an alarm system for the house that includes smoke and carbon monoxide detectors, which may or may not be separate from the smoke detectors; cameras that you can check remotely over the Internet; and smartphone apps that enables you to control lighting, entry doors, and so on. Figure 5-2 demonstrates the defense-in-depth principle, and although it may not depict a system used in larger organizations, it provides a basic understanding of how the layers of the system must rely on one another to be effective.

Security Categorization   Security categorization enables you to determine the level of security required for a system based on the information (or data) type the system uses or maintains. This book specifically addresses working with healthcare information, which includes sensitive information such as protected health information (PHI) and electronic protected health information (ePHI), personal health records (PHRs), personally iden-tifiable information (PII), and a number of other terms, depending on where you work (which can include the specific nation, continent, province, or state).

Figure 5-2
Simplified
defense-in-depth

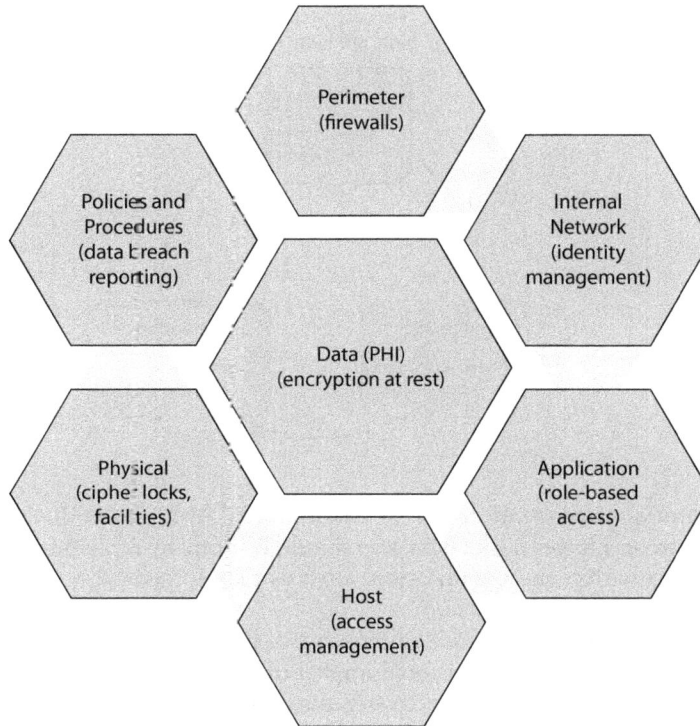

In determining the security categorization of a system, an application, or an orga-nization overall, you must first identify, or categorize, the type of information or data involved. You then review the security controls required, including those you have imple-mented and those that should be implemented (referred to as "planned"). Organiza-tions must determine the category, or categories, of information stored or used in their system, such as the healthcare information categories discussed in NIST SP 800-60, Vol. 2 Rev. 1, Section D.14.4. A similar system is shown in Figure 5-3. This method for security categorization can be adapted to fit any organization.

Note that one system may include multiple types of data—for example, your health information system may also store insurance data, billing information, employee records, and so on, which may be categorized differently than PHI and PII. To categorize a variety of data, based on the information type, the organization sets a "provisional impact level." Here's an example of how a healthcare security categorization system process might work:

If Confidentiality = Medium, Integrity = High, and Availability = Medium, the over-all security impact may be considered High if data integrity carries the most weight. An example in which data integrity might be weighted higher than the other informa-tion protection categorizations might involve a medical device like the linear accelerator used in precision radiology treatment of cancer. The data that informs the actions of the device must be protected from tampering, arguably against all other considerations so the patient does not get more or less radiation and the treatment is in the exact right area.

Figure 5-3
Categorizing
information for
security

For each: Is IMPACT
high, medium, or low?

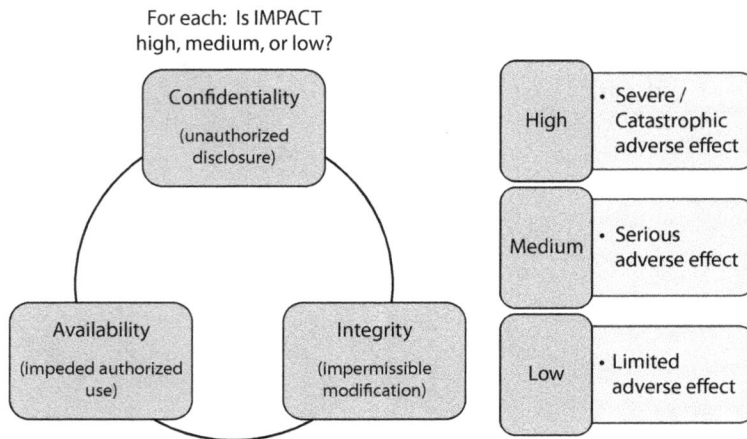

Confidentiality
(unauthorized
disclosure)

Availability
(impeded authorized
use)

Integrity
(impermissible
modification)

High
• Severe /
Catastrophic
adverse effect

Medium
• Serious
adverse effect

Low
• Limited
adverse effect

This initial categorization can be accomplished by an individual with knowledge of the data system. However, the next step should be done by representatives that serve different functions within the organization, such as IT, biomedical engineering, administration, patient care services, and so on.

The next part of the process involves two phases: the first phase involves reviewing the controls based on the provisional impact of High. In the second phase, the organization adjusts the controls based on its organization and systems. The organization also determines which controls are already in place (such as access control policies) and which ones are planned (such as training for system administrators).

In the final part, the organization finalizes the security categorization. Outside that process, the organization goes through the security controls and implements and documents how and if each control meets the criteria established.

Although this process may appear cumbersome, it is necessary to ensure that the organization adheres to security standards and can prove it to patients, government agencies, and other stakeholders. Healthcare organizations must develop strategies for protecting sensitive data. Security categorization supports developing processes, procedures, and policies as part of the organization's strategic vision. Categorization leads to effective implementation of established security standards. The result is useful documentation of the organization's security approach that guides the implementation of security controls in a tiered fashion, based on the systems operated and the data protected.

Identity and Access Management

An organization's IAM strategy defines and manages the roles and access privileges of network users and the circumstances in which users are granted or denied access privileges. NIST guidelines describe IAM as a set of critical cybersecurity controls that function together to ensure the right people and things have the right access to the right resources at the right time.[8] A successful healthcare IAM strategy must incorporate information use requirements with a complex technical environment and progressively demanding compliance requirements.

Although many technologies are available to help an organization create a general IAM strategy, each organization's IAM strategy must align with its particular requirements, especially with regard to accessing PHI, PHRs, and PII. Following are a few examples of IAM:

- **Password-management tools** These can be used to create complex passwords on request, and they provide a secure, encrypted repository for current passwords for retrieval as needed.

- **Privileged account management systems** For users and accounts with elevated levels of permissions, or for administrative accounts, these systems provide management assistance, often with automation, and an auditable record of account use.

- **Provisioning (and deprovisioning) software** As employees are hired, this software maps permissions and access to various resources based on users' roles or organizational policy (provisioning). User permissions and access are reviewed periodically, and when they're no longer needed (such as upon employee termination), the software supports removing the user's permissions and access (deprovisioning).

- **Certificate management** Certificates are digital keys used to secure data through encryption. Certificate management includes approval, issuance, inventory, distribution, controlling, suspension, and retirement. Certificates held by subscribers are documented by a registration authority, or responsible certificate authority, which is normally an external entity that issues trusted digital keys based on the authority's initial root certificate.

- **Single-sign on (SSO) applications** This access management solution enables secure authentication to more than one system managed by an organization using a single user credential. The underlying identity framework is usually the Lightweight Directory Access Protocol (LDAP) and the necessary LDAP credential databases to coordinate information services.

- **Multifactor authentication (MFA)** This additional layer of identification and access protection enhances the use of a password and user ID as credentials. MFFA requires two or more pieces of evidence, to include something you have (such as a key fob or smartcard), something you know (such as a passcode or PIN), or something you are (such as facial recognition).

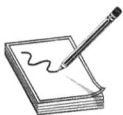

NOTE MFA is also referred to as two-factor authentication (2FA) because it requires at least two layers of identification. However, the use of two passwords does not constitute MFA or 2FA; the factors must be from different authentication components.

IAM helps the organization administer and secure credentials, privileges, and authentication processes in a consistent way. The various systems and tools that can be used to provide IAM can scale to the size of the organization and distribute access across multiple business and clinical entities. Centralized IAM models use Active Directory, which holds user credentials in one repository. Federated architectures use applications such as Ping-Federate to distribute user credentials across multiple systems with authentication requirements. Federated IAM may use single sign-on (SSO) to help reduce administrative fatigue from having to provide credentials for each system. The SSO solution would provide a level of trust that would be shared with each individual system even though user credentials are not stored in each. In any case, an IAM system provides a capability to guard against excessive authorization levels and protect against compromised user credentials.

The IAM security controls and mechanisms that accompany security processes constitute a valuable information protection resource to monitor and enforce policies and procedures in the healthcare organization. The processes of granting access, creating access roles, reviewing access periodically, and terminating access were once a manually accomplished, instance by instance, using rosters and spreadsheets that was a very labor intensive, frustrating process. Today, many IAM systems are available to help organizations automate and improve security by reducing human error and neglect due to the monotony of the required tasks.

Access Control

The ability to use a technical asset is defined as *access*. The term usually refers to a technical capability such as reading, creating, modifying, or deleting a file; executing a program; or using an external connection. The term access is often mistakenly confused with "authorization" and "authentication." Access control protects sensitive information and is made up of all of the actions and controls put in place to regulate viewing, storing, copying, modifying, transferring, and deleting information. Controlling access also includes limitations of time and situation. For instance, an end user may be allowed to access a system at a predetermined time, but not afterward, or for certain reasons, but not others. An example of situational access is provided in an emergency room, where physicians are given some access to a patient's behavioral health records at that point of care, but the same physicians would not have access to those records in a primary care setting.

Access control includes the following:

- **Authorization**   Policies and procedures for determining which permissions an end user will have and when (that is, a user's level of access).

- **Authentication**   The process used to verify the identity of end users and validate that they are who they claim to be.

- **Identification**   The act of indicating who a person is—in computing technologies, a person is usually identified by a username or identity code (for example, firstname, lastname). (Note that the identification does not include combining this username with a password, which is considered authentication, and combines a simple identity code with a verification code, or password.)

- **Nonrepudiation**   Use of identification authentication methods and tools in a digital transaction to provide indisputable or assured proof of who the sender and/or the recipient of the data is.

Organizations implement access controls to permit legitimate use by authorized personnel while preventing unauthorized use. Keep in mind that "legitimate use" can change depending on the situations at hand, however, so access control must occur at various levels and at key intervals of access. For instance, access control can be implemented at the operating-system level to safeguard files and storage media, and at the database level to guard against unauthorized access and potential corruption of data. In addition, well-designed applications and web services typically enforce several independent access controls to layer the protection, even if an SSO technology is used.

Access control is an effort to prevent unauthorized use, but it also allows for sharing of sensitive information at an acceptable level of risk to the organization. Without access controls in place, most organizations would consider it too risky to share PHI or PII, and that would prevent or degrade patient care in a digitized healthcare environment. For access control to be effective, an authentication process must support the controls.

Identifying personnel properly and granting them appropriate access levels can involve two types of authentication: The first, MFA, is present when at least two conditions are satisfied independently by the same individual who wants to access a network, system, or application. In many contexts, MFA and 2FA are synonymous based on how many conditions must be satisfied. When an organization implements proper MFA, the process is recognized as strong authentication. The second type, computer-based access controls, or logical access controls, determine who (a person) or what (a process) can have access to a category of data or a computing system. These controls may be built into the operating system; may be incorporated into applications, programs, or major utilities (for example, database management systems or communications systems); or may be implemented through add-on security packages. Logical access controls may be implemented internally in the computer system being protected or they may be implemented in external devices.

Logical access controls can help protect the integrity and availability of the following:

- Software applications that include EHR, as well as underlying operating systems, such as Windows and Unix, from unauthorized changes and misuses

- Sensitive information through management and limitation of access by people and system processes, which reduces risk of unauthorized access or disclosure

Access controls can be administered globally for access to an entire network or at a single system level. A single system access control could be implemented to restrict access to one or two people for the ER pharmaceutical cabinet, for example. Access controls augment and enforce the administrative and physical controls that work together to protect sensitive information and, in the case of the pharmaceutical cabinet, access to controlled assets.

EXAM TIP Know the exception to these access controls in HIPAA termed "break glass" procedures. This provision in HIPAA allows systems that include ePHI to be accessed in emergency situations, when, under normal conditions, access would be prohibited. The intention is to avoid patient safety or patient care adverse events resulting from lack of information and system availability.

Access control models are used to enforce authentication and authorization guidelines, and the controls used are automated. (Imagine how difficult it would be to check the credentials of each end user manually every time they desired access to data or to a system!) The common models for access control are mandatory, discretionary, role-based, attribute-based, and context-based. Some hybrid models combine features of each, but these are the most prevalent structures and approaches. You will recognize some overlap and common features in each and how they work together.

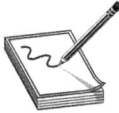

> **NOTE** Although these access control models are enforced by computer policies and configurations, some information security guidelines have provisions for overriding the policies and configurations, or for emergency access. The best example is the provision in HIPAA to provide "break glass" access in emergency situations. In other words, the system has a method for providing access to someone who may not have authorization or access under normal circumstances.

Mandatory Access Control

In mandatory access control (MAC), a central authority, such as the organization's chief information officer (CIO), creates the access control policy, which is implemented by the IT department. The actual access control is enforced at the hardware or operating system level as a technical control. Most often, MAC is used in organizations that handle classified information, such as the military and, in some cases, a healthcare organization, where rigid, centralized controls are used in some applications and networked resources. In this model, individual system or data owners cannot change the level of access allowed.

A MAC model depends on proper security categorization of information, because the access policy in this case most likely will be determined by the sensitivity of the information. In healthcare organizations, information confidentiality is vital, so the central authority can determine who is allowed access to information. Improperly categorized information can lock out individuals who may need access, or it may allow access to those who have no need to know the information. Neither case is desired. On the positive side, having a central authority enforce the access control makes standard, equitable policies possible.

Discretionary Access Control

A discretionary access control (DAC) model is used if access control is more decentralized or delegated to the owner of an individual system or to the owner of the data itself. Privileges are granted by the system owner or data owner to whomever he or she considers authorized to access the information. DAC is more flexible than MAC, but it introduces greater risk. For instance, once someone has access to view a file, the system owner has little control over whether that person decides to copy it and share it with others.

Role-Based Access Control

Role-based access control (RBAC) is probably the most prevalent type of nondiscretionary access control model, in which system owners determine the level of access based on a user's or group's job function or organizational role, versus individual attributes.

Role-based access is implemented to match access to data or systems according to the functional or structural role an individual plays within the organization. For example, a doctor who works in the emergency department will have the same access to data granted to another doctor in the emergency department, but this access would not be granted for a doctor who works in the ophthalmology department. In some cases, there may be one type of access control for physicians in pediatrics and another for nurses in the same department. An advantage to role-based access controls (RBACs) is that when a new doctor is assigned to the emergency department, the menus, access, and capabilities of another doctor in the department can be copied if the new doctor is to have identical privileges.

Rules-Based Access Control

Rules-based access control (RuBAC) uses of rules, policies, or attributes to set predetermined conditions for user access. RuBAC is a policy-based control that sets policies or rules that enable access and permissions to particular users, actions, objects, or contexts. RuBAC differs from RBAC in that RuBAC depends on established rules to grant access, rather than user roles. In RuBAC, for example, a rule could allow network or resource access to some IP addresses but block others. Rules require more administrative design and maintenance, as specific combinations of attributes are built to allow precise levels and conditions for access. Consider the scenario, for example, in which a newly hired physician is granted identical access as other physicians with the same role under RBAC. RuBAC can permit additional controls to increase or decrease access according to differences in the job functions or dynamic needs for access, such as time of day or location from which the physician desires information. RuBAC uses properties that are described to the access control engine and become preset rules.

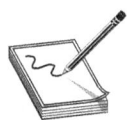

> **NOTE** RuBAC is related closely with another emerging model, the attribute-based access control (ABAC). In ABAC, based on very specific conditions or attributes, a high-precision policy or rule for access can be enacted. ABAC has shown promise in the healthcare environment, where patient privacy can be maintained in emergency situations. Role-based authentication may preclude access in some circumstances, particularly emergency situations, where it is more important to allow access based on environmental conditions than strictly the person's identity or normal job function.[9]

Context-Based Access Control

For context-based access control (CBAC), controls are not established at the user level but are based on settings within the firewall that control traffic flow based on application layer protocol session information. CBACs demonstrate that access controls are not always connected to a person. They are used to manage access by systems, services, and other computing assets. CBAC limits traffic using access control lists (ACLs), which implement packet examination at the network layer or at the transport layer. CBACs can inspect data at the network or transport layer but can also examine application layer protocol information.

Data Encryption

Encryption is another mechanism that can be used for logical access control, for both data in transit and at rest. This technical security control gives an organization the ability to limit who has access to sensitive data and to protect information confidentiality. Strictly speaking, encryption does not focus on protecting or providing data integrity or availability; however, cryptographic algorithms, called hashing algorithms, do provide for data integrity. Sensitive data, such as PHI and PII, must be encrypted under the prevailing information security regulations and standards, such as HIPAA and ISO 27001, to name just two. There are two basic states in which data can (and should) be encrypted: when it is at rest and when it is in transit.

Data at rest refers to data that is stored on any media and is not currently being processed or transmitted. If data at rest has been encrypted, media that is lost or stolen and recovered by someone unauthorized to view the data will be unusable or unreadable to the person who finds it, because that person does not have authorized access to it. In this case, the only people who can access the data are those who possess the cryptographic key to decrypt it. The principle concept is that the data is protected from unauthorized access and disclosure by being rendered unusable to anyone other than someone with authorized access. This type of encryption can be applied in two common ways: encrypt the entire volume of information on the disk with the same encryption key, or encrypt at the file level. Encrypting the entire volume of the disk has benefits in that human error is minimized, because users may forget or neglect to encrypt data if any part of the process is manual or discretionary, as file-level encryption can be. An advanced form of encryption of data at rest includes encryption of database files within the file at a table, column, row, or even individual cell level. At this advanced level, you will encounter the *tokenization* process, where the identifying data is encrypted and replaces the identifiable data within the file or database. A re-identifying key is stored separately to enable reinsertion of the column-, row-, or cell-level data in the original file or database. However, to satisfy most leading security standards and regulations, data at rest encryption for disk level and file level is sufficient.

With data in transit encryption, some sensitive data must be transferred via an e-mail message, while other data is transferred over a networked connection. During these transfer processes, PHI and PII data must be protected by encryption. The cryptographic key process is similar whether the data is at rest or in transit. To achieve encryption of data in transit, an encryption key is attached to a digital certificate related to public and private keys for each sender and recipient. The private key is secret, but the public key is not and can be used by anyone to encrypt the message. Only the private key of the intended recipient can decipher the message. These two keys are different, but they are related by a mathematical algorithm that makes this process possible. A certificate is the mechanism used to uniquely identify an encryption key and associate it with the asset owner, which assures confidentiality and prevents unauthorized disclosure.

It is important to note that the leading standard for encryption keys is included in NIST publication FIPS 140-2, *Security Requirements for Cryptographic Modules*. If an encryption key has been tested and certified under FIPS 140-2, it can be used to provide safe harbor protection under HIPAA in the United States. Keep in mind the distinction between HIPAA safe harbor and the former DPD safe harbor provisions, as described in Chapter 4. There are important resources that provide guidelines for implementation and use of encryption for data at rest and in transit. You will not need them on a daily basis, but you will use them to ensure that your configurations and solutions from product suppliers or developers meet your legal and local policy guidelines for encryption. The following are a few to consult:

- NIST SP 800-175B, *Guideline for Using Cryptographic Standards in the Federal Government: Cryptographic Mechanisms*
- NIST SP 800-111, *Guide to Storage Encryption Technologies for End-User Devices*
- NIST SP 800-52 Rev. 2, *Guidelines for the Selection, Configuration, and Use of Transport Layer Security (TLS) Implementations*
- NIST SP 800-77, *Guide to IPsec VPNs*
- NIST SP 800-113, *Guide to SSL VPNs*
- ISO/IEC 18033-*x*, *Information technology – Security techniques – Encryption algorithms* (This publication has multiple parts, indicated after the hyphen: Part 1 covers general techniques and more specific technologies are covered in later parts.)

Figure 5-4 depicts a simple e-mail transfer using encryption for data in transit. It illustrates components of public key infrastructure (PKI), which consists of all technology, personnel, and policies that work together to create, manage, and share digital certificates.[10] The encrypted information can be decrypted, allowing access only by those possessing the appropriate cryptographic key. This is especially useful if strong physical access controls cannot be provided, such as for laptops or mobile media devices. This ensures that if information is encrypted on a laptop computer and the laptop is stolen, the information cannot be accessed, because it is rendered unreadable without the decryption key. Encryption can provide strong access control, but it must be accompanied by effective key management.

EXAM TIP The cryptography described is public-key cryptography, also called asymmetric cryptography, where one of the two keys used is public and the other is private. In contrast, private-key cryptography is called symmetric cryptography, and both parties hold a private key known only to the key holders.

Figure 5-4
The transfer of encrypted data in transit

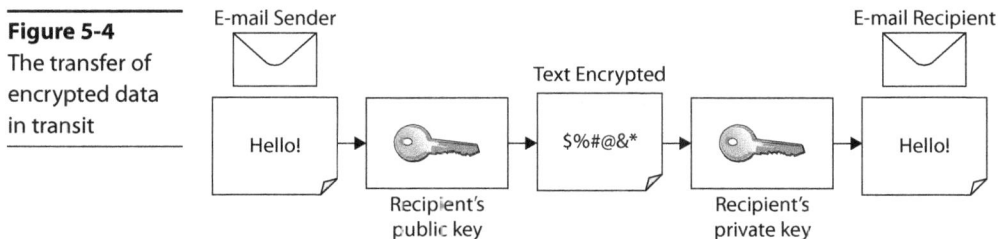

Training and Awareness

An active employee training and awareness program is one of the most cost-effective security controls that any organization can implement. Training and awareness can help prevent the breaches caused by employee mistakes and reduce complacency around handling PHI and PII. Training and awareness practices must be used in tandem to conduct a comprehensive workforce information security program.

Security training teaches employees skills and techniques that can help them be more successful at keeping healthcare information private and secure. Often, classes are delivered based on the end users' level of access, whether they are system administrators or standard end users, for example.

Training is most effective when it's delivered regularly. In fact, many required training courses are mandated for annual or more frequent recurrence, sometimes by law. This training is tracked, and compliance is reported to relevant leadership or to the appropriate government agencies. HIPAA, for example, requires that a healthcare organization provide training to all workforce members on relevant security policies and procedures.

Training can be especially effective when it's offered on an ad hoc or as-needed basis. A class on how to encrypt an e-mail containing PHI may be helpful as a weekly in-service topic for a specific audience, for example. The more often ad hoc trainings are offered on a variety of timely topics, the more effective they are at influencing proper information security behaviors.

Training can address many levels, from basic security practices to advanced or specialized skills, and often focuses on role-based access requirements. For example, a system administrator who manages a server farm with a specific operating system and desktop/laptop environment may need security-relevant training to perform her role. A network administrator who manages a network that uses specific vendor products also requires security training that is specific to the systems he manages, but this training would be quite different from that of the server administrator. Although these two examples are specific to technology, training is also important for employees with regard to specific duties performed in nontechnology roles. An example of such training could include payment card industry (PCI) requirements for staff who work in billing or cashiers in the insurance support areas of the healthcare organization.

Security awareness is the preferred outcome of training activities. Awareness is often incorporated into basic security training and can involve any method that encourages employee awareness of best security practices. Most awareness programs include marketing and communication of relevant information through information security campaigns using posters displayed in prominent areas, newsletters, banners that pop up during login, or announcements made in staff meetings, for example. Although delivery of security information could also be viewed as a form of ad hoc training, the targeted nature of the messages and the audience provide a distinction.

Awareness improves when all employees or certain groups of employees are regularly informed of proper security practices at work—such how to create appropriate passwords, what to do in the event of a virus or other security issue, or how and when to notify appropriate staff of a potential security violation. Many organizations require annual reviews of policies or procedures to test employee awareness. Awareness also improves employee security practices, such as logging off a computer system when it's not in use.

Sanction Policy

Even the best training and awareness programs cannot prevent every employee-caused security incident. To address employee violations of the organization's privacy and security practices and policies, a sanction policy is required. A sanction policy is a set of prescribed actions that management can take with regard to employee security violations.

Although some incidents are so serious that immediate termination is appropriate, the majority of incidents are accidental by nature. Therefore, the policy should outline progressive levels of discipline and provide for management discretion whenever possible. To facilitate this, the organization must categorize the types of infractions and match them against the various types of penalties to be considered. In the end, a good sanction policy will be fair and consistent, not only with regard to who commits a violation but also with regard to other organizational policies for human resource types of disciplinary actions.

As a part of the organization's training and awareness program, data from the sanction policy enforcement process is invaluable in determining trending issues and reasons for breaches, as well for aggregate reporting of outcomes. Research has demonstrated that informing employees specifically about the sanction policy and actions related to it help improve employee compliance with information protection policies in healthcare settings.[11]

Logging and Monitoring

Within the information security environment are many different event logs and types of logging. Basically, a log is a record that is generated by the processing of events on the network and on systems, applications, and end user devices. Each specific event is recorded. The logs that relate to potential security events, such as failed login attempts or denied access incidents at the firewall, can be helpful tools. One of the principle duties of an information security and privacy professional is to review logs actively. The information gained from logs is invaluable in supporting performance improvement, detecting abnormalities from a security perspective, supporting forensics, and responding to legal requests for historical data.

Monitoring and tracking the health and status of the system and its operations may require specialized training by staff members to understand what information is being collected, how to determine whether a potential violation or suspected event may have occurred, and how to identify issues up to and including vulnerabilities to a specific system or application. In short, logging and monitoring are functions of generating performance and security data and acting on any events that trigger alerts.

Reviewing logs is a daunting task, because the sheer volume and complexity of logs have increased over time. Manual review approaches are infeasible as the need to monitor the computing environment has increased in importance. Monitoring today requires automated methods, in which rules and/or parameters are set to distinguish normal network behavior from potential incidents or events. For instance, a good monitoring process would provide an alert when a simultaneous logon by the same end user occurs on the network inside the computing domain and on the organization's virtual private network. This incident would indicate the likelihood of spoofed or a stolen set of credentials. Although automated monitoring is the norm, administrators require the appropriate training and knowledge to set up the monitoring tools and to know and understand the complex rules of behavior, what normal behavior is, and what should alert action.

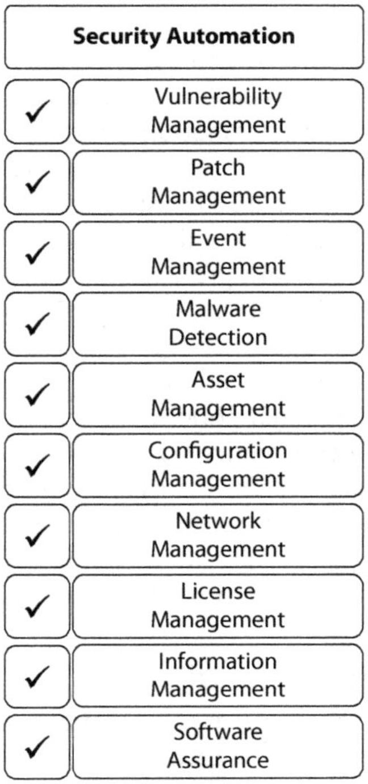

Figure 5-5
Security
automation
domains

A growing trend within logging and monitoring, because of improved automated tools and process in security automation, is information security continuous monitoring (ISCM). NIST SP 800-137, *Information Security Continuous Monitoring (ISCM) for Federal Information Systems and Organizations*, defines ISCM as the ongoing awareness of information security, vulnerabilities, and threats to support organizational risk management decisions. More important is that the directive outlines domains of potential automation and best practice philosophies around the domains, as depicted in Figure 5-5. Although this publication only introduces these domains, the key point is that logging and monitoring in these domains is increasingly automated and continuous.

Vulnerability Management

A *vulnerability* provides a description of a potential risk that exists within the organization and its information assets based on the state of a computing asset. The vulnerability makes it possible for a mistake by an internal employee or an attack to expose a security weakness. We often think of vulnerabilities when we assess systems and applications being up to date from a security perspective. But along with software and other technical controls, a vulnerability can be related to the lack of physical and administrative controls. For example, an unlocked office door could allow physical access by an unauthorized person, and the lack of a privilege access review process could lead to credential theft or misuse.

The measure of vulnerabilities is a central component of evaluating risk, particularly the likelihood of an event happening. Vulnerabilities are simply indicators that alert risk managers to consider actions and to balance risk, factoring in the likelihood of occurrence versus cost implications. Commonly, the cumulative impact of vulnerabilities increases concern and drives risk management priorities. In some cases, a single vulnerability could be significant enough that risk management actions are elevated to the highest priority. Figure 5-6 shows the interrelationships of vulnerability and risk.

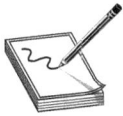

NOTE Updating systems and networks while they are operating in the production environment is important. However, a foundational component of vulnerability management starts before a system or network is put into operation. The concept of *system hardening* addresses this initial phase of vulnerability management. System hardening consists of configuration management that assures a baseline security level for any asset in production that includes industry-recommended security configurations and settings. For information about Windows baselines, or benchmarks, visit https://www.cisecurity.org/benchmark/microsoft_windows_desktop. This information can be helpful in hardening or securing an endpoint system using Microsoft operating systems, as recommended by the Center for Internet Security (CIS).

If we implement the proper safeguards, we can reduce vulnerabilities and mitigate the risks of most threats. Vulnerability management can never eliminate all vulnerabilities, however. Some threats will exploit a vulnerability that we are unable to manage by a security control or safeguard. For example, if a user is using an obsolete operating system that is no longer supported by the manufacturer, operating system upgrades and security patches are no longer feasible. If the outdated system is valuable or important to the business or clinical practice, the vulnerability may have to be accepted, and compensating controls such as network segmentation and limited access may be the best approaches to mitigating the risk, but not eliminate it.

Figure 5-6
Relationships among threats, vulnerabilities, safeguards, and assets

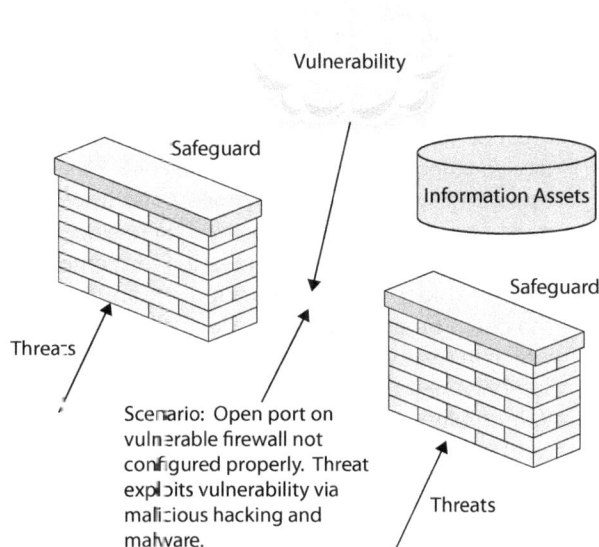

Vulnerability

Safeguard

Information Assets

Safeguard

Threats

Scenario: Open port on vulnerable firewall not configured properly. Threat exploits vulnerability via malicious hacking and malware.

Threats

The better an organization manages its implementation of safeguards, the less the chance that a vulnerability will affect its systems. In reality, however, there will always be new vulnerabilities leading to risk. The role of a healthcare information security and privacy professional is to design, implement, and enforce the security controls of safeguards that reduce risk of vulnerability exposure. To measure and evaluate whether the proper safeguards are in place and operating effectively and efficiently, a security controls assessment is a necessary part of your role.

The practice of vulnerability management includes the process of patching systems and applications with updated code or software changes. This patch management process is a technical control that is vital to maintaining a properly safeguarded network and computing environment. Operating systems and various applications all are designed and implemented with a secure configuration when they are introduced to the marketplace. However, vulnerability management, specifically patch management, is a dynamic, ongoing process that addresses current identified vulnerabilities in established application code. Sometimes the vulnerability is found through an exploitation, such as a hacking attempt or the introduction of malicious code. Other times, the vulnerability is discovered by software developers who bring the vulnerability to light before anyone exploits it (the preferred scenario, of course). In such cases, the patch required to fix the vulnerability is coded, developed, tested, and distributed to the marketplace as quickly as possible in hopes of preventing malicious activity.

You may have heard of a vulnerability being "in the wild." That indicates an active exploit in a production environment of one or more organizations. This is contrasted with creating a hack or exploit in a lab or research condition. "In the wild" exploits increase the criticality of patches, because the likelihood of further exploits for other organizations is increased significantly.

The process of patch management has benefited from security automation. Patches (once tested and validated) can be automatically distributed across a local area network and automatically updated on all networked resources. With some exceptions for types of operating systems, application compatibility, and patient safety concerns (see the following Exam Tip), this is efficient and effective.

EXAM TIP An example of where best-practice security in other industries must be tailored when applied to healthcare organizations is medical device vulnerability management. For FDA-regulated medical devices, the operating system patching process should *not* be automatic. Each patch must be evaluated and approved for use on all medical devices by that device's manufacturer before being implemented. In short, medical devices may be able to be patched, but the manufacturer must first test and approve the patch on each particular device. Otherwise, the addition of a patch, which in reality is a piece of third-party software, can result in a patient safety issue if the medical device malfunctions after the patch is applied. Vulnerability management for medical devices is improving all the time. Get familiar with the dynamic content at https://www.fda.gov/medical-devices/digital-health/cybersecurity to stay abreast of trends in this area.

Segregation of Duties

The segregation of duties is a sort of checks and balances system implemented to reduce the risk of accidental or deliberate misuse of information. It involves processes and controls that help create and maintain a separation of security roles and responsibilities within an organization to ensure that the integrity of security processes is not jeopardized, and to ensure that no single person has the ability to disrupt a critical computing process or security function. A segregation of duties policy, for example, prevents an individual from making system changes and then changing the audit logs so that there is no record of the changes. Or, for example, in another area of the healthcare organization's operations, an individual who is permitted to request a payment to a vendor or customer should not be the same person who issues the check for that payment.

Vulnerabilities are not always technical in nature. The ability of one individual to cause unauthorized changes or disruptions, inadvertently or intentionally, is an example of a nontechnical vulnerability to the overall information security program.

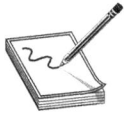

> **NOTE** Segregation of duties in the financial sector is bolstered by a required policy that forces employees in designated critical positions, such as elevated access and authorization privileges, to take mandatory time off, commonly for five consecutive business days. This practice is meant to increase the organization's ability to detect insider threats. Some healthcare organizations also use this practice as well as job rotation, which also minimizes the control a single individual can have by forcing breaks in duties periodically and moving employees into other roles on the team.

Least Privilege (Need to Know)

The term "least privilege" may be more familiar to many of us as the "need to know" principle. Least privilege refers to each user having only the permissions, rights, and privileges necessary to perform his or her assigned duties, and no more. In addition, users of information should be granted access only to the information they need to perform their duties. Least privilege does not mean that all users have extremely limited functional access. Some employees will be granted significant access to data if it is required for their position. Following this principle can decrease the risk of and limit the damage resulting from accidents, errors, or unauthorized use of system resources.

Many of the concepts within information security (and privacy) relate to avoiding too much access or too much disclosure, where such access or disclosure is not needed. Generally, least privilege or minimal use concepts must support every information protection program. It is an imperative to protect information from individuals who have no need for it, have no reason to use it, or no longer need it. Limited access policies go hand-in-hand with least privilege policies. These policies require that only as much information as needed should be disclosed, transferred, used, and stored, and as soon as the information is no longer required, it should be destroyed.

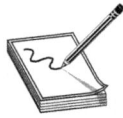

NOTE It is important to ensure that the implementation of least privilege is complemented by a plan for substitute or rapid granting of access to other personnel when an authorized individual is not available. Without careful planning, access control can interfere with contingency plans and ultimately, patient safety.

One of the distinctive elements of providing information protection in a healthcare environment is that least privilege concerns can be highly dynamic. For example, a physician may have access to records one day because she is dealing with a specific patient's case or a specific responsibility, but the next day that access may be restricted if her duties change. This commonly happens as physicians see patients in emergency situations, such as when a behavioral health patient arrives in the emergency room. Another example is that sometimes, for peer review under medical records management processes, physicians may be granted temporary access to pediatric records, where their normal clinical duties would not include children under the age of 18. This process is important within a healthcare setting for continuity of patient care.

Business Continuity

Business continuity, or continuity of operations, includes all the actions taken to enable a healthcare organization to perform clinical and business services with minimal to no interruption or degradation. The organization must be able to perform certain activities in an effort to continue its mission should an unforeseen event occur. The ability to deliver medical care, for example, could be affected by electrical outages, weather-related events, community-based events such as riots, accidents, or even a serious outbreak of a virus that affects staffing levels. The healthcare organization must plan for and have procedures in place for such events.

Few industries are required to function 24/7, but in healthcare, this is a must. Not only is this affected by regulatory pressures, but many governments at the national, provincial, and state levels also require reporting procedures when a healthcare organization is not functioning. For our purposes, we concentrate on information asset functioning, so network or application downtime is the primary issue. In the United States, healthcare networks are included in the NIST publication *Framework for Improving Critical Infrastructure Cybersecurity*, which includes rigid guidelines to help assure continuity of operations.

As with all security controls, business continuity plans also include time-related elements that help ensure that a facility can recover from an issue quickly. Having a continuity of operations plan (COOP) for disasters is a preventive aspect of security control, and monitoring network activity is a detection function. Once a disaster happens, the optimal method for business continuity is a redundant system or an alternative source of recovery. For example, if an electrical outage occurs, a healthcare organization may switch temporarily to power provided by generators running diesel fuel. This helps ensure that patient care and business processes are not likely to be interrupted. When network resources are not available, because of power outages or for another reason, manual processes should be implemented. As an example, a lab system that processes samples using bar code technology may also have a manual process that uses hand-written intake forms. Personnel should be trained and able to implement the manual forms in the event that the bar code–scanning system is unavailable.

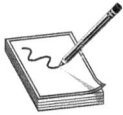

> **NOTE** Most organizations have implemented and rely upon advanced information technology solutions. In some cases, the manual processes once used are no longer possible. Consider, for example, a healthcare facility that currently uses a computerized system to order patient lab procedures. If the system goes down, healthcare workers would need an alternative way to order labs, such as using paper lab request slips with checkmarks, signatures, and so on, for the applicable tests to be conducted. However, if there is no supply of those paper slips, ordering the appropriate lab procedures would be difficult, if not impossible. Or perhaps the medical staff has not been trained in how to access and use those paper slips if the computerized system goes down. These examples illustrate that we tend to rely on the technological improvements to the point at which certain manual processes can no longer be relied upon or accomplished.

Disaster Recovery

Disaster recovery is another important security control that supports business continuity. The ability to recover systems, specifically information technology systems, is a vital aspect of operations in any business, but in healthcare organizations, especially, it can mean the difference between life and death.

Power outages, weather events, or other incidents can cause damage to the data center where the systems are housed. Even if the system itself is not damaged, restarting or configuring the system is an important consideration in a disaster recovery plan. Once a system has been remediated (and after the threat is no longer present), a process for bringing the system back online is needed. This is true for every system or application. For example, if a database server is corrupted by an attack, the server must obviously be tested and evaluated prior to putting it back into the production environment.

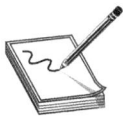

> **NOTE** Disaster recovery procedures must be in place to prioritize operations and restore systems in a staggered process. Following a total network outage, restarting all systems immediately and simultaneously can result in unintended failures at some network locations, which can result from electrical surges or load balancing issues, for example.

The best COOP, specifically for system recovery, includes a plan for a scheduled, prioritized system restart. Clinical systems and business systems would be restarted first. Then additional systems could be started, while the impacts of the restarts are monitored. Depending on the duration of the outage or system failure, a significant amount of new and sensitive healthcare information may have been collected. That data will need to be integrated into the entirety of the patient record and related business records.

System Backup and Recovery

System backup processes and recovery capabilities are fundamental components of a healthcare organization's resiliency. To illustrate, a University of Texas researcher estimated that large hospitals' losses can reach $1 million per hour during an unplanned outage of their EHR.[12] Having secondary or duplicate copies of data, high-availability systems, and alternate operating locations are all part of a robust resiliency program to ensure the availability of data and reduce downtime.

Events such as ransomware attacks or natural disasters may cause primary systems or sources of data to be unusable. System backups and recovery plans alleviate the impact of these risks. Backups are needed for other reasons as well, such as for audits, forensics, and other regulatory information requests. For the most part, we will concentrate on the use of backups and recovery as part of a security control to maintain the CIA triad. Factors that determine the strategies for system backup and recovery include the sensitivity of the information, the risk tolerance of the organization, and operational requirements.

Backup Storage Approaches

There are several types of backup approaches with distinct purposes. With advancing technology such as cloud platforms and cloud storage solutions, you will encounter variations in these approaches. Learning the traditional basic backups cycles will be a good start, however, so we will cover the most traditional forms here—full backups, incremental backups, and differential backups:

- **Full backups**   Backups should include a full copy of the entire system, including the entire database, operating system, boot files, and an exact copy of the system drive. Usually, the first backup copy is a full backup. Subsequent backups are usually not full backups. Storage requirements are a significant concern if previous backups are not deleted. To be safe, full backups are good practice before any major upgrades or migrations of systems occur. This backup can be used to fully restore the last known good copy of the system files. The restore process from a full backup is the slowest of the options presented here.

- **Differential backups**   This process backs up only the changes made since the last full backup and copies those changes in each subsequent backup. The system accumulates updates periodically with a collection of all modifications and variations in multiple, subsequent copies. Differential backups occur each day until another full backup occurs. Differential backups help to compress the time it takes to restore a system, but depending on the frequency of differential backups, storage costs can become a problem. To restore from a differential backup, you would normally use the latest differential copy and the full backup copy together.

- **Incremental backups**   An incremental backup copies only the files, data, and system information that have changed from the previous backup. You can run incremental backups more often because of the relatively small storage requirements and the cost-effectiveness of the solutions. Restoration from incremental backups would include the last incremental backup and the last full backup.

Backup Storage Locations

Related to the ability to restore backups and operate during a business disruption is the location of backups. A risk assessment and business requirements evaluation will help determine which location approach the organization should use. The correct choice depends on how much downtime the organization can accept, any pertinent regulatory requirements, and which solution or combination of solutions offers the best options regarding data availability.

The most secure locations for data storage during a catastrophic event are offsite locations, particularly because onsite data centers may be unusable or destroyed. There are three types of offsite configurations:

- **Hot site**   A hot site is a computing environment that is almost identical to the onsite environment. This is the best choice for critical systems. To minimize disruption of services, the hot site runs concurrently, along with the main production environment. The use of a hot site is the costliest of location options, because these sites continuously operate and secure data assets. System backups at a hot site may occur via two main approaches: If the hot site is intended to serve as a high-availability solution, backups are continuous or a secondary data flow in real time. In this scenario, hot site systems provide a redundant capability to maintain uptime requirements to a level close to 99.999 percent. More than likely, hot sites require daily backups so the site can be made operational in a very short amount of time, usually measured in a few hours. A good hot site would be located far enough away from the source site to be outside of any shared risks, such as earthquakes, hurricanes, and so on.

- **Warm site**   Warm sites are locations with adequate equipment, such as hardware and software, that can be accessed fairly quickly when needed. The warm site normally has electricity, telecommunications, and networking infrastructure at a minimum. Backups are stored there in case they are needed for recovery. In the event of a disaster or cyber incident that causes disruption at the source site, the warm site would be brought to full power. There would be a short delay to production levels for critical systems, because immediate recovery is not expected.

- **Cold site**   The least costly option is a cold site. A cold site includes the bare minimum and may store nothing but backups, or backups could be transported or transferred to the cold site when required. A cold site would take the longest to power up and bring to production levels.

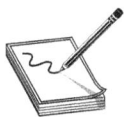

NOTE   An emerging alternative to physical production environments (on-premises) system backups are cloud solutions that can act as hot and warm sites. An availability zone can provide an isolated, logical data center in the cloud environment. Backups can be transferred from the physical site and stored in the availability zone, which can be used as the alternate production environment, to be initiated as needed. Using the cloud can be a more reliable and cost-effective solution than physical facilities for data storage and backups.

Configuration, or Change Management

To help ensure integrity within the parameters of the CIA triad, organizations establish a configuration, or change management process. This process is part of an organization's overall information governance approach and a valuable security control measure to ensure consistency in how changes are made to the network, systems, and applications. The goal of change management is to establish standard procedures for managing changes efficiently to control risk and minimize disruption to IT services and business operations.

A change management process is a critical best practice that's included in the Information Technology Infrastructure Library (ITIL) framework. ITIL recognizes the value of an efficient, organized methodology for taking new products or updates of existing products from design to operations without adding risk.[13]

In the realm of healthcare, a change management process may affect a laboratory department that, for example, wants to purchase a new information system for processing lab results. The new system would require network access and must interface with current systems, including EHR. Imagine the result if the acquisition and implementation of this new system did not include a formal, management-level review of the operating system, interfacing requirements, physical installation environment, and other significant factors. Without a change management system in place to ensure that the new acquisition is consistent with existing systems, results could be disastrous: the new system might fail to be interoperable with existing systems, chiefly the EHR, or the system may not work at all.

Other considerations for change management could involve required changes to perimeter security defenses, such as border firewalls. If a networked system needed to communicate with external entities across the Internet, the data traffic devices would exit the organization's network through the firewall via distinct ports using specific protocols. Outside of the ACL's approved ports and protocols, all other traffic would be blocked. Special-purpose computing systems, such as medical device systems, may require the use of a port not on the current ACL. To request or ultimately make changes to perimeter defenses, a formal change management process is required.

Incident Response

Incident response is effective as a corrective measure that occurs after a security incident. A successful incident response strategy can limit the duration and impact of an exploited vulnerability. Today, as data breaches seem almost inevitable no matter how well you implement security processes and controls, the one security control that may make the most difference is your incident response strategy. NIST SP 800-61 Rev. 2, *Computer Security Incident Handling Guide*, provides direction for establishing a solid incident response program that accomplishes detection, analysis, prioritization, and handling of security events, such as data breaches. According to Stroz Friedberg (Aon), a leading global cybersecurity service firm with specific expertise in incident response, "The way an organization responds can be the difference between exacerbating the reputational and financial damages from a breach, and mitigating them."[14] A solid incident response strategy will be based on significant regulatory requirements regarding notification, with HIPAA and HITECH in the United States, and internationally with the European Union's DPD, for example.

Understanding Privacy Concepts

As an HCISPP, you are expected to have a solid understanding of privacy concepts. Some concepts are used independently of security controls. However, as the healthcare industry becomes ever more digitally based versus paper based, the integration of privacy and security controls also increases. The significance of privacy cannot be overstated. Worldwide, the emphasis on privacy as a human right can lead to enforcement under criminal law. In this section, we examine how various privacy frameworks incorporate privacy concepts. Another current aspect of privacy is the ability to provide privacy in the face of social media, public surveillance, and information sharing.

Within healthcare, the roles and responsibilities of those who are charged with protecting information converge around distinct roles that may or may not have previously involved working with digital or electronic information. Some roles originate from traditional privacy or legal roles in health information management, with a shift from paper-based information storage to digital storage; others come from IT support backgrounds, such as local area networking, application management, and end-user support, where new concerns over protected health information are relevant. Still others may come from the clinical engineering or biomedical technology professions, where the interconnectivity of medical devices and to internal and external networks is rapidly evolving. Figure 5-7 depicts the intersection.

For these previously distinct and somewhat separated communities, this section provides a primer in privacy compliance for those with stronger backgrounds in security, and in security compliance for those with stronger backgrounds in privacy. It offers

Figure 5-7
Convergence of healthcare competencies with information privacy and security responsibilities

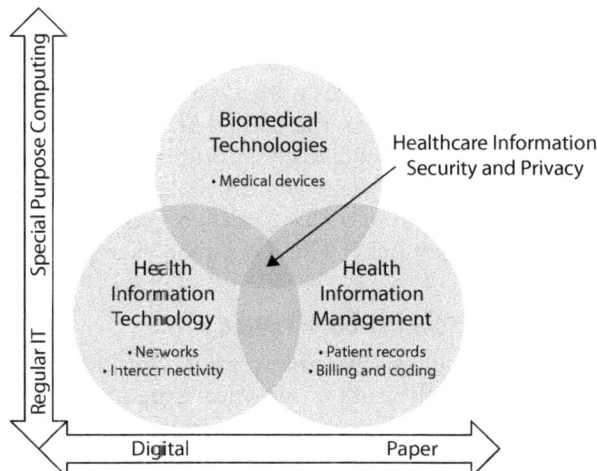

guidance to those who have a responsibility for complying with information privacy in healthcare, as well as those with traditional privacy or legal compliance roles in healthcare, who have increasing roles in protecting digital information through information security management.

> **EXAM TIP** The distinction between privacy and security has begun to narrow. Some advocate that privacy is a concept embedded in the practice of providing information security or cybersecurity. However, for purposes of this text and the exam, we will maintain a distinction: Information privacy concerns what is being protected and why. Security addresses how an organization can protect the private information.

The following concepts and definitions are found in the leading privacy frameworks and regulations. Minor differences may exist, particularly where terms are combined to make one principle rather than two distinct principles in the framework. Refer back to Chapter 4 to review these terms in the context of the framework that advocates them.

US Approach to Privacy

The United States does not apply a uniform data privacy policy across all industries and data collectors. Because of a variety of factors, and to maintain a free-market economy, the United States approaches data privacy from a sector, industry, or functional perspective. The central principle in this approach is that government does not set a singular policy that transcends industries. Instead, each industry is governed by a combination of self-imposed guidelines and government-originated regulations specific to that industry. What results is incremental legislation that is focused on specific concerns. Examples include the Electronic Communications Privacy Act of 1986, the Children's Online Privacy Protection Act (COPPA) of 1998, the Fair Credit Reporting Act, and the 2010 Massachusetts Data Privacy Regulations.

To understand how the United States approaches privacy law, you must consider the US Constitution and that the establishment of the federal government included an intentional reluctance to influence or meddle in private business and the economy. In this case, the result is a reluctance (at least initially) for the federal government to legislate privacy. Additionally, privacy in the United States tends to be limited by what society is willing to accept, and that can change significantly over time. Privacy laws have emerged and are enforced within industries at a federal level, such as HIPAA in healthcare, and at the state level, where some states have relatively stringent privacy laws. The recent California Consumer Privacy Act (CCPA) is a good example.

European Approach to Privacy

The European Union approached the concept of privacy from a very different perspective than the United States. Because of historical experiences such as the Nazi regime, many Europeans have a natural suspicion and fear of intrusive, unnecessary, unfettered access to personal information, which has led to the creation of stringent privacy protection laws.[15]

This is not only reflected in the overarching data protection approach in the DPD, which has been updated to the GDPR, but also in how the European Union sees data transfer to non-EU nations. Additionally, there is a variation between the European Union and other nations in what identifiers are considered personal information. For instance, the European Union includes race, ethnicity, and union status as protected, sensitive information. The impact of identifying someone based on this information was once the catalyst for secret denunciations from neighbors and friends in the 1930s. This led to detentions of targeted individuals and groups (for example, members with Jewish heritage) that sent friends and neighbors to work camps and concentration camps.[16] The European Union favors stringent and widespread privacy protections for its citizens and has led the world in establishing and enforcing data protection laws.

Consent

In the privacy context, consent is a voluntary action by an individual to allow collection and sharing of their personal information for purposes that are disclosed to them beforehand. For consent to be legitimate, a few conditions must be satisfied: Individuals must provide consent voluntarily and must also be informed about their rights, one of which is that it is okay to change their minds after they provide consent. Of course, individuals must also be able to understand these conditions and be capable of communicating their decisions.

According to the HIPAA Privacy Rule, a healthcare organization must obtain authorization for the exchange of information, with a general exception for information needed for purposes of treatment, payment, and operations. Consent can be *informed* or *granted* by a competent individual. In granted consent, a competent individual such as a family member can provide consent when the patient cannot do so. This can happen when the patient is heavily medicated or injured and is unlikely able to make a rational decision. When complying with HIPAA guidelines and using or disclosing PHI for purposes of treatment, payment, or healthcare operations, a healthcare organization does not have to obtain consent. However, the organization may opt to obtain consent where practical.

For other uses and disclosures, such as for research and third-party population health analytics, additional patient consent may be required. Under the DPD, data should not be disclosed without the data subject's consent. That provision extends to GDPR as well. The DPD addresses both informed consent, where the subject has sufficient information before making their decision, and specific intent, indicating the subject is advised of the precise nature of the data and purpose for which it is collected. There is no differentiation under the DPD as to the purpose such as treatment, payment, or healthcare operations.

Choice

Choice is defined under various privacy standards. Choice provides an individual the option of whether to provide the information freely or withhold it. The distinction between choice and consent is that choice is about providing options, whereas consent is about providing permission. The choice offered to an individual must be between legitimate options, and the options must be presented in a clear manner without deception.

Choice is offered through opt-in and opt-out provisions. One version of opt-in or opt-out provisions for legitimate data collection and sharing is a healthcare organization that provides a statement to patients about their choice to provide personal information or withhold it. An organization can structure its opt-in and opt-out processes in multiple ways to obtain patient choice. If the individual does nothing, it can be an implicit opt-in or opt-out choice by default; if the individual makes an active choice (by selecting or unselecting an option), it is an explicit choice. When collecting sensitive information, it is best to require the individual to make an explicit opt-in or opt-out choice. Examples of implicit and explicit opt-in and opt-out statements are shown in Figure 5-8.

With the growing adoption of EHRs, the opt-in or opt-out choice can have a profound impact. When providing consent to receive care, patients should be offered an informed choice if that information is collected into the EHR and then automatically shared as part of a health information exchange (HIE). This additional sharing may be outside of what the patient may expect. Therefore, additional consent may be required. To receive such informed consent, either by a patient opting in or opting out, healthcare organizations may have to provide notice to thousands of patients, which is logistically difficult and costly.

The DPD mandates that an individual can exercise free consent, which is identified using the term "choice." This enables the data subject to be able to exercise a real choice, and there should be no deception, intimidation, coercion, or significant negative consequences if the subject does not consent. The DPD does not, however, mention the right to withdraw consent. With the recent enacting of GDPR, individual choice is still preserved as consent requests must be easily understood and accessible; the intended uses of the information must be made to the individual and in plain language.

Per the HIPAA guidelines, the term "choice" is more routinely associated with the right to revoke an authorization that was previously granted at any time. This revocation must be in writing and is not effective until the covered entity has received that revocation. The Privacy Rule requires that the authorization must clearly state the individual's right to revoke. There are two permissible ways a healthcare organization can satisfy the mandatory communication of the revocation process to the individual. Either they provide it as part of the authorization process or they include the revocation process in the notice of privacy practices. In either case, the revocation process must be described in clear terms that the individual can understand.[17]

Figure 5-8
Examples of implicit and explicit opt-in and opt-out statements

Preselected (must be unselected to indicate choice):

☑ I understand the privacy practices terms and conditions. (Opt-in, implicit)
☑ Do not share my information with third parties. (Opt-in, implicit)

Not preselected (must be selected to indicate choice):

☐ I understand the privacy practices terms and conditions. (Opt-in, explicit)
☐ Do not share my information with third parties. (Opt-in, explicit)

The explicit statements are best when collecting or using sensitive data.

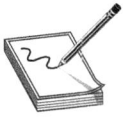

NOTE It is easy to confuse the appropriate use of the terms *opt in* and *opt out*. For instance, a patient portal web site may provide a choice for patients to opt in to the healthcare organization's data collection and storage system by selecting a checkbox that reads, "I agree to the terms and conditions found in the hospital privacy statement." In this case, the checkbox should not be prechecked, because a preselected, affirmative statement would be more appropriately defined as an explicit opt-out choice—that is, the patient would have to physically uncheck the checkbox to opt out.

Limited Collection

A principle common across data protection best practices and regulations is the collection limitation principle. This principle basically asserts that organizations can collect only what is necessary and nothing more. In accordance with the DPD, any personal data that is collected must be used for a specific purpose that is disclosed to the individual, and the collection must be limited to the specified use of the data. The HIPAA Privacy Rule has a similar provision that defines a limited data set as a collection of data elements that comprise only the required protected health information. All other identifying information is removed.

This following list represents a sample of some of the identifiers of the individual or of the individual's relatives, employers, or household members that would be removed under this principal:

- Name
- E-mail address
- Certificate or license numbers
- Web URL
- Address
- Social Security number
- Vehicle identification number/license plate
- Device numbers and serial numbers
- Telephone numbers
- Medical record numbers (patient ID)
- Account numbers
- Biometric identifiers, including fingerprints, retina scans, and voice prints
- Fax numbers
- Health plan beneficiary numbers
- Full face photographic images/comparable images

Limited collection is a safeguard that helps assure individuals that data collectors, such as healthcare organizations, do not collect too much information because it is easier than specifying data that is required or because it could be used for other reasons, such as marketing. It is also helpful to guard against overcollection, which can result in problems if data loss occurs. Numerous data breaches are caused or exacerbated by persistent data that was never really needed but was nonetheless collected, stored, maintained, and ultimately lost. Think about the forms patients fill out while waiting to see a doctor, or the web forms customers fill out prior to gaining access to an online service. If all of that information is required—or relevant, as the collection limitation principle generally states—then the requests probably follow the collection limitation principle. However, if some of that information is not needed, or the data collector uses it for a purpose other than that understood by the individual providing it, the practice is inappropriate.

Legitimate Purpose

If healthcare organizations are to state the purpose of the data collection, collect it in a lawful or fair manner, and use the data only for the stated purpose, they must also ensure that the collection purpose is a legitimate one. Legitimate purpose is a principle that takes collection limitation a step further. Under HIPAA, it is a legitimate business purpose for which an organization requires the information to perform its mission. The HIPAA Privacy Rule allows public health authorities and providers to collect and disclose health information relevant to their public health responsibilities as a legitimate purpose. In this case, legitimate purpose is aligned with the importance and public interest in identifying threats to the community and individual well-being. A healthcare organization in the United States must collect patient information only as that information assists in the provision of treatment, payment, or operations. If the organization is sharing that information, it must still limit disclosure to reasons that are defined as legitimate under the law. One such provision is in public health information disclosure.[18] To carry out public health and safety responsibilities, healthcare organizations are permitted to provide data access to public health authorities and those who have a public health mission. This provision extends to third parties who handle PHI for the healthcare organization. If the third party is required to disclose PHI to public health entities, that disclosure possibility should be stated in the business associate agreement.

Legitimate purpose is present in the EU DPD, which allows personal data to be processed only for specified explicit and legitimate purposes. The DPD mentions a related privacy concept, fair processing, which instructs the data collector to obtain an additional or updated consent from the individual if the processing of the data changes from the legitimate purpose originally presented to the individual.

Purpose Specification

The purpose specification explicitly states that individuals should be informed of why their information is needed and how it will be used. If the purpose changes, new consent and choice options should be provided to the individual. The principle of purpose specification protects data subjects or individuals by also setting limits on the collection and further processing of their data. Combined with legitimate purpose, this concept makes it necessary for data collectors to disclose the specific reasons or intentions for collecting patient data. When an individual provides personal data to a company or another organization, that person usually has a right to know, and can choose to consent to, the purpose for collection and use. Purpose specification may also include disclosure of reasons or ways the information will not be used—for example, sold to third parties.

Disclosure Limitation

Disclosure of information must be controlled by limitations. Disclosure of healthcare information is limited to treatment, payment, and operations. Leading privacy frameworks generally limit disclosure but also provide specific exceptions where public safety and health considerations outweigh the need for individual privacy. Dramatic examples are cases of child abuse or some communicable diseases. There are also provisions for disclosure to be permitted when that use is clearly provided in authorization forms signed by the individual or outlined in privacy practices notifications. Disclosure limitation can be further reduced based on an individual's desire and request. Although the provider does not need to agree to the additional limitations, they may accept limits above the legal requirements. If the provider voluntarily agrees to the additional limitations, it is then obligated to honor the patient's request. In short, privacy frameworks may authorize disclosures, but they do not mandate them. The data collector and individual can establish additional limits.

Transfer to Third Parties (or Countries)

HIPAA allows for third-party transfer or sharing of PHI for the purposes of healthcare payment, treatment, or healthcare operations. The law also mandates a special type of contract between the covered entity and the third party, called a business associate, under a business associate agreement (BAA). As you'll recall from Chapter 1, BAAs should include the possibility of transfer of PHI with business associates. The healthcare organization can inform the individual that the business associate is legally obligated to protect the information using applicable security controls to maintain confidentiality for as long as they have the data. The BAA will also have terms and conditions to outline the appropriate uses of the information by the business associate, such as prohibiting any further transfer.

Disclosure limitation includes concerns for data being transferred to third parties in other countries. The European Union uses the term "third countries" to refer to foreign nations that are third parties in information sharing transactions. Disclosure limitation to third countries is a component of adhering to the "onward transfer" principal included in DPD, GDPR, and the Organisation for Economic Cooperation and Development (OECD). EU laws such as DPD and the GDPR place clear responsibility for onward transfer to third countries on the EU data controller. The EU country must ensure that the third-country entity provides information privacy protections at the same level as the DPD or GDPR. Under the DPD, that assurance could come from working with a third country that was vetted under safe harbor. Today, that assurance comes from designation on the privacy shield list of countries under GDPR.

Transborder Concerns

Electronic information transfer and advancing technologies such as cloud computing have surfaced transborder information privacy concerns. The central issue in the transfer of personal data across international borders is the assurance that each nation provides an equal amount of protection to its citizens' sensitive information. The ability to transfer electronic information internationally is generally viewed as a positive, though varying privacy approaches and lack of jurisdiction hinder or prevent such information flow. This can be legislated, as in the case of DPD and GDPR, where specific authorizations must be in place before data transfer is allowed, such as safe harbor and privacy shield.

Although HIPAA does not specifically prohibit transfer of electronic PHI, healthcare organizations must understand the risks in sharing information with third parties outside of HIPAA jurisdiction. The guidance from the US Department of Health and Human Services (HHS) on this topic includes recommendations to have the cloud service provide enter into a BAA, document the risks in the covered entities' risk assessment, and implement reasonable and appropriate technical security controls.[19] This is not always aligned with how a cloud service provider configures its environment, however.

Cross-jurisdictional or transborder transfers should be accepted only when the clinical or business requirement is substantial. Cloud service providers have begun to recognize the reluctance for healthcare organizations to take the risks of transborder transfer. You will see international cloud services, such as those provided by Microsoft or Amazon, offering solutions that store and transfer data within the United States only and entering into BAAs, easing the transborder concerns of US healthcare organizations.

Access Limitation

Limiting access to data follows the concept of allowing only the minimum access necessary. Healthcare organizations must implement and enforce reasonable levels of control over PHI to permit access only to those individuals with a legitimate need. This requirement may include certain adjustments of physical controls in addition to technical safeguards. For example, locking doors to rooms where data is kept or installing ID badging systems with video surveillance to data centers are considered reasonable controls, based the data's sensitivity. Technical measures such as passwords, intrusion detection systems, user behavior monitors, and identification management systems are relevant technical solutions to help control and restrict access.

Access limitation can extend into an individual record as well. An example is an individual's medical record that includes substance abuse information, as well as recent emergency department visits and pharmaceutical prescriptions. Some of that information may be needed by an authorized healthcare provider, but other portions of the records—in this case, the information related to the substance abuse—may be unrelated to the emergency department visits and therefore should be unavailable to an attending physician. Although not always possible, many record systems can be configured to provide that level of granularity of system access and authorization. In smaller organizations, such as a medical group of a few associated healthcare providers, it may be infeasible and unnecessary to be so restrictive based on the sophistication of their IT and continued use of paper-based records. It is always necessary to provide training and awareness regarding access limitations. If technical and physical controls are not reasonable, training and awareness is even more important.

Accuracy

As covered in previous chapters, the accuracy of data (referred to in security as *integrity*) is vital to the health of the patient, and it covers the entire scope of the overall healthcare record. A patient (or, for that matter, anyone, including care providers) who determines information within the record is in error has the right to request an amendment to the record or entry. The right to request the change is in effect as long as the healthcare organization maintains the record. The healthcare organization may decline the request for amending the record if any of the following conditions are present:

- The healthcare organization did not create the entry. If the individual who is the subject of the information can demonstrate that the entity that actually created the information no longer has the ability to make the changes, the healthcare organization may be in the position to accomplish the amendment.

- The healthcare organization established that the data in question is not included in what the organization defines as its "designated record set."

- The information is not subject to review under the HIPAA Privacy Rule.

- The healthcare organization decides the information is, in fact, accurate and verifiable.

One final note, even as a healthcare organization does not need to make the change or amend the record if the conditions support not honoring the individual's request, it must inform the public about its right to ask. The healthcare organization is required to disclose through its Notice of Privacy Practice or another notice document that satisfies relevant regulatory authorities that an individual has the right to request amendment to their records and how to do so.

Completeness

Data must be accurate and current according to the principle of completeness. This principle is found in HIPAA, DPD, and GDPR, as well as many other leading frameworks. The requirement consists of using reasonable measures to ensure that the data remains up to date based on the purpose for collection and use. EU member states and US healthcare organizations are required to take steps to erase or fix incorrect data when they learn about it. There is an increased responsibility for completeness for organizations that intend to share the information. They must assure completeness before sharing the information.

Quality

Certainly in our healthcare organizations the term "quality" has a multitude of meanings and uses. With respect to privacy, it likely has different meanings based on what part of the organization you may be supporting. Quality of data has an association with the quality of care, and knowing who is responsible for the quality of the data is also of value. The concepts of data integrity align with assuring the quality of data, underscoring the continuous integration between privacy and security. The more assurance the organization can provide that the data it manages has a high quality, the more capable it is of ensuring that the information is complete and accurate as well as to be used for the reasons stated when it was collected.

Management

This privacy framework principle identifies the importance for an organization to establish a function to build, implement, enforce, and document the processes to assure confidentiality of sensitive information. A central component of management is the governance structure that must be present to include assigned accountability that shows the privacy program's policies and procedures are working effectively.

Management of privacy is dependent on involvement and support from all senior leaders of the organization, not just senior leaders who are accountable for privacy or security. The tone from the top of the organization structure is associated with the behavior and culture of the entire organization. Without support from the senior leaders, employees are likely to give privacy practices less priority, and processes may be circumvented. Additionally, management at all levels must support the reporting of privacy-related incidents and monitor the effectiveness of the program through ongoing measurement of important indicators. If you can find evidence of senior-leader involvement, privacy reporting, and documentation of program requirements that are communicated to the organization, you can be confident that this privacy principle is being met.

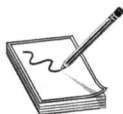

> **NOTE** You should be familiar with the concepts of privacy by design and privacy by default. These approaches instruct organizations to integrate and engineer privacy into relevant processes such as design, purchase, implementation, and decommissioning of systems as well as vendor selection and all aspects of patient care. Privacy by design and privacy by default have long traditions and are written into recent regulatory guidance such as GDPR. See https://iapp.org/resources/article/privacy-by-design for additional resources on Privacy by Design.

Privacy Officer

Regardless of where you are in the world and which regulatory requirements you must comply with, most privacy regulatory requirements require the designation or assignment in writing from management of a privacy officer, and most require specific experience or training of such individuals. While the individual's title may not be that of privacy officer, the intent is to create a role that ensures compliance with specific requirements. In the United States, the requirement to designate a privacy official is a primary requirement of the HIPAA Privacy Rule. GDPR mandates the assignment of a Data Protection Officer, with similar responsibilities. The privacy official is responsible for establishing a privacy program with the required policies and procedures to comply with regulatory direction. The privacy official will manage and oversee several specific tasks:

- Develop and publicize the notice of privacy practices (covered later in this chapter in the section "Notice").

- Make sure patients are provided and acknowledge receipt of the notice of privacy practices.

- Authorize exceptions for disclosure of information when warranted for purposes such as research, marketing, and fundraising.

- Administer patient requests for amendment of their records.

- Assess the need to apply additional information protection controls to increase privacy of sensitive records.

- Serve as the focal point for any internal employee complaints concerning regulatory guidance (such as HIPAA Privacy Rule) and compliance.

- Handle inquiries from patients and patients' families for information about privacy practices and access to information.

If you are employed in a large healthcare organization or facility, the privacy officer role may be a senior management level professional. They typically require staff support just to handle all these administrative tasks. In a small clinic or practice, privacy officer responsibilities may be only part of an individual's job responsibilities. In these scenarios, the privacy responsibilities are likely added to job requirements for managing medical records, security, and patient administration. You can infer that this complexity is not always helpful for strong privacy practices.

The person selected to be a privacy officer may seem to face a difficult role, whatever the size of the organization. The privacy official must also understand and implement a program following other regulatory requirements such as existing requirements of state or other local laws and professional codes of ethics. The most important part of a privacy official's job is to develop a culture in the organization that considers privacy protection as part of everyone's role and responsibility, not just the privacy official.

Supervisory Authority

The supervisory authority is an independent, nongovernment entity that is required by each EU member state to oversee compliance with DPD and GDPR. This entity is responsible for overseeing the effectiveness of data protection within its jurisdiction. The supervisory authority works with government agencies to govern data protection including legal enforcement for any noncompliance and violations of the regulations. The supervisory authority is also focused on aiding the secure transfer of information within the European Union. Individuals who think their privacy rights have been violated bring their complaints to the supervisory authority for legal action. Data controllers interact with supervisory authorities by providing notice before collecting personal information. This transaction is recorded in a public register.

Processing Authorization

Processing authorization refers to the function of data controllers to restrict the use of information to minimize the risks to individuals as much as possible. The supervisory authority reviews transfers and use before processing and provides an evaluation. The authority's decision may come with requirements for measures to further reduce risk, including additional safeguards needed before information processing. Data controllers also must ensure that processing is not done unless there is prior written authorization between the data processors that adheres to the purpose of data collection and outlines any transfers to other third parties on behalf of a processor. If this sounds complicated, think of the relationship between US covered entities, business associates, and business associates of business associates. The downstream sharing of data must be controlled through specific authorizations.

Accountability

As discussed earlier in the chapter, although accountability generally not considered part of the basic principles of security, it is relevant and should be included as a principle of privacy. Accountability can be described as the ability to determine a responsible party for an action taken regarding privacy or security. Accountability is demonstrated by an organization through processes to assign responsibility for the effective operation of privacy controls. The responsibility should be irrefutable, and individuals should be able to determine who controls their sensitive information that is collected and used. Accountability can be associated with the liability of healthcare organizations for adhering to regulations and laws, such as HIPAA, DPD, and GDPR. Fines and penalties are potentially levied, because authorities view healthcare organizations as accountable to follow basic principles of privacy (and security).

Training and Awareness

As with information security training and awareness as a security control, educating the workforce on privacy principles is a cost-effective way to protect personal information. One of the key differences you may find in privacy training and awareness is the need to educate employees on the regulations that govern data privacy. In comparison with information security, which of course is regulated by legislation, data privacy is steeped in national and local (state) laws, while information security is guided more by standards, such as NIST SP 800-53, which deals with security and privacy controls. Consider the impact and focus of international laws such as DPD, GDPR, and the Personal Information Protection and Electronic Documents Act (PIPEDA) have in relation to privacy of data. The fact that the HIPAA Privacy Rule came first and has been in effect since 2003 illustrates the approach to assuring data privacy has been a legislative approach. Training and awareness programs need to focus on the laws and regulations that enact and enforce data privacy.

Good training and awareness programs on data privacy also focus on how employees should comply with local policies and procedures. It helps to create training content that informs people about why keeping sensitive information confidential and using it for the purposes it was collected helps compliance. Perhaps the most important aspect of training is providing clear and relatively easy ways for employees to report privacy-related incidents as they happen. Reducing administrative barriers to reporting, such as providing a hotline or direct reporting system, and minimizing fear of retribution for reporting, are important components of the incident reporting process.

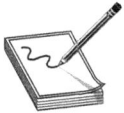

> **NOTE** A valuable topic to cover in privacy training and awareness curricula is recognizing threats to data privacy. Excessive use of information by employees, for instance, can be presented in scenarios that employees may otherwise consider business as usual based on who is sharing the information and conditions in the healthcare setting.

Openness and Transparency

Openness and transparency are principles that emphasize that trust in the collection and use of sensitive information, such as the exchange of electronic health information, can best be established in an open and transparent environment. Each component stresses the importance for individuals to know and understand what personal information is being collected and stored. It also applies to how that information is used and disclosed, as well as how reasonable choices can be exercised with respect to that information. Openness and transparency work together to support the important privacy requirements of choice and consent. It is infeasible to conclude that an individual can provide explicit or implicit choice and consent without knowing and understanding the actions of the data collectors and processors.

Openness

The concept of openness enables any member of the public who has a legitimate interest to be provided with information about the processing of personal data. Although this does not imply access to the data itself, it does mean that the organization should disclose how the data it maintains on behalf of others is kept secure, processed, or shared. According to the Organization for Economic Cooperation and Development (OECD) privacy principles, organizations are advised to maintain a policy and procedure approach that exemplifies openness in all practices and decisions related to the use of sensitive personal information. An organization should be able to demonstrate or provide answers to an individual about the type of information the organization maintains, how it is safeguarded, and how it is used.[20] Of course, openness would include disclosing all purposes for collecting information and the intended uses before collection.

Transparency

In general, transparency, while related to openness, refers to permitting an individual who has data maintained by an organization to be aware of specifically how that data is maintained, processed, or shared. In fact, in many regulations, such as DPD, specific notice must be made when data is being processed to keep the data subjects informed of how information is maintained, processed, or shared. Data controllers must demonstrate transparency by requesting approval that certifies the processing of the information is fair. Transparency supports the right of data subjects to access all data related to them and request deletion or correction of any data that is not accurate or that is being used outside of prior consent. Another aspect of transparency is the willingness of organizations to share information about the policies and procedures that govern the information sharing. PIPEDA is a good example of a regulatory framework that includes transparency in disclosure of policies and procedures as a part of privacy best practices.

Proportionality

Proportionality addresses assurances that personal data that is collected and shared is limited only to that which is necessary and used for the intended and described purpose. Proportionality is included in the Articles of the DPD, which adds the need for data to be accurate and current to meet the intent of this principle. The GDPR has carried the principle forward in its data processing guidance. This principle would, for example, advise against collection of sensitive genetic information through a mouth swab to establish and collect identification data when the sufficient personal information could be obtained from a government-provided identification card.

Proportionality also refers to the level of risk to maintaining and using the information. In the Generally Accepted Privacy Principles (GAPP) framework and DPD law, the principle cautions against holding information longer than is needed would fit within the definition of excessive data collection and use. The OECD privacy principles warn against transfer of information when risk of unauthorized use and disclosure exceeds the benefit of the transfer.

Use and Disclosure

The DPD includes particular direction with regard to how data is intended to be used and how long it can be retained. The data collector must follow the principle specification principle and use the data only for its intended purpose, as disclosed to the data subject. The data should be retained for only as long as needed to fulfil its intended purpose. At that point, the data must be erased. Data can be maintained for analysis, but laws such as PIPEDA direct organizations to make the data anonymous. Entities that want to adhere to GAPP must use data collected only according to what is disclosed in the notice they provided to individuals. Under HIPAA, PHI can be used for treatment, payment, and operations, as well as research and other specified purposes, as long as there is informed patient choice and consent. Use of PHI for reasons outside of these conditions is prohibited.

EXAM TIP You should be aware of the right to be forgotten, or right of individuals to request erasure of their personal data. GDPR strengthened the DPD principle for use and retention. There is, however, a caveat for EU healthcare providers that allows retention of health data in spite of an individual's request when the data is needed and the healthcare provider protects it according to the legal obligations.

Use Limitation

When disclosing PHI, the amount or content of data provided must be limited to what is required to satisfy the request and nothing more. Although the additional data might be useful at a later date or for another purpose unrelated to the patient's current visit, that data should not be collected.

The use limitation requires that the healthcare organization first determine that the disclosure does not violate the disclosure limitation principle, and then it must disclose only the minimum necessary information. Even with legal use or consent, the healthcare organization is obligated to limit use to the volume of data and content that is required for the intended purpose. For instance, if an audit log is required by law enforcement because a hospital employee is suspected of snooping in a medical record, producing an entire access log for all personnel on a certain day, showing all accessed or modified patient information, would be inappropriate because it would involve not only disclosure of the name of the hospital employee and the PHI he or she accessed but possibly also a tremendous amount of PHI irrelevant to the investigation.

A permitted or required use or disclosure does not absolve an organization from excessive use if reasonable efforts are not made to restrict access or control subsequent handling of the information. Privacy principles and laws typically include provisions for use without consent for specific law enforcement and legal proceedings, such as the OECD and HIPAA.

Access

Whether you are referencing the PIPEDA in Canadian law, the DPD or GDPR in European law, or the HIPAA Privacy Rule in US law, you will find provisions regarding the rights of individuals to request access to their personal information that the organization collected. Furthermore, individuals should be given the ability to correct, or rectify, any information that they believe to be in error.

In a healthcare setting, changing some information may not be permissible under other governing medical-legal considerations. However, an annotation of the individual record can be made to highlight the alleged discrepancy. In other cases, if the record can be corrected, provisions must be in place to do so.

In the European Union, data subjects have the right to demand that the data controller notify all third parties that received the data in error, in order to correct the record. With the havoc that medical identity theft can have on an individual's life and financial state, it's easy to see that having the right to access health information and correct a health record is a very important thing. Imagine the issues that could occur to a person whose insurance rates increase because an imposter is receiving care under his or her identity. That individual may initially be the only one to suspect something is wrong, so having the right to access his or her personal information in a timely manner and without excessive cost can limit personal distress and the damage caused by fraud.

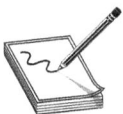

NOTE Accounting of disclosures is a concept related to the right of access under HIPAA. Along with a right to access the record, the individual has the right to know to whom their PHI was disclosed.

Individual Participation

One of the central tenants of all privacy principles is the acknowledgment that privacy works best when the affected individuals are active and involved in the use of their data. The OECD privacy principles clearly outline the privacy expectations individuals should have in this regard, many of which are reflected in subtopics such as notice, consent, choice, and access and correction, which are covered in this chapter.

HIPAA, for example, was enacted in 1996 in large part because the use and disclosure of a patient's health information was too often deemed the privilege of the healthcare organization, without the individual's participation in such disclosure. HIPAA helped to rectify this by clearly outlining the rights of the individuals to have access to, and to participate in, the use of their healthcare information.

Using the OECD privacy principles as a comprehensive illustration, individual participation charges data collectors to do the following:

- Provide data collected to individuals or attest to not having such data in the data collector's control.

- Respond to individuals in a timely and reasonable manner that the individual can understand at a fair cost paid by the individual.

- Explain why a decision to access information is rejected and provide instructions for appealing that decision.

- Permit individual requests to erase, fix, complete, or amend data pertaining to them. Where the challenge is appropriate or correct, the data collector should change the record accordingly.

Notice

Those who have experienced healthcare treatment in the United States have become painfully aware of the requirement to sign a document each year (and it seems like every visit) indicating that we understand HIPAA. In fact, however, what a patient is signing is a statement that he or she understands the *notice* of privacy practices of your healthcare provider or organization. The ability to provide choice and consent is related very closely to the organization's responsibility to provide notice to the affected individual. Under the HIPAA Privacy Rule, US healthcare organizations must not only provide notice at the point of care, but they must also display the notice of privacy practices on their web site, if they have one, in a prominent, easy-to-find way.

Healthcare organizations should obtain a signature from each patient to indicate that a copy of the notice of privacy practices was received and understood. To complement the process, the notice should be posted in plain view onsite at the organization. If a patient wants a copy, it should be relatively easy to provide one. In the United States, healthcare organizations are required to provide notice to patients upon enrollment, at the time of the first appointment, when receiving healthcare services (for example, before undergoing procedures), and any time a patient asks to see such documentation.

The notice is generally in paper form and presented to the patient at the required occasions. Notice, as a privacy principle, is satisfied when the patient signs an acknowledgment of understanding of the notice of privacy practices published by that healthcare organization, which contains the following:

- An explanation of how the covered entity's protected health information may be used and disclosed (if the healthcare organization is required to use it in any other way, the patient must consent to this first)

- The healthcare organization's acknowledgement of its duties to protect health information privacy

- The patient's privacy rights, which include the right to view the information on hand, the right to file a complaint with the federal government (specifically, HHS) if a violation is suspected, and the right to request an amendment to the record if it is incorrect

- Contact information relative to the privacy practices and complaint process

In contrast to a healthcare privacy framework, the data privacy framework of the DPD seeks notice every time data subjects have their data collected. Depending on the individual's preference for the content and frequency of these notices, the DPD allows for a data collector to provide a choice to data subjects to opt in or opt out of notices based on various criteria. This permits the individual to decide on the level of detail or frequency they prefer for data collection.

Events, Incidents, and Breaches

The terms "events," "incidents," and "breaches" are probably not words you want to hear or use on a daily basis. However, with the increase in cybersecurity attacks and the sophistication of attackers, preparing for and responding to them make up a major portion of your responsibilities.

Events and incidents are seemingly synonymous data protection terms, but the difference may be in what characterizes them. According to NIST SP 800-53 Rev. 4, an event is simply and broadly defined as anything that happens in an information system that is observed. Under that definition, it could be a reading from a logging record or an informational alert from a monitoring system. An incident, however, is much more complex and related to risk. The publication describes an incident as an occurrence that actually or potentially impacts the information security of an information system or the sensitive information used by the system. An incident may result in or progress to a violation of policy or procedures. In short, an event can lead to an incident. From an incident, you may experience the next step, a breach. A breach is an unauthorized disclosure, regardless whether it was caused intentionally or unintentionally. Measures for dealing with breach notification may be specific to country, state, and other jurisdiction. Understanding these measures is important as you prepare yourself to protect data in a healthcare organization.

CAUTION Be aware that you need to establish a balance in how you approach data breach notification. You can be negligent in failing to notify individuals and regulators within adequate, required timeframes, and fines and penalties result in most countries for such negligence. You can also contribute to "data breach notification fatigue" if you overnotify. This can open your organization to undue scrutiny and needless bad publicity. Remember that data breaches have an impact on the financial bottom line of organizations, on patient care, and on organizational reputation. Knowing the rules and actions to take, therefore, will likely position you in a key role in your organization's data breach notification procedure.

Notification in the United States

To comply with HIPAA as it has been amended most recently by the Omnibus HIPAA Final Rule (2013), healthcare providers have very specific notification requirements.[21] First, the threshold for when to notify is very clear. A healthcare organization must measure against a risk of disclosure standard established in this regulation. For instance, when a healthcare organization suspects that health information may have been disclosed in an unauthorized manner, it must determine how great a risk exists that the information was actually viewed or used by an unauthorized recipient. An unencrypted e-mail sent to a valid recipient was not likely a reportable breach if the e-mail was not intercepted or sent to other unauthorized recipients. In that case, there is no risk of unauthorized disclosure, and no additional reporting is required. If the information may have been disclosed (for example, as a result of a lost, unencrypted laptop), however, the healthcare organization would be required to promptly notify affected individuals of a breach. If a breach involves more than 500 individuals, the organization *must* notify HHS and the media. Where the breach affects fewer than 500 individuals, the healthcare organization is required to report these in aggregate on a yearly basis.

Notification in the European Union

Although many European nations have experienced breaches, data breach notification traditionally has tended to depend on the rules established by each independent nation. That is beginning to change, however. The latest amendments to the DPD and enactment of GDPR strengthen compulsory obligations to inform EU regulators when data breaches occur across the European Union. The report must be immediate. With a few exceptions, the report must be filed within 24 hours of a security breach of personal data. The directives standardize the data breach notification process across EU member states.

EXAM TIP As discussed at the beginning of the chapter, because privacy principles differ from location to location, you should familiarize yourself with the specific requirements of other nations and locations. In other words, study the DPD and GDPR if you are non-European; study Canadian and EU requirements if you live in the United States. The (ISC)[2] exam is likely to include material on regulations not specific to your home country.

Notification in Canada

Canadian breach notification rules vary across national privacy guidance rules (PIPEDA) and provincial-level privacy rules. Where provinces have guidance that is considered substantially similar to PIPEDA, Canada's federal law, the provincial guidance is sufficient according to federal regulators. That said, PIPEDA currently has limited requirements for notifying individuals. However, some provincial laws do have mandates. Those that require data breach notification are Ontario's Personal Health Information Protection Act, Newfoundland and Labrador's Personal Health Information Act, New Brunswick's Personal Health Information Privacy and Access Act, and Alberta's Personal Information Protection Act.

The Relationship Between Privacy and Security

Security is focused on protection of information from unauthorized disclosure as well as the capabilities needed to detect, respond, and recover from events that become incidents. The focus of privacy is restricting and managing the authorized access to sensitive information and making sure individuals provide personal information only after they are informed of and understand their rights. In performing your role as a healthcare information security and privacy professional in your organization, you must be familiar with certain general and specific areas, but it's also important for you to know how these areas relate to one another. For example, you must understand how consent relates to authorization, how openness relates to transparency, and how legitimate purpose relates to purpose specification. Knowing how HIPAA, DPD, PIPEDA, and other regulations differ is also important.

Privacy and security have evolved over time to become a combined general category of "information protection." The progression was natural, as we find more and more texts and seminars on healthcare privacy and security with the terms used synonymously. However, there is still a distinction between the two that you need to understand. Primarily, information security will never focus on privacy principles such as notice, consent, and accounting of disclosures, for example. Privacy, it can be argued, will focus on more than just digital assets; it will also fulfill obligations to the patient. For example, the organization's promise in the notice of privacy practice may indicate obligations it has that are not related to ensuring confidentiality, integrity, and availability of the data. Maybe its obligations are focused on ensuring the relevancy of the information it collects. This consideration may not have any impact on information security concerns for the same information.

Granted, the domains of privacy and security are closely related, and increasingly so. However, it is unlikely we will ever get to a point where they are indistinguishable and synonymous. We can be relatively certain that for privacy to be effectively provided, security controls must exist and operate effectively. With that in mind, there are a few concepts that demonstrate the interconnected nature of privacy and security, particularly in healthcare, where an unbreakable bond exists between the two: these concepts are dependency, integration, and ownership.

Dependency

The relationship between security and privacy has developed into one of dependency. To achieve security in the healthcare industry, there are certainly elements of privacy that must be addressed. Security controls are more effective and efficient when privacy principles such as data retention or purpose are followed, which reduce the need to protect data that is not required and can be potentially breached. At the same time, privacy is often provided through one or more information security controls.

Within the regulatory process for protecting privacy of personal information (for example, under HIPAA), encryption is seen as an adequate information security control for ensuring the confidentiality of the information transferred via e-mail. Integrated within this security control is the ability to make sure that the person to whom you want to send the e-mail is authorized to view it. The patient experiences the dependency of privacy on security in that the confidentiality they expect is usually regulated by access controls and detection of unauthorized use, as examples. In short, information security tools are used to protect unauthorized disclosure from a privacy perspective.

Privacy depends on good information security practices to preserve the right of individuals to choose who has access to their information. In fact, maintaining the right to refuse to share the information at all is an element of privacy that information security is designed and implemented to protect. In the use of EHRs, identification, authentication, and access management technologies serve to allow credentialed access to defined amounts of data. Without proper credentials, access is denied. Based on the patient's choice and consent, access is even more defined. For example, when patients choose to disallow any requests for their patient status, information found in the EHR cannot be shared with friends, family, or individuals calling the reception desk. Of course, there are usually additional instructions provided to allow specific family members or powers of attorney to receive patient status updates.

Integration

Privacy and security depend on each other, and that dependence results in an integration of the two. In other words, providing information security may involve privacy issues. Conversely, providing privacy can introduce unintended information security concerns that may have nothing to do with whatever privacy protection is being implemented. For example, a number of security safeguards (surveillance cameras and facility access logs, for example) require monitoring people or collecting personal information. These safeguards introduce privacy concerns, because not only do they keep data and people more secure, but they collect personal data in the process. So, while initially you may be concerned with unauthorized access to a patient portal, you may end up having an additional concern with privacy controls. As information privacy and security professionals, we must balance such information security measures against the privacy impacts of collecting personal information, constantly assessing risk. Almost daily, we see integration of privacy and security processes. The goal is to ensure that we understand the implications of privacy and security actions on one another as well as on the problem we intended to address.

This is not to say that integration necessarily produces a negative consequence. Most integration of privacy and security is positive in nature. Information security controls in a digital environment successfully provide privacy as they automate routine processes such as access management. They also reduce errors in enforcement that would exist in paper-based environments, where policy adherence or human action is the only line of defense. For instance, a network firewall or access control list programmed into a router is certainly less fallible than a records room clerk in charge of clearing individuals for facility entry. Moreover, privacy is the intended consequence of many information security practices. Where organizations enforce role-based access configuration of their EHR systems, the privacy of each individual's information is protected by allowing access only to those providers who have a requirement to use the data. In a paper-based records system, this level of data segmentation and constrained availability is nearly impossible. Eavesdropping and easy access to data in plain view is too likely. In the context of integration of information protection, it is relevant to reiterate that the introduction of HIT often improves privacy and security concerns, even as we examine the impacts to information protection HIT capabilities generate.

Another example, and a timely one, of how privacy concerns are integrated with information security involves bring-your-own-device (BYOD) initiatives. While healthcare organizations are increasingly allowing individuals to bring their own smartphones, laptops, tablets, and mobile devices to work, under these initiatives, they are also instituting information security policies and procedures to protect the PHI and PII on their networks—the same networks these devices are accessing. One such procedure is *data wiping*. In the event an employee quits or is terminated, and that person used his or her own device to access the organization's network resources, the BYOD policy likely gives the organization the right to remotely and completely erase everything on the device. This would include the work-related information along with any potential PHI or PII. It could also include pictures, personal information, and personal property.[22] Because of this, the healthcare organization's effort to protect privacy through information security may actually infringe on the privacy of the employee. When implementing the BYOD policy, the integration of privacy and security issues should be considered.

Ownership of Healthcare Information

When it comes to healthcare, traditional expertise grew independently around privacy (such as protecting identity) and information security (such as protecting resources). Over time, both disciplines evolved and developed into specific competencies found in the workforce.

Today that reality has changed. Privacy and security have been integrated into an almost singular competency that every person handling PHI or PII requires. The reasons for the integration have already been discussed—the digitization of health information, networking of medical systems and devices, and regulatory pressures to safeguard health information, to review a few. This is a global reality.

Let's examine the impact of privacy and security from the perspective of information use, beginning with a quick look at health information ownership according to international law and customs, with a focus on the key concern of ownership of the information once it is collected by a healthcare organization. This concern is addressed differently in different countries, based on each country's views on data ownership and laws. Recognizing how authorities view this concern helps you understand how relevant guidelines, laws, and customs affect the overall privacy and security approaches the country expects healthcare organizations (or data collectors) to take.

United States (HIPAA)

True ownership of health information is hard to determine. If we try to make a comparison between how the United States regulates property rights against a notion of data ownership, the comparison is flawed. To clarify, the issue is what level of control a patient in the United States actually has with regard to the use of their private information. Property rights offer owners control as to how their property is used or not used. The rights enforced by US laws provide guidance about how the information is used, but patients don't have ownership rights in that some nonconsensual PHI uses are authorized, such as use for public health reasons or for use under purview of an institutional review board (IRB).

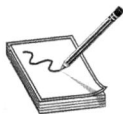

NOTE An IRB is an internal organization in an academic healthcare environment where research is conducted and is in place if clinical trials are performed with the use of human subjects. The IRB governs some baseline consent and authorization guidelines that would not necessarily include additional input from the patient.

Patients do have the right to know what information is collected about them, the right to access that information, the right to request amendment when the information is believed to be incorrect, and the right to know who else has seen the information. Once the data is collected, however, the healthcare organization owns the information in the recorded format, whether written or electronic, such as a file folder or a digital file. The legal responsibility to safeguard the information under HIPAA stems from a perspective of proper caretaking of the data, but the law favors healthcare organization ownership.

European Union (GDPR)

In the European Union, GDPR makes it very clear that the individuals who provide their personal information are the data owners. Data collectors have a responsibility to protect sensitive information continually, but the rights individuals have over their information do not change as the information changes hands. There are strict provisions for gathering personal data, which allow collection of data only for legitimate purposes. Once data is collected, the healthcare organization must respect the rights of the individuals as the data owners. Chief among the rights of data owners under GDPR is the right to complain and obtain redress if an individual believes his or her information is not being used in a way the data collector indicated. In fact, as mentioned earlier in the chapter, as the data owner, the individual has the right to be forgotten from that organization's databases.

United Kingdom

Because healthcare is funded and provided almost exclusively by the National Health Service (the United Kingdom's government healthcare system), health data and medical records in the United Kingdom are seen as government property. Controls must be in place to safeguard the information, of course. There are provisions for patients to view and address perceived discrepancies in their records, but the philosophy of ownership leans toward the government. The overall responsibility for the records lies in the authority of the Secretary of State for Health.

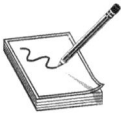

> **NOTE** The UK implementation of GDPR includes a national data opt-out, which became effective in March 2020. Under this provision, individuals can choose not to allow their sensitive information to be used for research and healthcare planning.

Germany

Germany is presented here outside of the governance of the GDPR, because Germany passed its own law, known as an *implementing law* for GDPR. The Federal Data Protection Act (FDPD), effective as of May 25, 2018, was enacted the same day as the GDPR. Germany was the first EU member state to issue its own implementing law.

One of the most important focuses of the FDPD is extensive provisions on the processing of personal data of employees. The law serves to clarify and strengthen the obligation of the provider not only to safeguard the information, but to document all health information completely. For example, the provider must document information such as patient history, diagnoses, treatment, and prognoses. The law mandates that the provider properly maintain the records (whether paper or digital) and preserves ownership with the individual. For example, the law mandates that any and all information be made available for the patient upon his or her request. However, there is some ambiguity in the implementation law about secondary uses of health data. A debated issue is that data controllers in special cases may process the health data for a purpose that is different from the original one. FDPD references GDPR, which has an exception that permits the processing of data for scientific or historical research, or statistical purposes, without consent.

Understand Sensitive Data and Handling

The process of collecting, recording, storing, and exchanging data electronically introduces risks of disclosure, but understanding how healthcare data might be impacted by the method in which you handle it is an important aspect of your role in protecting that data. Most individuals obviously do not want their healthcare records disclosed to others without their permission. Confidentiality is essential to privacy, which is essential to patient care. Confidentiality practices are in place to protect the dignity of patients and to ensure that patients feel free to reveal complete and accurate information required for them to receive the correct medical treatment.

EXAM TIP You should be familiar with recent breach reports from the Internet about healthcare data disclosures, even if your organization has never experienced one. While you review the reports, make an effort to read the details and determine, even when it's not part of the report, what aspect of security failed the organization. This will help you prepare for scenario-based questions on the exam.

Sensitivity Mitigation

Personal information, especially PHI according to HIPAA, is sensitive because of what the information contains and how the information can be misused. Identifying information is often unchangeable, and disclosing it in an unauthorized way invades a person's privacy and can affect their safety. People have a right, or at least an expectation, that employers, the community, or family members do not need to know certain sensitive details about their personal lives. With healthcare data, the fact that the information cannot be changed easily means that fraud and identity theft based on medical information can be almost impossible to undo. As a certified HCISPP professional, you must recognize the critical importance of protecting sensitive information and take every reasonable precaution in reducing the risk of unauthorized data use. Some of the methods to mitigate the sensitivity of the information are to anonymize it or de-identify the data sets. In these ways, the information remains useful for healthcare research or data analytics but cannot be attributed to an individual. When we remove sensitive information from a data set so that it can be useful, but it no longer is attributable to an individual, we preserve privacy.

Anonymization

By definition, the anonymization of data is a process of replacing PII and PHI with a string of X's or some other values that render the data unreadable, yet maintain the location for the data. For example, in a database, the record may have a field for Last Name. The actual last name can be replaced with several X's. The original data is lost, but a data field for last name remains in the database schema. Some identifying data may be useful to include, such as the patient's address postal code, and this useful information can be retained while achieving anonymization. Your analysis of an anonymization procedure should factor in details specific to the context. For example, some small geographic locations may provide identifiable information based on postal code only, so this should be factored into your analysis. In unstructured data, such as a provider's note section, the use of X's could replace the actual last name but still allow analysis of the information.

If you need to re-identify the data later, you can use related and similar processes of pseudonymization and tokenization. Pseudonymization calls for using a fictitious value in place of the original data. Tokenization includes using encryption of the data to create a unique value for each data element. Both processes require a key or code to re-identify the data. The value provided by using pseudonymization and tokenization is that the data is still useful for data analysis and data processing because the data attributes are maintained, and re-identification is possible, unlike in anonymization.

De-identification

De-identification is a sensitivity mitigation process by which data is considered not unique to a specific person and, therefore, not subject to regulation such as the HIPAA Privacy Rule. Using the HIPAA Privacy Rule as a guide, there are two ways to achieve de-identification: the safe harbor method and the expert determination method.

The safe harbor method involves removing all data elements, or direct identifiers, that constitute individually identifiable information. Safe harbor is achieved when the 18 data elements listed in the HIPAA Privacy Rule are stripped from the record. As long as you are clear on which data elements are applicable, this method is probably the easiest to satisfy. Here are those direct identifiers from HIPAA:

- Names
- Addresses (first three digits of a postal code excluded in large communities)
- Most dates related to the individual (such as birth date, except for year)
- Telephone numbers
- Vehicle identifiers and serial numbers, including license plate numbers
- Fax numbers
- Device identifiers and serial numbers
- Personal e-mail addresses
- Universal resource locators (URLs)
- Social Security numbers
- Internet Protocol (IP) addresses
- Medical record numbers
- Biometric identifiers, including fingerprints and voice prints
- Health plan beneficiary numbers
- Photographs and images of the entire face
- Account numbers
- Certificate/license numbers
- Other unique identifying number, characteristic, or codes that may apply if they are likely to identify a specific person

The expert determination method for de-identification is a bit more nuanced. The expert determination process uses a statistically proven method that removes both direct and indirect identifiers and requires an expert in the process of de-identifying sensitive information to assess the risk of anyone re-identifying the data based on the data that remains in the database or record. Here's how it works: Some data sources include direct identifiers and indirect identifiers. Indirect identifiers are bits of information that can be pieced together to identify a single individual—such as race, ethnicity, hair color, and occupation. As mentioned, postal codes can also fall in this category when the population within one postal code is small enough to allow re-identification based on a combination of data elements. Think of this effect as describing someone based on attributes that they may share with a population. As you combine these indirect identifiers, it may become possible to identify who you are describing in that population.

The general outcome of sensitivity mitigation is de-identified data, whether established using a safe harbor approach or an expert determination method. If the organization needs to reinstate the identity of the individuals in the future, re-identification is the reversal process. A code or key is created to link the de-identified data to corresponding PII and PHI. That code or key is protected by the organization and maintained separately, sometimes in a literal safe or a software application. De-identified and anonymized data have beneficial uses in healthcare, as public health, data analytics, and population health efforts are enabled by being able to examine large data sets. Because the de-identified or anonymized data sets are not subject to the HIPAA Privacy Rule, they can be used and shared more broadly to assist research and marketing as well.

Categories of Sensitive Data

As you know, personal healthcare data is internationally protected by regulation or law. Almost every privacy and security framework includes specific direction for healthcare data. Within the general category of healthcare information (for example, PHI), there are some noteworthy subtypes that bear mentioning, because they have additional or even separate handling provisions for those that require access or use. As a representative sample, the following subsections present EU public health information protection requirements and some US-specific requirements.

European Union

The DPD gave EU member states' data collection agencies the authority to deviate from regular handling procedures for privacy-protected information where there are concerns for the welfare of the public and public health and safety. GDPR has continued that. The DPD allowed for special handling considerations for health data that should be disclosed in the interest of public safety. The directive also clearly outlines an acceptance of member states that decide to deviate from normal processes for the purposes of scientific research, gathering of government statistics, and settling claims for benefits and services in the health insurance system. However, data collectors must otherwise continue to provide safeguards for protecting sensitive data from other, unauthorized disclosure.

United States

Although it is possible to assume that HIPAA contains the complete set of regulatory concerns and controls relative to healthcare, this is not completely accurate. Other regulatory laws and sets of controls exist with special purposes relative to specific patient populations.

Substance Abuse Healthcare organizations that treat patients for drug and alcohol abuse must not only comply with HIPAA, but they must also comply with the Confidentiality of Substance Use Disorder Patient Records, updated in 2017; the Comprehensive Alcohol Abuse and Alcoholism Prevention, Treatment, and Rehabilitation Act of 1970;

and the amended language of the Drug Abuse Office and Treatment Act of 1972. The considerations addressed by these regulations center around providing additional confidentiality. Even providers that treat a patient in one care setting, such as primary care, have to obtain an additional privilege to access the drug and alcohol treatment records from another care setting, such as a drug and alcohol treatment center, if that record is relevant to the primary care treatment. Typically, substance abuse treatment and records are regulated under behavioral health laws, and additional access clearance is required to access them

Education Records of Minors The Family Educational Rights and Privacy Act (FERPA) governs the use and disclosure of the PII of minor students and, where applicable, PHI. For the most part, FERPA disallows an educational entity from disclosing any information to a third party without parental consent. While FERPA would not at first seem to have any relationship with HIPAA, it does overlap because schools in the United States commonly employ a nurse or healthcare provider. The data collected by these individuals is covered under FERPA, even if the school has no obligation under HIPAA. The HIPAA privacy and security rules exclude from additional or redundant governance any PHI collected by school healthcare providers. FERPA is generally considered sufficient to protect the health information of minor students as part of securing the defined education record. In short, properly safeguarded information under FERPA would be compliant with HIPAA if the school is under HHS regulatory control.

HIV/AIDS The accidental disclosure of HIV/AIDS records can be a particular source of distress for patients. You can read summaries of complaints and investigations from the HHS that document mistakes and errors that resulted in sensitive HIV/AIDS disclosures to unauthorized recipients.[23] The HIPAA Privacy Rule is applicable to protecting HIV/AIDS records. However, the confidentiality of these diagnoses was also protected using the Rehabilitation Act of 1973 and the Americans with Disabilities Act of 1990 before HIPAA. The dilemma with HIV/AIDS historically is that healthcare organizations have to weigh public health concerns with individual patient confidentiality. This is a serious decision with impacts, as patients with HIV/AIDS have been discriminated against over the years. Unauthorized disclosure of this category of PHI has potentially devastating consequences to many patients and their employment, health insurance, and in the communities they live.

Mental Health Mental health treatment by a qualified healthcare provider will result in a special type of medical document called psychotherapy notes. These are kept separate from a patient's regular medical record. There are many provisions for healthcare providers to share mental health information for the care of an individual, but stringent controls over this information are warranted because of the sensitivity of the information and the risk that unauthorized disclosure can cause unwanted effects, such as causing the patient delay or stop seeking the care they need. Special consent may be needed by the individual to release contents to the psychotherapy notes. Because of the risk of harm to themselves and others, HHS and Office of Civil Rights have published clarifying guidance that relaxes disclosure rules when the provider thinks a patient is in imminent danger. This also includes notification of law enforcement and specific individuals who may be the target, such as the spouse, of a patient. These exceptions are outside of regulated requirements for patient consent.

Genetic Information   As technology improves in collecting and using genetic information, there is little doubt that this data will be clinically significant and useful parts of the comprehensive medical record. However, the potential to misuse this information exists. For example, employers and health insurers may discriminate based on potential conditions or predispositions to disease or disability indicated in a person's genetic code. To begin to address these unwanted actions against people, in 2009 the United States enacted the Genetic Information Nondiscrimination Act (GINA). Without controls to protect an individual's genetic information, including specific notices of privacy practices and obligating informed consent documents, individuals would be reluctant to participate in pioneering research and genetic studies.

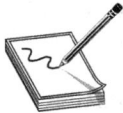

> **NOTE**   Pregnancy information also requires special sensitivity handling. Normally, pregnancy is not a diagnosis with similar stigma to other situations covered in this section, but a history of pregnancy must be kept confidential and cannot be used to discriminate against women. In addition, pregnancy cannot be used as a pre-existing condition for health insurance purposes, and employers must offer maternity care as part of any insurance plans that are a benefit of employment.

Chapter Review

This chapter introduced security objectives and attributes. The evolution from information security to cybersecurity reflects the evolution of healthcare from a paper-based system to a digital one. Responsibilities to protect health information have increased now that duties include or involve electronic information security (cybersecurity) roles and responsibilities as well as traditional, paper-based information. The information in this chapter is central to your overall understanding of healthcare information security and privacy. There are many types of security controls, such as access models, encryption, business continuity, data disposal, and incident response, to name a few. Each control focuses on preventing, detecting, or correcting data incidents, or any combination of those. Mastering implementation and management of information security controls is fundamental, yet the skills required can be complex and challenging.

Under most regulatory requirements, including national, state, and local requirements, organizations are tasked with designating privacy officers, who are responsible for assuring the privacy of data, for assisting customer patients with issues or complaints, and for monitoring the quality and coordination of security within the organization. One of the many duties of the privacy officer is processing authorizations for certain kinds of research, marketing, fundraising, and other issues that are not directly health related. Use relates to the intended use of the data at the time of collection. Retention relates to the time for which the data must be accounted for and kept secure. Chapter 7 will address what should happen when required retention periods end.

If privacy data is disclosed in an unintended or unauthorized way, regulatory requirements include measures to advise those affected by the loss or breach. Openness enables any member of the public who has legitimate interest to be provided information about the processing of data, while transparency refers to permitting an individual who has data maintained by an organization to be aware of specifically how their data is stored, processed, or shared.

Under the HIPAA Privacy Rule, use limitation states that covered entities must reasonably safeguard protected health information to limit incidental uses or disclosures made pursuant to an otherwise permitted or required use or disclosure. Access limitation covers the topic of limiting access to protected health information to those in the workforce who need access based on their roles. Under the OECD privacy principles, individual participation requires that individuals be permitted to obtain the status of data related to them, communicate with the data controller, and challenge data related to them. In sum, the integration and dependency between information privacy and security are fundamental components that you, as an HCISPP, must understand and master.

Questions

1. A healthcare provider is examining a new patient with complaints of severe back pain. The provider suspects substance abuse and dependency on pain medication based on her initial observation. She requests access to previous substance abuse records. That request is denied to protect patient privacy by the health information management director who controls access to the electronic health record. He claims to be following governing law and ethical practices. Which of the following principles is impeding patient care?

   A. Confidentiality

   B. Integrity

   C. Availability

   D. Accountability

2. In a healthcare office environment, which of the following applications may possibly have sensitive data included within its storage media?

   A. E-mail

   B. Scheduling

   C. Billing

   D. All of the above

3. Which of the following are elements of business continuity?

   A. Continuing mission capabilities after a power loss

   B. Continuing contact with a patient who moves from the care area

   C. Keeping in contact with a former business associate

   D. Preparing for an external assessment while continuing to see patients

4. Which of the following describes the ability for a user to do something with a computer resource, such as permission to review, edit, or delete?

   A. Least privilege

   B. Logging

   C. Monitoring

   D. Access control

5. Which of the following is defined as a condition or weakness in (or absence of) security procedures or technical, physical, or other controls?

   A. Threat

   B. Risk

   C. Vulnerability

   D. Exploitation

6. The principles of security, often referred to as CIA, are

   A. Confidentiality, integrity, accountability

   B. Contingency, integrity, accountability

   C. Confidentiality, integrity, availability

   D. Confidentiality, interoperability, availability

7. To protect health information in an e-mail sent to a colleague, which would be a proper security control?

   A. Logical controls

   B. Strong authentication

   C. Encryption

   D. Least privilege

8. Based on some concerns you have with the organization's firewall, you export a report of a data packet transfer during the last 15 minutes. You see evidence of packet loss and a stalled data transfer. Which of these terms best defines the type of information you are reviewing?

   A. Incidents

   B. Breaches

   C. Events

   D. Alerts

9. According to many leading privacy principles and regulations, which concept would be followed to make edits or amendments to the record should a mistake be identified after a patient requested a copy of her last medical procedure?

   A. Accuracy

   B. Access

   C. Individual participation

   D. Openness

10. Which of the following is not an element of the limited data set under HIPAA?

   A. Social Security numbers

   B. First three digits of your postal code

   C. E-mail address

   D. Bank personal identification number

Answers

1. **C.** Because the director will not make the patient's data available, it is likely to impact the treatment of this patient negatively. A, confidentiality, is incorrect. Under some circumstances, such as substance abuse, additional provisions are necessary to maintain the confidentiality of patient identification, but this is not the case in this scenario of a legitimate medical need for access. B and D are incorrect because the security principles of integrity and accountability are not at issue with disclosing previous prescriptions and potentially abuse of pain medication in this scenario.

2. **D.** Even though an organization may have policies in place that prohibit the use of e-mail for communications with the patient and others about specific sensitive healthcare diagnoses, users and patients could be including this information in their e-mail communications. As a result, you should assume that e-mail data should be stored with the same security controls as other sensitive data systems. Clearly, patient scheduling and billing data contain personally identifiable data as well as protected health information.

3. **A.** Business continuity addresses the organization's ability to deliver its mission (healthcare, for our purposes) when it may be affected by electrical outages, weather-related events, or community-based events such as riots, accidents, or an outbreak of a virus that affects staffing levels. Although maintaining contact with former patients or business associates and preparing for external assessments are part of doing business, they are not part of business continuity.

4. **D.** Access control defines the technical ability to perform a function with a computer resource. Although A, least privilege, does cover the level of access, it defines an overall scope and is not specific to a user or role. B is incorrect because logging describes the process of capturing the system information that relates to the asset, not setting any privileges. Likewise, C, monitoring, is a passive activity that is defined by oversight of system activity, usually through review of logs.

5. **C.** A vulnerability is a condition of weakness that can be exploited by a threat. Although it can be exploited and is a risk to the system or organization, only vulnerability matches the definition. A, threat, is an action or a condition that presents a source of concern for the security of an organization, like a phishing attack. B, risk, is a measure of a negative event happening based on mitigations, the frequency, and impact of that event. D, exploitation, is the result of a risk realized; an attack that exposes a weakness and results in a successful security incident.

6. **C.** The principles of security are confidentiality, integrity, and availability. Although accountability, included in A, is an often-mentioned principle, it is not considered a component of the CIA triad. Likewise contingency, included in B, especially in the healthcare setting. D, interoperability, is also discussed, but it is not a primary principle.

7. **C.** Encryption is the technical security control that satisfies the safe and effective transfer of sensitive information via e-mail. A is incorrect because logical controls include access controls, which may be incorporated into the operating systems to permit a technical capability such as reading, creating, editing, modifying, or deleting within an application or system. B is important to gaining access to the system in general but would not protect the information from unauthorized access during data transfer. Least privilege, D, is also not the best answer as the concept is associated as a control for access and authorization to the information, not the secure transfer.

8. **C.** Events are all the observable items or entries that describe activity on the network or within the device logs. These observable details are not necessarily a problem, as further investigation can determine whether an event is in fact an incident. A, incidents, are events that describe an information security item that requires you to take action against and possibly remediate. This scenario does not describe a breach, B, because the review has only determined traffic flow that failed before leaving the organization through the firewall, and there is no mention of the data being sensitive. D, alerts, is incorrect because the scenario does not include a mention of those events triggering a notification to you as the security professional.

9. **A.** Accuracy is the appropriate principle. Providing patients with the ability to request corrections to their records helps ensure records' accuracy. The scenario does imply access, B, by honoring the patient's request to view her record, but the scenario contains a more significant element of using the access to achieve accuracy. C, individual participation, is incorrect for a similar reason, in that knowing the information exists and getting access is individual participation,

but the scenario describes accuracy of the information. You could assume the organization does follow the principle of openness, D, but it is not explicit in the scenario that the patient knew and understood the policies that were actually followed.

10. **B.** The first three digits of your postal code are not part of the limited date set under HIPAA, because that result could include thousands of people. A, C, and D are incorrect: Social Security numbers, e-mail addresses, and bank PINs are all part of the limited data set because they have a connection to your health record.

References

1. Dean, B. 2017. Privacy vs. Security: Do today's models work with the Internet of Things and its cousin, big data? *SecureWorks* blog, March 23, https://www.secureworks.com/blog/privacy-vs-security.

2. Lewis, K. 2017. Security Policies and Plans Development. In *Computer and Information Security Handbook* (pp. 565–570). Morgan Kaufmann.

3. Stine, K., R. Kissel, W. Barker, A. Lee, and J. Fahlsing. 2008. *Guide for Mapping Types of Information and Information Systems to Security Categories: Appendices.* NIST SP 800-60 Vol. 2 Rev. 1, Section D.14.4. https://csrc.nist.gov/publications/detail/sp/800-60/vol-2-rev-1/final.

4. Government of Canada. Canadian Provincial Privacy Act (R.S.C., 1985, c. P-21). http://laws-lois.justice.gc.ca/eng/acts/P-21/index.html.

5. Borland, S. 2014. "2,000 NHS patients' records are lost every day with more than two million serious data breaches logged since the start of 2011." February 14, Daily Mail.com, http://www.dailymail.co.uk/news/article-2559876/2-000-NHS-patients-records-lost-day-two-million-data-breaches-logged-start-2011.html#ixzz3CgQ3zTL9.

6. European Parliament and the Council of the European Union. 1995. "DIRECTIVE 95/46/EC OF THE EUROPEAN PARLIAMENT AND OF THE COUNCIL of 24 October 1995 on the protection of individuals with regard to the processing of personal data and on the free movement of such data." Chapter VI, "Supervisory Authority and Working Party on the Protection of Individuals with Regard to the Processing of Personal Data," Article 28, Section 7. http://eur-lex.europa.eu/legal-content/EN/TXT/PDF/?uri=CELEX:31995L0046&from=en.

7. McBride, T., M. Ekstrom, L. Lusty, J. Sexton, and A. Townsend. 2017. Special Publication (NIST SP 1800-11, Draft). *Data Integrity: Recovering from Ransomware and Other Destructive Events.* Available for download at https://csrc.nist.gov/publications/detail/sp/1800-11/draft.

8. NIST Information Technology. 2020. "Identity and Access Management." https://www.nist.gov/topics/identity-access-management.

9. Afshar, M., S. Samet, and T. Hu. 2018. An Attribute Based Access Control Framework for Healthcare System. *Journal of Physics*: Conference Series 933. https://iopscience.iop.org/article/10.1088/1742-6596/933/1/012020/pdf.

10. Breaux, T. 2014. "Encryption and Other Technologies." In *Introduction to IT Privacy: A Handbook for Technologists*. Portsmouth, NH: International Association of Privacy Professionals, p. 126.

11. Yang, C. and H. Lee. 2016. A study on the antecedents of healthcare information protection intention. *Inf Syst Front 18*, 253–263. Can be purchased at https://link.springer.com/article/10.1007/s10796-015-9594-x.

12. Ziegler, A. 2018. Hospitals, Doctors and Patients Impacted by Unplanned EHR Downtime. *Healthcare IT Today* (online). https://www.healthcareittoday.com/2018/06/18/hospitals-doctors-and-patients-impacted-by-unplanned-ehr-downtime.

13. UCISA (University of Oxford). 2019. "ITIL – Introducing service operation." http://docshare01.docshare.tips/files/21461/214619725.pdf.

14. Aon. nd. "Is Communications Planning Part of Your Incident Response Plan?" Reprinted from E. Strotz, July 2016, at securityroundtable.org. https://www.aon.com/cyber-solutions/thinking/develop-breach-response-communications-plan.

15. Onitiu, D. 2019. "'The Duty to Remember v the Right to be Forgotten: Holocaust Archiving and Research, and European Data Protection Law': Notes from Arye Schreiber's seminar hosted by NINSO, the Northumbria Internet & Society Research Interest Group." Northumbria Legal Studies Working Paper No. 2019/01. Download from https://papers.ssrn.com/sol3/papers.cfm?abstract_id=3343476.

16. Black, E. 2001. *IBM and the Holocaust: The Strategic Alliance Between Nazi Germany and America's Most Powerful Corporation*. New York: Crown Publishers/Random House.

17. US Department of Health and Human Services Office for Civil Rights. 2018. "Guidance on HIPAA and Individual Authorization of Uses and Disclosures of Protected Health Information for Research." https://www.hhs.gov/sites/default/files/hipaa-future-research-authorization-guidance-06122018%20v2.pdf.

18. US Department of Health and Human Services. 2003. HIPAA Privacy Rule, "Public Health," 45 CFR 164.512(b). https://www.hhs.gov/hipaa/for-professionals/special-topics/public-health/index.html.

19. US Department of Health and Human Services. 2017. "Guidance on HIPAA & Cloud Computing." https://www.hhs.gov/hipaa/for-professionals/special-topics/cloud-computing/index.html.

20. Gerber, B. 2020. "OECD Privacy Principles," Organization for Economic Cooperation and Development (OECD). http://oecdprivacy.org.

21. Holloway, M. 2013. "HHS Finalizes HIPAA Privacy and Data Security Rules, Including Stricter Rules for Breaches of Unsecured PHI." Lockton blog, https://www.lockton.com/Resource_/PageResource/MKT/01232013_HHS%20 Finalizes%20HIPAA_Data%20Security_Unsecured%20PHI.pdf.

22. Alotaibi, B., and H. Almagwashi. 2018. "A review of BYOD Security Challenges, Solutions and Policy Best Practices," *2018 1st International Conference on Computer Applications & Information Security (ICCAIS),* Riyadh, 2018, pp. 1–6.

23. US Department of Health and Human Services. 2020. "Health Information Privacy Enforcement Examples Involving HIV/AIDS." https://www.hhs.gov/civil-rights/for-providers/compliance-enforcement/examples/aids/cases/index.html.

Risk Management and Risk Assessment

This chapter covers Domain 6, "Risk Management and Risk Assessment," of the HCISPP certification. After you read and study this chapter, you should be able to:

- Understand risk management concepts, leading frameworks, and relevant processes
- Be able to assess risk management controls for effectiveness and efficiency
- Differentiate between quantitative and qualitative approaches to measuring risk
- Conduct risk management activities relevant to role and position in the organization
- Evaluate risk and support risk treatment decisions such as risk avoidance, mitigation, or transfer of residual risk in the organization

Healthcare information privacy and security has evolved from solely the pursuit of regulatory and standards compliance to risk reduction and information protection controls maturity. Compliance with laws and standards are still important, but our profession has advanced to be better aligned to clinical and business enablement. That requires a proficiency in risk management.

The concept of risk in healthcare organizations has several definitions depending on where you work. From a clinical perspective, risk is the measurement of the quality and safety of healthcare provided. Risks that put patients at harm are identified, and actions are taken to prevent or control the risks. Because we are concerned with information protection, risk is the measure of the potential harm caused by a purposeful or accidental event that negatively impacts the confidentiality, integrity, or availability of information assets. Information risk can also result in patient harm.

As you read this chapter, note that the use of the term "risk" will apply to information risk unless otherwise specifically mentioned. We cover the organized, systematic approach to managing risk and decision-making in information protection. There are several frameworks for doing this important work. Once you understand what your risks are, you can begin to decide what you want to do about it. We cover several approaches to managing risk. For example, organizations must decide whether to mitigate, accept, or transfer risk. We'll also introduce a few other approaches to managing risk. In the end, your role is to measure the risk and communicate the alternatives to leadership with regard to how information protection integrates with business strategy, clinical practices, and third-party relationships.

Understand Enterprise Risk Management

Making decisions about managing information risk requires a systematic and organized approach. Otherwise, emotions or personal preferences can influence actions and may even increase the chances of an event happening or increase the extent of the impact. In a healthcare setting, we see this when clinical expediency is not balanced against risk of unauthorized information disclosure. There are many frameworks and a few different methodologies to use to assess and measure risk to help you make decisions. It is important to determine which fits best in your organization.

Before we introduce some of the leading risk frameworks, we need to define the following terms that are used in discussing frameworks and methodologies:

- **Threat**   A source of potential information loss or damage relevant to your organization
- **Vulnerability**   A weakness that may expose the organization unnecessarily to a threat
- **Probability**   The likelihood that a threat can happen (increased based on vulnerability)
- **Impact**   The extent of damages expected by a threat event happening
- **Mitigation and controls**   Actions or processes put in place to either prevent (control) or lessen (mitigate) the impact of exploited threats

Figure 6-1 introduces the overall concepts underlying decision-making using risk measurement to choose between alternatives; this is a foundational concept behind any information risk management framework.

Measuring and Expressing Information Risk

We have to admit there is no perfect security strategy that eliminates all chances that an organization will experience an event. Some say it is not a matter of "if," but "when." Therefore, we focus on reducing the risk of adverse events as much as possible. To do that, we have to measure and express risk in an understandable format. Here are some risk equations you may be familiar with:

Risk = Likelihood × Impact

Risk = Threat × Vulnerability × Impact

Risk = Probability of Event × Measures of Consequences

These risk equations do not imply that risk is always measured in objective terms (numbers, percentages, data results, and so on). These measures relate to quantitative risk

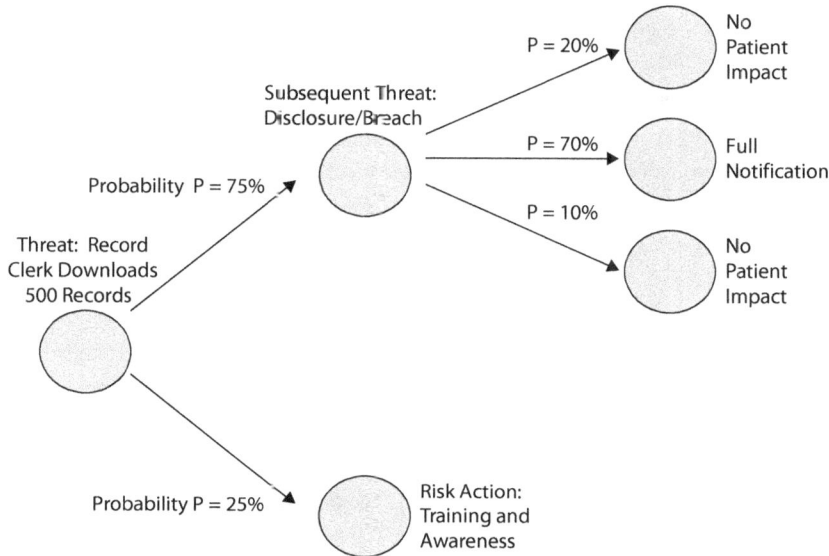

Figure 6-1 Simple risk-based decision tree

evaluations. Risk can also be expressed in subjective terms, such as a management value or priority measurement (low, medium, high, and so on). In healthcare, the impact of risk may be measured in monetary cost, reputation loss, and (most importantly) adverse patient events. As an illustration, an organization called Open Web Application Security Project (OWASP) is a leading body of standards-setting organizations and experts from around the world. The organization uses a combination of simple measures to calculate risk. Based on subjective values (0–9, with 9 being the highest), assessments are made against threats and vulnerabilities to achieve an estimation of impact.[1] These notional values are plotted on a chart to help you quickly identify the level of overall risk severity of the issue (Figure 6-2).

Generally speaking, the common points made by almost all credible information risk management frameworks highlight these important steps:

1. Identify a person or people who are responsible for privacy and security issues.

2. Perform an information risk assessment (using a standards-based framework).

3. Have up-to-date policies that cover the proper use of sensitive information assets.

4. Charter a formal board or committee that oversees information risk management.

5. Communicate findings and remediation progress through that group to senior leadership (and the entire organization, as needed).

6. Manage third-party risk by assessing their proper use of sensitive information.

7. Maintain an active privacy and security awareness training program for employees.

8. Have an obvious incident reporting process for employees to follow.

Figure 6-2
OWASP
methodology
for making risk-
based decisions

	Overall Risk Severity			
	High	Medium	High	Critical
	Medium	Low	Medium	High
Impact	Low	Note	Low	Medium
		Low	Medium	High
	Likelihood			

Your organization can take several approaches to measure and evaluate risk. Many organizations may opt to combine approaches based on their mission, asset valuation, risk tolerance, or cost–benefit of conducting the analyses. We will discuss these approaches throughout this chapter. For now, here is a quick introduction to these approaches to demonstrate the types of outcomes you may have using risk evaluation and measurement tools and techniques:

- **Quantitative approach** This includes the use of objective data such as financial impacts, revenue losses, historical frequency and probabilities, and risk scores associated with vulnerability management. Because data can be difficult to obtain, this approach is sometimes used in conjunction with qualitative methods.

- **Qualitative approach** The components of the risk equations are valued at levels such as high, medium, and low. Subjective factors are used to measure and evaluate risk. This approach is particularly useful when the assessment must be made in a short period of time or the assessors are familiar with the subjects of the assessment (such as systems, processes, vendors, or applications).

- **Hybrid or semi-options** In some scenarios, a combination of both qualitative and quantitative approaches is used together. These approaches may be used sequentially. For example, a qualitative assessment begins the assessment, and a quantitative assessment follows to provide projected financial losses or magnitudes of severity of a threat. Alternatively, the approaches can be used in tandem with frequency, for example, being quantified while impact on intangible assets being assessed on a qualitative scale of high, medium, and low.

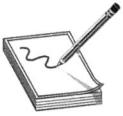

NOTE The use of quantitative or qualitative approaches is not a choice between quality or value. Collecting data for a qualitative or quantitative assessment includes interviews of stakeholders and subject matter experts across the organization, reviews of historical records, and observations by the assessors of controls, processes, and behaviors. Both assessment and evaluation methods can lead organizations to proper risk responses.

Identifying Information Assets

To begin an assessment and measurement process to evaluate risks to the organization, you must identify the information assets to be assessed. In this effort, you should be concerned with hardware and software for systems, devices, and appliances owned and operated within the organization. This will include identifying locations of systems and data storage for electronic protected health information (PHI). Both GDPR and HIPAA require organizations to have and maintain data inventories. With this information, you can initiate those healthcare information risk assessments that consider the threats or impacts to sensitive healthcare information.

The regulations do not prohibit manual approaches to establishing an inventory. Depending on organization size and complexity, you may be able to document asset inventory using project archives, interviews, and physical location by observation. More realistically, most organizations will need to use technology in the form of asset scanning tools to identify information assets. Numerous tools are available to perform different functions. A couple of examples of tools and scanning approaches you may consider for use are listed here:

- **Passive scanning** The approach typically scans network traffic for metadata contained in the packets that identify the assets and particular attributes of the assets. This information populates the inventory. Passive scanning does not adequately identify assets that do not communicate but are attached to the network. It can also miss some network and security appliances that operate only at the physical or data link layers.

- **Active scanning** On-demand scanning of the network can improve inventory of assets and information about the assets. This approach attempts to reach every asset on the network regardless of whether or not the asset is communicating. A downside to this approach is the risk of creating downtime as the network resources are taxed, or the individual assets possibly crashing as a result of the scan.

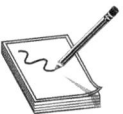

NOTE Related to scanning of networks for asset inventories, scanning tools can be part of an asset discovery process that identifies unauthorized additions or changes to the expected inventory or configuration of the assets. For example, asset scanning is one method of identifying an unauthorized Wi-Fi hotspot or rogue access point.

Asset Valuation Methods

Information asset valuation is a process that ascribes worth to data and technologies within the organization. Assets in a healthcare organization support important areas such as patient care activities, the operations of the organization, and research initiatives. The value of the assets will be specific to the organization as variables such as sensitivity, criticality, and strategic benefit will factor into the level of protection the assets require. Part of the measure of an asset's value is the cost or other impacts to the organization if the asset is lost or unavailable for a period of time.

To begin an asset valuation exercise, we have to explore a couple of ways of gathering the data about the assets. When we discussed risk assessments earlier in this chapter, we featured two approaches, quantitative and qualitative. In conducting asset valuation, there is a similar differentiation in approaches—one is based on objective measures and the other is based in subjective analysis. Here are the two basic approaches:

Descriptive Approach

This subjective approach is obtained through structured and unstructured data collection tools such as interviews, surveys, checklists, and comment forms. The values may also come from focus group sessions with subject matter experts and stakeholders to establish baselines and develop indicators to monitor that value is gained. This type of valuation estimates the following:

- **Intrinsic value** This describes how accurate, comprehensive, beneficial, and exclusive the assets are.
- **Business value** This measures the relevancy of the assets and their usefulness for business purposes.
- **Performance value** This refers to the utility of the assets to drive key business or clinical indicators and initiatives.

Metric Approach

These measures are objective, or based in statistics, financial data, historical records, clinical outcomes, or economic rates. Calculations may come from external sources such as the costs to replace the assets, or from regulatory actions such as fines and penalties. Other sources of this data are asset logs, annual expenditures, return on investment calculations, or depreciation rates. Here are some of the categories of metric asset valuations:

- **Cost value** This is the cost to the organization resulting from loss of the asset and the associated expense of replacing it.
- **Market value** This is associated with the worth of the asset (such as a system, data, or technology) based on selling it or providing it as a service to another organization.
- **Economic value** This relates to the importance or direct influence the asset has on increasing revenue or reducing costs.

Using Valuation Approaches with Tangible and Intangible Assets

Assets can be categorized as tangible or intangible. You can use descriptive and metric approaches to measure each of these categorizations. Let's take a closer look.

Measuring the Value of Tangible Assets   Tangible assets are generally things you can touch. The word "tangible" means perceptible to touch. Assets such as office buildings, hardware, data centers, and some computer systems are often tangible assets.

To measure the value of these, a primary approach is a metric evaluation of original cost of the asset minus depreciation. Depreciation is a valuation of the reduction in value of an asset as it is used over time, presuming assets lose value even with normal use. Normally, an asset is valuable at least until the depreciation reaches a zero financial balance. Some assets exceed that timeframe, however, and can remain valuable for more years.

You can also determine tangible asset value by assessment of replacement costs. Those values can be obtained through market comparisons of competing suppliers and other sellers of similar products.

Measuring the Value of Intangible Assets   These assets are property of the organization but are not physical assets, though they do have value and are often subject to regulatory requirements that necessitate investment in safeguards. Examples of intangible assets are goodwill, reputation, brand, licenses, patents, trademarks, and copyrights.

Healthcare organizations can generate a tremendous amount of intellectual property in clinical practices, research outcomes, and business models that have tremendous value. Most importantly to our learning in this area is that PHI is a source of intangible value to the organization in that it can be used to improve the clinical practices, reach research outcomes, and help develop new business models.

Measuring intangible asset values is difficult. There may not be a true original cost, depreciation estimates are not applicable, and replacement costs are not a possibility, particularly where the intangible asset is unique to the organization (such as patents, reputation, business process). Several approaches can be used to value intangible assets, including the following:

- **Cost**   When applicable, the original cost of the asset can be compared against replacement cost. The drawback is that an intangible asset is usually worth much more than the cost required to develop or obtain it. Replacement costs generally do not provide a true representation of comparative value. This may foster risk assessment decisions to accept more risk than the high value of the asset would require.

- **Capitalization of historical profits**   Intangible assets can lead to increased revenue and market share. Accounting for the costs of the intangible assets are changed from an expense to an asset and spread out over time associated with the returns on the investment. You can also refer to this approach simply as an income approach to valuation of the asset.

- **Cost avoidance or savings**   Reputation or favorable brand recognition provides a good example of an intangible asset benefit that can be measured in the reduced risk of a data breach, a reduction in potential fines and penalties, and the prevention of lost revenue from abnormal patient churn to competing healthcare organizations.

- **Market**   Some intangible assets are similar between organizations, such as copyrights or franchise licenses. If there is enough similarity, one company can estimate the value of its intangible asset based on the terms of a sale of a similar asset between two other companies.

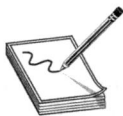

NOTE   Intangible assets can have a definite expiration period, or an indefinite expiration period. Patents and trademarks that are not renewed are examples of definite intangible assets. Brand and reputation are some examples of indefinite intangible assets, because the organization intends for the value to continue without end.

Risk Components

The components of risk are the separate factors that can be measured to help predict the chance, cost, and magnitude an adverse event may have. It may be obvious, but risk is specific and unique to each organization. To sufficiently evaluate risk, apply adequate security controls, and treat the risks appropriately, all components need to be included. Think about a risk evaluation that includes an estimate of $4M due to a flood. The chance, however, of a flood in the location of the hospital is a once-every-100-years occurrence. Without the inclusion of frequency or likelihood, the impact of a $4M loss might be overestimated. Each component can and should be assessed individually as well as multiplied together to reach a measurement that can be trusted and useful. In these next sections, we will discuss important factors of information risk.

Exposure

Exposure is related to the concept of vulnerabilities in the context of information security. An exposure is a measure of the potential for occurrence as part of a vulnerability. You may see this term expressed as a predisposing condition in sources such as NIST SP 800-30 Rev. 1, *Guide for Conducting Risk Assessments*. As an HCISPP, you will understand that the environment you work in involves the use of PHI with a high degree of information sharing. This is an example of a predisposing condition or an exposure that will help you risk assess various vulnerabilities. Other sources view exposure, in part, as the existence of misconfigured systems or defects in software applications that can increase likelihood and impact of a vulnerability that an attacker exploits.

Likelihood

The probability, or likelihood, that a vulnerability will be exploited is an important component of the risk equation. We can evaluate the likelihood from the perspective of the attacker or adversary. This view includes consideration of adversary attributes, including capabilities, skills, persistence, and objectives that increase or decrease the chance the attacker could exploit a vulnerability. Another angle to use to measure likelihood is through historical data. For example, the likelihood that natural disasters could occur can be predicted based on past occurrence of the events. You could add a measure such as service level agreement (SLA) compliance with patch management to a likelihood measure. If the organization typically does not meet SLA requirements, the likelihood of vulnerabilities being exploited increases without any increase in adversary attributes.

> **EXAM TIP** Test scenarios may appear to depict high levels of risks because a vulnerability exists. If the weakness has never been exploited, the real risk may be low. However, the sense of urgency can be exaggerated because of the estimated negative impacts. Make sure to consider real likelihood in exam scenarios (and in reality).

Impact

Risk decisions cannot be made without a realistic estimation of the effects or consequences of a security event. Overestimation can lead to overly restrictive and costly actions to avoid or minimize the outcome of a security risk. Underestimation can have the opposite effect, as the organization may not prepare adequately. Think of impacts such as having to limit healthcare operations to emergency care only because computing capabilities and access to data are blocked by a successful ransomware attack. Natural disasters, such as hurricanes and tornados, can render information technology unavailable and data access impossible. During such events, the unavailability of data to healthcare providers poses a significant negative impact on patient care and patient safety.

Impacts are measured by the quantitative and qualitative harm they bring to the organization. As a reminder, quantitative measures, such as financial losses, are objective. Qualitative impacts could be loss of reputation, a subjective assessment. Keep in mind that assessing impact is unique to each organization. An impact to one organization may not be equally harmful to another. Decision-makers will differ in accepting or rejecting projections of the harm the organization assets will sustain.

Threat

Threats are dangerous events or circumstances that are caused by a source attempting to exploit a security vulnerability. A threat exploits a vulnerability to cause impact. Cyber-attackers, malicious insiders, and untrained employees can all pose information security threats. Natural disasters are also potential threats to the protection of information. For example, firewall security logs (or, more likely, the dashboard reporting of the firewall tool of your choice) identify significant traffic coming from geographic locations that are known cyber-espionage havens. Those IP addresses may belong to nation-state actors who are threats to your organization. In the same way, because untrained employees are more likely to click links in phishing e-mails, they can serve as threats to the security of the organization.

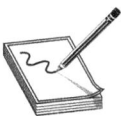

> **NOTE** Different threats can result in the same impacts. A phishing attack resulting in malicious software execution and a disgruntled employee may cause the same outcomes: unauthorized access, unintended changes to data, and loss of availability to information and IT resources.

Vulnerability

If you have worked in IT and security for any amount of time, you've most likely heard about vulnerabilities. We will formalize that understanding as a component of risk. In simple terms, a vulnerability is a weak point in software applications or program codes that can be exploited by a threat. A vulnerability can also be an area of susceptibility for the organization, such as a lack of tested disaster recovery plans. In the event of a natural disaster, the vulnerability is exploited—not by an attacker, but by the natural threat event happening.

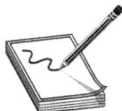

NOTE As this chapter contains a heavy emphasis on definitions, you would benefit from becoming familiar with the general sources that privacy and security professionals use for definitions and concepts related to risk. One such source that is publicly available is NIST SP 800-30 Rev. 1, *Guide for Conducting Risk Assessments*, available at https://csrc.nist.gov/publications/detail/sp/800-30/rev-1/final.

Evaluating Risk Components

We have introduced equations to determine risk earlier in this chapter. We have defined each of the components that make up risk. When you pull it all together, you can see how risk is a measure, quantitative or qualitative, of how likely a threat is to expose a vulnerability in an organization, and to what extent a successful event will result in negative consequences. You should be familiar with a couple of other topics related to risk as well.

First, information risk is an independent subcategory of overall organizational risk, also known as enterprise risk. However, in the subcategories of enterprise risk, information security is often a consideration. For example, in operational risk, revenue projections may be at risk for a variety of factors, one of which could be information security events. We have discussed earlier how information security events can impact the organization's reputation. That said, information security events are one component of the overall reputational risk factors (such as a malpractice lawsuit).

Another topic within information risk, a strategic view of information of risk includes a process to assign prioritization of assessed risks. Budgets, time, and staffing are limited. Along with treatment of risks, which we discuss a little later in this chapter, information risks that the organization decides to mitigate must be prioritized. Related to prioritization, some risks are related to others, or a mitigation of one is also a mitigation of the other. This is particularly true when individual risks are low priority by themselves, but when several risks are considered together, the cumulative risk elevates the priority. Aggregation of specific risks can improve cost effectiveness in reducing risk—for example, reducing risks in vulnerable software, network monitoring gaps, and inconsistent service account management through investment and corrections to the IT asset management system.

Employing Security Controls

To protect information, the organization must employ security controls, such as standards or technologies that are generally accepted as effective at reducing information risk. Cost is a concern in that a security control is not effective if it costs more to implement and maintain than the value of information asset it protects. Controls outlined in HIPAA, NIST guidance, and ISO publications meet the requirement for properly implementing security controls.

The nature or function of these controls is organized into the following categories:

- **Administrative**   Also termed management, these controls are focused on operation of an information security program with governance implementing and enforcing required policies and procedures.

- **Technical**   Also called logical controls, these controls are technologies including hardware, software, and other IT solutions used to ensure information protection capabilities.

- **Physical**   These controls are barriers, deterrents, and impediments that prevent or alert against unauthorized entry or access to property and information assets.

- **Operational**   Sometimes referred to as procedural security, these controls are characterized by people conducting some routine, practice, or technique. Examples of operational controls are incident response plans, clean desk policies, and disaster recovery plans.

Another way of categorizing the security controls is according to the security phase the control is meant to impact. To illustrate, here is a list of security control phases and their benefit:

- **Direct**   Describe what the expected user actions are.

- **Deter**   Discourage attacks and violations.

- **Prevent**   Attempt to avoid the incident.

- **Detect**   Identify the event as it happens.

- **Correct**   Rectify the situation as quickly as possible.

- **Recover**   Restore operations safely.

- **Compensate**   Provide alternative or complementary controls.

You will notice that leading security control frameworks have thousands of security controls. When you have knowledge of the sources, categories, and benefits of security controls, you have a foundation for making decisions about which of the thousands of security controls are applicable to your organization. Trying to implement all of them will fail, and some controls are not applicable to every organization based on mission, size, and risk tolerance, to name a few considerations. At this point, you have the context for how to shape, or incorporate, information safeguards in an organization with these overarching concepts and taxonomies. Figure 6-3 depicts these groupings of security controls as well as their overlap with regard to integrating and serving multiple control functions.

Compensating Controls

In healthcare, it is often the case that prescribed controls and even alternative controls are not feasible to implement. One of the most prevalent examples of this scenario occurs within medical device management. Some medical devices are imperative in diagnosing and treating patients, yet these devices may not adhere to some of your information security requirements.

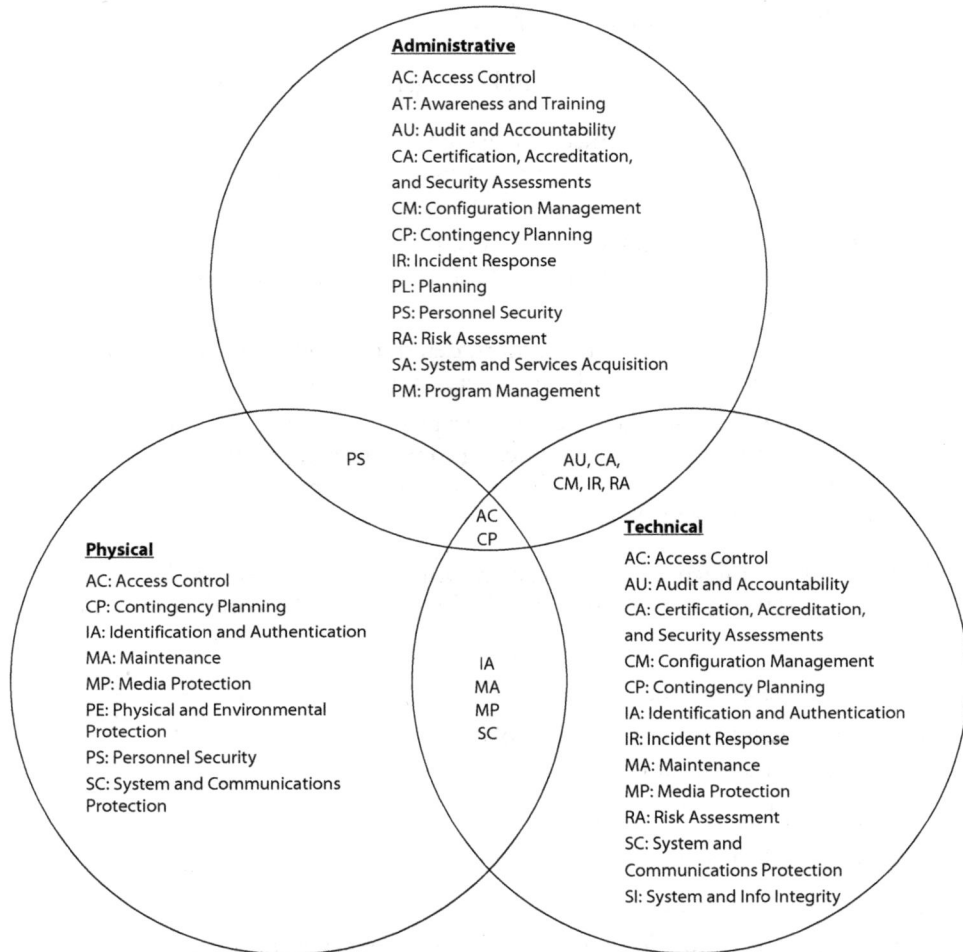

Administrative
AC: Access Control
AT: Awareness and Training
AU: Audit and Accountability
CA: Certification, Accreditation,
and Security Assessments
CM: Configuration Management
CP: Contingency Planning
IR: Incident Response
PL: Planning
PS: Personnel Security
RA: Risk Assessment
SA: System and Services Acquisition
PM: Program Management

PS

AU, CA,
CM, IR, RA

AC
CP

Physical
AC: Access Control
CP: Contingency Planning
IA: Identification and Authentication
MA: Maintenance
MP: Media Protection
PE: Physical and Environmental
Protection
PS: Personnel Security
SC: System and Communications
Protection

IA
MA
MP
SC

Technical
AC: Access Control
AU: Audit and Accountability
CA: Certification, Accreditation,
and Security Assessments
CM: Configuration Management
CP: Contingency Planning
IA: Identification and Authentication
IR: Incident Response
MA: Maintenance
MP: Media Protection
RA: Risk Assessment
SC: System and
Communications Protection
SI: System and Info Integrity

Figure 6-3   Overlap of security control categories and functions

In some cases, the device manufacturer has evaluated and approved only one version of an operating system that is considered obsolete for regular office automation. Additionally, the same medical device may not be able to accept software vulnerability patches because they negatively impact the device. In this case, the healthcare organization cannot knowingly allow the medical device to operate on the local area network. Disconnecting the device or upgrading it without manufacturer approval is also not an option for the healthcare organization. This example demonstrated the need for compensating controls.

A compensating control is a safeguard or a combination of approaches used in place of a prescribed security control. Compensating controls are valid deviations. They are neither shortcuts to compliance nor approaches used to help avoid implementing a control. Before implementing a compensating control, you should conduct a risk analysis to document the legitimate need for a deviation (legitimate technological or documented business constraint). In the medical device scenario, the alternative controls of private network segmentation and manual patch management would be legitimate deviations. In addition to these examples for medical devices, other examples of compensating controls are backup generators, hot sites for continuing IT operations, and sensitive information server isolation. The intent of the original, prescribed control is met, but the bona fide considerations are addressed to balance both information protection and patient care.

In sum, a valid compensating control offers several distinct elements:

- It satisfies the original requirement and is as thorough as the prescribed control.

- It provides a similar level of defense as the original requirement.

- It is acceptable if the compensating control is actually more stringent than the prescribed control.

- If any additional risk is present because of the compensating control, the compensating control must meet cost–benefit or risk–reward criteria.

- If the compensating control is temporary, it should be removed when no longer required.

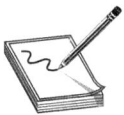

> **NOTE**   It may be relatively obvious, but after compensating controls are evaluated and implemented, they are usually more difficult or more costly to implement than the prescribed control.

No one should view compensating controls as a shortcut to compliance. In healthcare, nevertheless, it is common to meet resistance to implementing compensating controls. Some clinicians and healthcare providers will argue that a prescribed information asset control "negatively impacts patient care," so it should not be implemented. Although negative impact is always a primary concern in the cost–benefit analysis of any information protection decision, that does not excuse a reliance on overly relaxed controls or standards. The goal of having a healthcare-specific information privacy and security curriculum is to learn to integrate the valid concerns of caregivers with the imperatives of providing healthcare information privacy and security. This balancing act makes understanding the proper use of compensating controls a key skill to master.

Next Generation Cybersecurity Approaches

In Chapter 5, we introduced the concept of defense-in-depth within the discussion of security controls and security categorization. Although defense-in-depth is rooted in traditional layered approaches to implementing security controls, it is static compared to the dynamic risks we face in healthcare information privacy and security today. There are two emerging approaches with which you should become familiar: assumption of breach and SecDevOps.

(continued)

Assumption of breach transfers emphasis from perfect identification and protection investments in firewalls, intrusion detection systems, and antimalware applications to better detection, response, and recovery capabilities. Its philosophy is that no prevention strategy can be flawless. Given enough time and persistence, the adversary will get in. In short, cybersecurity incidents are not a matter of *if*, but *when*. Assumption of breach is related to an agile defense methodology that focuses on minimizing impact of an intruder or unauthorized access and having resiliency in the systems and processes. This does not minimize or reduce effectiveness of prevention or protection controls and solutions. Assumption of breach simply prepares security professionals to improve risk management across the entire cybersecurity attack sequence.

SecDevOps is a combination of security, development, and operations. The term is derived from a perspective that application and software development today is best accomplished using continuous integration and continuous delivery (CI/CD) principles rather than traditional methods. In the past, development was a process of milestones, version releases, and quality assurance checks that increased development time and cost. CI/CD ushered in the integration of development with operations, hence DevOps. Add security built into the DevOps timeline and you have a fully integrated, incremental SecDevOps process that enables security to be an integral part of requirement setting, design, and delivery in more frequent iterations.

Security Categorization

To determine what controls should or should not be implemented, the organization must shape its approach around the types of information it collects and uses. According to FIST PUB 199, *Federal Information Processing Standards: Standards for Security Categorization of Federal Information and Information Systems*, security categorization is a process of evaluating the information against confidentiality, integrity, and availability (CIA).[2] You can use a simple low, medium, or high valuation reflecting the importance of each component to determine a subjective score. For example, if you believe availability is the most important component of CIA for PHI, you might use an equation like this:

Security categorization = Confidentiality (low) + Integrity (low) + Availability (high)

This valuation may lead an organization to provide controls that ensure availability, such as investing in a generator and providing continuous power to information systems. In this case, investment in confidentiality and integrity controls may be secondary and more conservative. Figure 6-4 illustrates a simple process to provide information security categorization. To determine the security categorization in healthcare, you can use the equation for PHI and for personally identifiable information (PII) after you identify where this data is and how it moves through the organization. At that point, the information is categorized and you can determine the level of protection that is required.

Now that you have a basic understanding of how information security levels are categorized, it's important to acknowledge the complexity of the categorization process.

Figure 6-4
Categorizing
information for
safeguarding

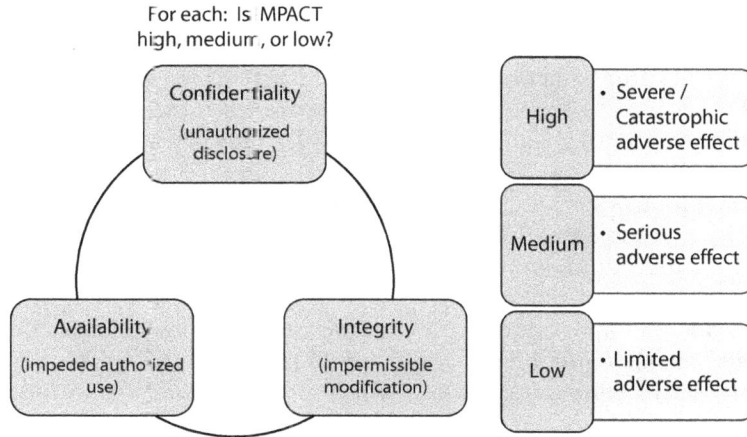

As noted in NIST SP 800-60 Vol. 1 Rev. 1, *Guide for Mapping Types of Information and Information Systems to Security Categories*, a certain system may actually use various types of data with multiple levels of impact to the organization if the data is breached.[3] The electronic health record (EHR), for instance, includes PHI, insurance data, and contact information. Some occupational health services will even include employment records in PHI. The categorization formula remains the same: using the categories of confidentiality, integrity, and availability, the organization must assess each type of information in the same way, albeit independently for high, medium, and low values, depending on their criticality in each of these three areas. When it comes to an organization's EHR system, this is a team effort. Representatives from clinical service departments, finance, IT, and clinical engineering (medical devices) should be included to ensure the best outcome. Categorizing information security is a means of taking inventory for sensitive data and facilitates other risk management activities.

Assessing Residual Risk

A *residual risk* is a portion of a risk that remains after a risk assessment has been conducted and mitigated to the best extent possible. It is important to note that some residual risk may be accepted, while other residual risk may be transferred or avoided. To help you understand the response to risk an organization will take, a key factor to remember is the *residual risk tolerance*. In short, this is the level of comfort an organization has for the likelihood and potential impact of a threat that exploits a vulnerability. Closely related to risk tolerance is the concept of *risk appetite*. You should understand the slight differences between the two because each has usefulness in managing information risks:

- **Risk tolerance**   The degree of risk or uncertainty that is acceptable to an organization, usually defined at the operational or system level.[4]
- **Risk appetite**   The types and amount of risk, on a broad level, an organization is willing to accept in its pursuit of value. It is generally defined at the organizational level.

Among the considerations are how the response to the risk fits with the organizational mission and objectives. A point we make often in this book is that the healthcare industry is different from other industries with information privacy and security concerns. Residual risk tolerance is a prime example of where this is true. For instance, in managing networked computing equipment, a proper risk management approach is to load software, particularly antivirus management software, on devices as part of a standard configuration. With this software, vulnerability patches can be pushed out remotely and automatically by system administrators. Computing devices stay at protected levels, keeping risk of virus infiltration low at a reasonable cost to the organization. However, with medical devices such as digital X-ray systems and smart infusion pumps also connected to the network, it's important that any additional software not be loaded on the machines. Each device manufacturer must test and approve software additions, updates, and deletions to these special computing devices, which typically cannot be included in the automated patch management process. This does not mean they cannot be secured, however. There must be an alternative process available that reflects the concept of residual risk tolerance, because the organization accepts that one size does not fit all. Perhaps the medical devices can be segmented into a private networking scheme or enclave. Maybe software patches can be loaded manually only. This may inflate cost and level of effort, but it is an effort required within a healthcare-savvy information protection program. An organization may have to accept more risk, or a higher risk tolerance, for medical devices as a trade-off for the patient care benefits provided by the technology.

Based on the residual risk tolerance, you can take several approaches to address the risks found in the risk assessment:[5]

- **Avoid** The least tolerance for these categories of risk causes the organization to try to sidestep the risk completely. Alternatives to the original process or technology must be found and implemented. As a simple example, imagine a healthcare organization that assesses the risk of a legacy IT system as high or above the established risk tolerance level. To avoid the risk, the healthcare organization would upgrade or replace the legacy system to address the risk.

- **Transfer** Two approaches to this category are prevalent. First, the organization shifts the risk to a third party. This is usually as a function of a contractual document or language in an agreement that holds harmless the healthcare organization from any exploitation of a risk. This risk transfer process is termed *indemnification*. The second risk transfer approach is to buy an insurance policy to cover the financial costs relative to the impact of the breach. In US healthcare organizations, cybersecurity insurance is used to help defray the financial burden of conducting investigations, notifying patients, and doing things such as providing credit monitoring patient credit histories. In fact, depending on the type of cybersecurity insurance, the coverage can include paying fines and penalties. Of course, cybersecurity insurance cannot reimburse an organization for costs related to lost business, damaged reputation, and time wasted on breach remediation. All of this must factor into the approach to addressing risk.

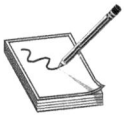

> **NOTE**   A business associate agreement in the United States is an example of an administrative control that transfers some risk to the third party that handles the protected health information on behalf of the healthcare organization.

- **Mitigate**   If you cannot avoid the action that increases risk, you may choose to mitigate the chances of negative impact. Implementing administrative, physical, and technical controls such as those discussed in in NIST SP 800-53 Rev. 4, *Security and Privacy Controls in Federal Information Systems and Organization,* enables you to use information privacy and security to mitigate risk. There is no way to eliminate risk completely through the use of security controls. Mitigations will always lead to a level of residual risk that the organization will have to accept, albeit a low level well under risk tolerance thresholds.

> **EXAM TIP**   For exam purposes, NIST SP 800-53 Rev. 4 is current. However, NIST SP 800-53 Rev. 5 is in final public draft status as of May 2020. For a comparison of Revision 4 and Revision 5, refer to a matrix authored by MITRE Corp at https://csrc.rist.gov/CSRC/media/Publications/sp/800-53/rev-5/draft/documents/sp800-53r5-draft-fpd-comparison-with-rev4.xlsx.

- **Accept**   There are situations in which you can accept risk. After considering avoidance, transfer, and mitigation options, you must simply accept some risks. This may even happen when the residual risk exceeds the risk tolerance levels, though these cases should be rare. Nevertheless, when the benefit of accepting the risk outweighs the potential for harm, risk can be accepted. When an organization chooses to accept risk, it still must document this measured decision and continue to assess the risk as options change or risk increases.

Accepting Risk

A risk acceptance decision is a conscious choice to expose the organization to negative impacts based on a comparison of the risk assessment with the benefits that are expected. Unless a risk is avoided, you will always have some level of risk acceptance after transfer and mitigation efforts are implemented. Risk acceptance must be based on informed decision-making through a process to identify the risk and assess the options. When all of these factors have been addressed and it has been determined that the risk is acceptable, assignment of risk ownership and documentation is needed.

Risk is dynamic, as we have noted. Over time, risks can increase or decrease. Ownership of the risk is a process of assigning the responsibility to maintain any conditions that permitted acceptance of the risk. For example, consider a limited use of videoconference capabilities as an acceptable information security risk when they are used only for a small pilot group involving no transfer of PHI. Ownership of this risk may be assigned to the marketing team that wanted to use the technology to conduct focus groups for a new clinical service in development. The team would be primarily responsible for acceptable use of the technology. If the team expanded its use of the collaboration tool, as the risk owner, it would be responsible for initiating a new assessment. Not reviewing the conditions and increasing exposure and risk would be a violation of security controls.

Understand Information Risk Management Framework

A risk management framework is effective only if it drives organizational decisions and behavior. Running decisions through the framework to categorize information assets and identifying levels of risk are the first steps. This data must progress to the next steps. The organization needs to identify and prioritize the actions it will take to address the risk it has identified. An organization that stops at this point of identifying risk is probably going to be considered negligent by regulators. In the event of data loss and one or more of the identified risks being exploited when the organization failed to implement a response to the risk, the organization can expect increased fines and penalties.

At a high level, NIST builds a risk management framework around the activities of a risk management program. The best use of the information in this chapter about risk management frameworks is to recognize how each framework approaches one of the most foundational concepts of healthcare information privacy and security: information risk. You will see that no matter what tool you desire to use, the objective is to measure risk by identifying vulnerabilities, assigning a likelihood of occurrence, and assigning a value of the impact to your organization. From there, you can begin to design and implement controls to mitigate the likelihood of risk, minimize the impacts, and thereby manage risk.

NIST Risk Management Framework (RMF)

One of the most commonly cited risk management sources is the risk management process defined in NIST SP 800-39, *Security Risk: Organization, Mission, and Information System View*. However, that does not preclude the use of other credible sources. The choices depend on your organization's mission, scope, and tolerance for information risk. NIST approaches risk management as a holistic process that must take the entire organization into account. At a high level, NIST builds a risk management framework around the activities of a risk management program.[6] Over the years, the risk management framework that NIST has developed has evolved from a concept of ideas that should work for all organizations to a well-defined framework that is malleable to be used in most sectors. Following are high-level steps identified by the NIST RMF:

- **Framing risk** What is the organization's risk tolerance, and how does it make decisions about risk?
- **Assessing risk** What are the values for the risk equation, and what are the results?
- **Responding to risk** Based on the organization's risk tolerance, what alternatives will be chosen to address risk?
- **Monitoring risk** How will the organization oversee changes and respond to any impacts of risk mitigation activities? This is a continuous process.

Keep in mind that these four steps are interconnected by as much information and communication flow as possible. The process is continuous, so the information and communication flow must contain feedback and improvement concerns.

A second source you should be familiar with is NIST SP 800-37 Rev. 2, *Risk Management Framework for Information Systems and Organizations: A System Life Cycle Approach for Security and Privacy*. While the guide is intended for use in US federal agencies, the concept of a risk management framework is important to commercial businesses, including healthcare organizations. The NIST RMF is a disciplined, organized, and repeatable process for achieving information protection of information systems. When comparing the information in NIST SP 800-37 Rev. 2 with a similar framework in NIST SP 800-39, *Managing Information Security Risk*, for example, you can see overlap. Both are lifecycle concepts with continuous monitoring and improvement as a central concept. NIST SP 800-37 Rev. 2 specifies as one of its stated purposed that senior leaders must be provided "the necessary information to make cost-effective, risk-based decisions with regard to the organizational information systems supporting their core missions and business functions."[7]

The two models presented in SP 800-37 Rev. 2 and SP 800-39 are not redundant and can work in tandem. The more detailed nature of the RMF enables flexibility to adapt the framework to industry-specific standards and guidelines. In sum, the RMF provides organizations with the flexibility needed to apply the right security controls to the right information systems at the right time to manage risk adequately. In the United States, many of the HIPAA Security Rule standards and implementation specifications correspond to the steps of the NIST RMF.[8] Approaching risk management using these NIST frameworks will help any healthcare organization comply with its risk management strategy.

Within the NIST RMF are specific steps organizations should take to manage their risk, not only at system and application levels, but also organizational level risks associated with the collective risk from systems and applications. In NIST SP 800-37 Rev. 2, the RMF consists of six steps, as displayed in Figure 6-5. Each step has multiple tasks that should be completed in the order outlined to meet the requirements of a fully effective risk management process. Organizations historically did not fully implement all aspects of the framework, resulting in unidentified or unmitigated risks caused data loss or exposure. Effective implementation is not always easy, inexpensive, or even understood by all functional areas in an organization. The organization must have a governance structure that supports this effort.

EXAM TIP Know the differences between NIST Cybersecurity Framework (CSF) discussed in Chapter 4 and NIST Risk Management Framework (RMF) discussed in this chapter. The CSF is voluntary and intended for commercial activities, and the RMF is mandatory for US federal agencies. Another key difference is the steps in each framework. Though they include many similarities, the CSF does not have steps to "implement" controls and "authorize" controls as the RMF does. In addition, both frameworks can be used together. More detailed guidance for using both frameworks is available in NIST Interagency or Internal Report (IR) 8170, *Approaches for Federal Agencies to Use the Cybersecurity Framework*, available at https://nvlpubs.nist.gov/nistpubs/ir/2020/NIST.IR.8170.pdf.

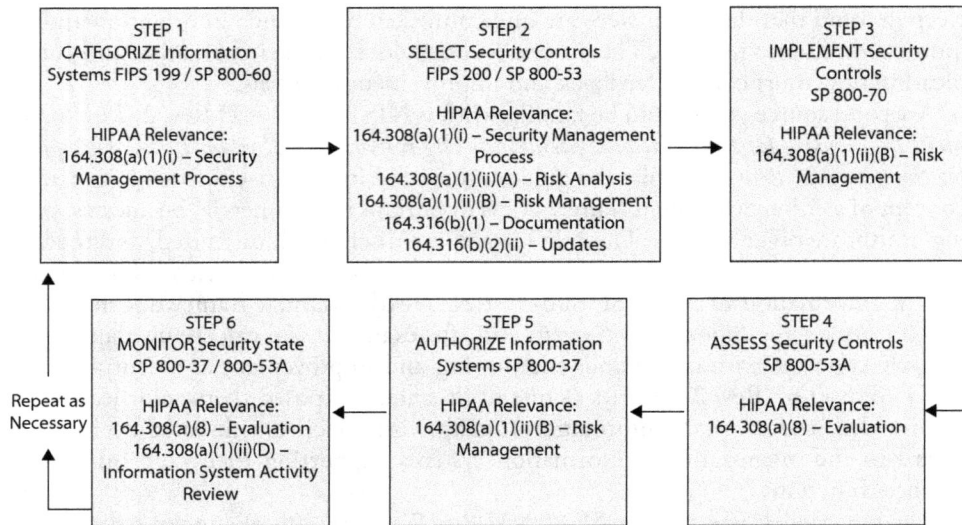

Figure 6-5 NIST risk management framework steps and tasks

International Organization for Standardization

We discussed the International Organization for Standardization (ISO) earlier in Chapter 4 in the context of its role in developing governance guidelines. Here, it is discussed in the context of how it approaches information risk management. For those who work outside of the United States or in US healthcare organizations that do business internationally, having an awareness of ISO standards is important. Since 1947, when the ISO was created, the organization has published 19,500 standards for business and technology industries.

From an information risk management perspective, two leading standards apply. The first, ISO/IEC 27001, *Information security management*, presents best-practice information about security management principles, a framework, and a process for managing risk. These guidelines are applicable to any organization or mission regardless of its size, activity, or sector. This standard approaches risk by focusing improvement of objectives by identifying opportunities and threats. From there, the organization can allocate resources to deal with the risk effectively. If you use ISO/IEC 27001 or any of the ISO/IEC 27000 family of standards, you will learn to define risk not as a chance or probability of loss, but by means of the effect uncertainty has on your objectives.

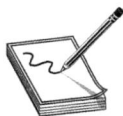

NOTE In Chapter 4, we mentioned ISO 27799, *Health informatics – Information security management in health using ISO/IEC 27002*. ISO 27799 uses ISO/IEC 27002 and augments the requirements of ISO/IEC 27002 with healthcare-specific considerations for information security management.

The ISO 27000 family of standards also introduces the final step in the risk management process: risk treatment. Adapting risk treatment actions from this guidance, you will realize that you have some familiar risk mitigation options for your organization to address risk:

- **Avoid**   Do not do the action causing the risk.
- **Accept**   The probable cost of the occurrence is less than the value of the objective.
- **Retain**   Provided informed consent and potential loss are minimal, you can budget for risk.
- **Remove**   Eliminate the vulnerability or source of risk.
- **Change**   Adjust the likelihood of occurrence or the consequences (mitigation).
- **Share**   Transfer the cost through insurance, contracting, or other third-party agreement (outsource).

The second major ISO source for information risk management is ISO/IEC 27005, *Information technology – Security techniques – Information security risk management*. Every source of risk management guidance should have risk assessment at the core of the processes. However, keep in mind that risk assessment is only a piece of the entire risk management process. ISO/IEC 27005 focuses on risk in information systems and expands on effectively and efficiently conducting just the risk assessment. Starting with selecting the proper risk assessment techniques, this standard guides the assessor through the proper steps.

You should be familiar the following information regarding the risk assessment steps according to ISO:

1. *Define the risk method you will use.* There is no specific template to follow, but you will need to make sure you have security benchmarks, risk measurement values, risk tolerance levels, and what the ISO/IEC 27001 terms a "scenario-based" or "asset-based" risk assessment.

2. *Inventory your information assets.* This is particularly important for an asset-based assessment. Document information assets including IT hardware, software, intellectual property, and medical devices.

3. *Identify threats and vulnerabilities.* As with other frameworks for risk assessment, you need to understand what manmade and natural threats are possible. Vulnerabilities that can result in those threats being realized must be cataloged too.

4. *Estimate the likelihood and impact amounts.* This is another common step among frameworks. It is important to estimate the potential for a threat to happen and the resulting consequences.

5. *Reduce risk through mitigation to acceptable residual risk levels.* ISO/IEC 27001 includes a variation of the risk handling taxonomy. To avoid risk is to terminate it. Applying security controls is to treat the risk, compared to mitigating it. ISO/IEC 27001 also uses the term "transfer" to describe shifting risk to a third party. The action to accept risk is called "tolerate."

6. *Assemble reports to communicate risks.* Two examples of reports that are used for compliance with ISO/IEC 27001 as well as certification are a Statement of Applicability (SoA) and a Risk Treatment Plan (RTP).

7. *Review, monitor, and audit.* A continuous risk assessment process with revisions to improve the processes is required to stay current with ever-changing elements that determine risks.

Going back to the risk management process focusing on objectives, risk assessment helps risk managers recognize the risks that could affect the achievement of objectives as well as the adequacy of the controls already in place. Keep in mind that like all good processes, the system needs constant communication to and from stakeholders, and it is cyclical. Once the last step of the risk management process, risk treatment, is completed, it is time to begin again with establishing the baselines. In all of the better risk management processes, always start with a baseline assessment or an inventory. As you can see, the ISO/IEC 27001 and ISO/IEC 27005 standards are no different.

A component of ISO guidance that differs from other frameworks is that certification is available by qualified assessors. Organizations can voluntarily choose to achieve ISO/IEC 27001 certification to demonstrate compliance and competency. It is possible that certification helps to assure customers of trustworthiness of the organization to protect information.

Centers for Medicare and Medicaid Services

The Centers for Medicare and Medicaid Services (CMS), an operating division of the US Department of Health and Human Services (HHS), combines the oversight of the Medicare program, the federal portion of the Medicaid program and State Children's Health Insurance Program, the Health Insurance Marketplace, and related quality assurance activities. This represents the healthcare coverage for more than 100 million people in the United States.[9]

CMS Risk Management

The Centers for Medicare and Medicaid Services has developed its own risk management framework, which closely follows the NIST framework.[10] Because CMS is specifically a healthcare-sector support agency, it has worked to ensure that compliance with HIPAA and other legislative requirements applicable to healthcare are addressed in its framework. Much like NIST, the framework follows these steps:

1. Categorize the system based on the information (data) types in use.

2. Select security controls.

3. Implement security controls.

4. Assess security controls.

5. Authorize the information system.

6. Monitor security controls.

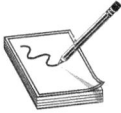

NOTE CMS has created a library of documents in support of its risk management framework. The Information Security and Privacy Library is available online to all organizations, and although it was established as a method to meet the Federal Information Security Management Act (FISMA) guidance for government systems, it is a great resource for all organizations.[11]

Understand Risk Management Process

Whatever process you determine fits your organization and satisfies any regulatory requirements, your risk management process must accomplish a full assessment of risks and minimization of uncertainty. In healthcare information privacy and security, we want to use a risk management process that integrates security, privacy, and enterprise risk. Outcomes will include proper decisions for control choices and risk treatment. Starting with an authoritative source such as NIST SP 800-30 Rev. 1, *Guide for Conducting Risk Assessments*, the process for managing risk consists of four phases:[12]

- **Framing** The strategy for how risk decisions will be made in an organization. The process is related to the organization's perceived tolerance for risk.

- **Assessing** The determining of risk based on a measure of the threats, vulnerabilities, likelihoods, and impacts the organization faces.

- **Responding** The generation and implementation of options to address assessed risks based on how you decide to frame risk decisions.

- **Monitoring** The continuous observance of the effectiveness of risk management activities in place and adaptation to changes in the environment. This phase includes ensuring that risk management approaches are aligned with industry standards and regulatory requirements.

These four phases are guided by continual information flow throughout the process. Each phase is connected and integrated. In fact, information is shared to inform each phase. For example, in the framing stage, the board of directors may indicate a low tolerance for financial and regulatory risks. That information is very important to inform how the organization may respond to risks; it may opt for more stringent controls above regulatory requirements. Another example, given the same risk tolerance levels, auditing of security controls with findings of ineffective operations may need elevation to the board as significant. In organizations with a higher tolerance for risk, those same findings may not receive the same sense of urgency.

When structuring a decision that measures risk around these components, you can use a risk management framework, discussed earlier in this chapter, to weigh cost against benefit or risk versus reward. In all cases, you can ensure that you are implementing controls that are relevant and cost-effective to the assets you are trying to protect.

Risk management processes are the combination of three key activities. Those distinct activities are assessment of risk, management or treatment of risk, and monitoring of risk. In healthcare, information risk management is so important because in addition to financial and operational risks, healthcare risk management must include patient care and patient safety risks. The process must include stakeholders from departments throughout the organization, not just information security personnel. The results must be shared throughout the organization as well to reduce risk, improve patient care, and enhance business processes. A good definition of the risk management process includes prioritization of risk treatment options.

Quantitative vs. Qualitative Approaches

You have been introduced to approaches to measuring and expressing information risk in this chapter. In the section "Measuring and Expressing Information Risk," we differentiated between quantitative and qualitative approaches. Here we examine more specific uses of the two approaches.

Starting with a quantitative approach, you remember that objective data such as financial measures or historical trends are the goal. Here are some common financial variables to consider:

- **Exposure factor (EF)**   Expressed as a percentage between 0 and 100 percent. It estimates the value of an asset that is lost due to a risk occurrence.
- **Single loss expectancy (SLE)**   The asset value multiplied by the exposure factor as a one-time occurrence.
- **Annualized rate of occurrence (ARO)**   The likely occurrence per year of an incident. If the threat may occur once every five years, the ARO is 0.2. If the threat happens five times in one year, the ARO is, of course, 5.
- **Annualized loss expectancy (ALE)**   This equation is derived from the others. It is the SLE multiplied by the ARO.

Let's take a look at a fictitious example. If a ransomware attack risk is being calculated, the variables could include a database asset that is valued by the organization at $100,000. In a ransomware attack, we can imagine a 50 percent loss of the asset due to incomplete backups for this scenario. In this organization, the estimate is one successful ransomware attack in any five-year period. Therefore, we can provide a quantitative risk assessment that indicates the following:

- Exposure factor (EF): = 50%
- Single loss expectancy (SLE): $100,000 × 0.50 = $50,000
- Annualized rate of occurrence (ARO): = 0.20
- Annualized loss expectancy (ALE): $50,000 × 0.20 = $10,000

Now we can examine an approach using qualitative analysis. This example includes information from the Common Vulnerability Scoring System (CVSS). You may be familiar with CVSS, the open framework for vulnerability ratings that is used by the

National Vulnerability Database (NVD). The NVD is a joint effort between NIST and the US Department of Homeland Security. The CVSS consists of three metric groups that you can use to make a qualitative assessment of a specific risk factor:[13]

- **Base metric**   Components that are able to be exploited and impacted
- **Temporal metric**   Vulnerability attributes that may change over time
- **Environmental metric**   Unique vulnerabilities relevant to a single organization

We can use another fictitious scenario to construct a qualitative assessment and score it with the CVSS. We will illustrate the base metric here. In practice, the base metric score is often sufficient to make our point and for you to make a threat assessment that can be used with other variables to come to a good risk decision. The base metric is fundamental and unchanging over time to determine severity. If you desire, you can expand the use of CVSS to examine mitigations using a second component, the temporal metric formula. The third component, the environmental metric, can also be added to assess the pervasiveness of a vulnerability throughout the organization. For purposes of illustrating the use of a validated qualitative risk management processes, we will spare you the increased complexity of the CVSS calculator.

> **CAUTION**   CVSS is described as a measure of vulnerability severity, but it is not a risk management tool. Severity is a component of assessing total information risk and information risk management decisions. That said, the tool is still applicable in this risk management discussion about qualitative risk measurements. In fact, it is offered here to provide an example that is much more complex than the usual qualitative measurement discussions that use simple high, medium, and low values.

Take note that this CVSS example shows that qualitative or subjective values can be associated with numerical values to provide a semi-objective measure rooted in expert opinion or observations; this helps to address perceptions of qualitative measures as less reliable or less valuable in decision-making as quantitative measures. As you remember, there are times when quantitative values are best to use and other times when qualitative measures are more appropriate. Sometimes, a combination of both could be the best option.

In our next scenario, an organized group of cybercriminals constructs a multiple-source botnet attack that can overload and organization's public web pages and results in an embarrassing and costly distributed denial of service (DDoS) attack. Figure 6-6 depicts the choices and selections that are available in the CVSS calculator for the basic metric.

Presuming that selections made in the basic metric area could be based on opinion or subjective estimation, you may differ with the responses indicated in the figure.

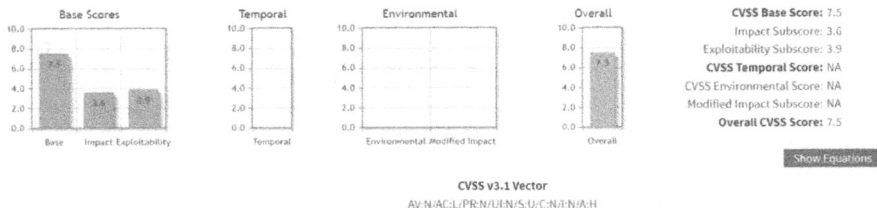

Source: https://nvd.nist.gov/vuln-metrics/cvss/v3-calculator

Figure 6-6   CVSS calculator example of assessment score

As noted in the figure, all of the base metric components are required to achieve a base score. Here's an explanation of the base score metrics:

Exploitability Metrics

- Attack vector (AV) = Network (AV:N)
  A DDoS attack is remotely conducted against a network, although no network access is required.

- Attack complexity (AC) = Low (AC:L)
  The attacker does not need special access or tools. Repeated attacks can be expected to also be successful.

- Privileges required (PR) = None (PR:N)
  The attack is initiated by an unauthorized actor.

- User interaction (UI) = None (UI:R)
  In our scenario, no user needs to be involved for a successful attack.

- Scope (S) = Unchanged (S:U)
  The attack is concentrated within a single organization.

Impact Metrics

- Confidentiality impact (C) = None (C:N)
  There is a low risk of loss of confidentiality due to a disruptive DDoS attack.

- Integrity impact (I) = None (I:N)
  No data or system integrity is expected.

- Availability impact (A) = High (A:H)
A successful denial of service would be highly likely to cause complete loss of data and system availability over a period of time.

Included in the figure is a set of graphs of each base metric and their respective scale (0–10). Additionally, within the calculator, each component becomes a vector. In this case, the vector is AV:N/AC:L/PR:N/UI:N/S:U/C:N/I:N/A:H. From the vector, the CVSS calculator is able to execute an algorithm to result in a total CVSS score of 7.5 based on our scenario and subjective assessment of each component of the base metric elements. To interpret the significance and risk level of a score of 7.5, you would consult with the CVSS standards user guide that is available.[14]

Intent

Whether you choose to implement a risk management process that is entirely quantitative or totally qualitative in focus or a combination, the intent of the process is the same. You can determine that one assessment framework works better for your organization over another. However, the objective is constant. A risk management process is meant to minimize risks to the organization by understanding threats, vulnerabilities, likelihoods, and impacts and reducing or mitigating potential negative outcomes. Keep in mind that the three principle reasons information risk management is so important to you as an HCISPP is that the process is your central competency to help your organization:

- Stay current with regulatory and legal requirements, as risk management is a necessity.

- Apply and enforce security and privacy controls to ensure confidentiality, integrity, and availability of information.

- Provide relevant and essential input to influence and support risk management decisions.

Information Lifecycle and Continuous Monitoring

Risk management has to be integrated into the entire lifecycle of information technology and data assets. In general, information goes through several phases, and in each phase there are privacy and security requirements. Assessing and managing risk must occur when information is created or received, shared, handled, stored, and disposed of when it is no longer needed. For example, in the last chapter, we discussed security categorization, which is a process that should occur no later than in the creation or receipt phase of the information lifecycle. Destruction of a computer hard drive with PHI stored on it would occur in the disposal phase, for example.

In each phase, risk management actions are required of the information owner. As a security professional, you probably are not the information owner, but you will have a significant role in assessing risk levels, informing risk decisions, and assuring that risk treatment is accomplished by the information owner. Within a healthcare organization, the chief executive officer (CEO) or authorized delegates are designated formal information ownership responsibility. That may seem excessive, but the formal assigning is in reference to international standards and regulations such as the GDPR that define information owners and are explicit on accountability at the most senior levels of the organization. In the United States, you may find information ownership assigned at different levels in the organization. However, this does not devalue the roles and the impact they have on risk management during the information lifecycle. Information owners are expected to do the following:

- Provide for the privacy and security of the information under their control.
- Understand the value of the information and replacement costs.
- Estimate the impact of information loss or tampering.
- Maintain appropriate safeguards to protect the information.
- Report incidents in a timely manner upon occurrence.
- Allow access on a strict business or clinical "need to know" basis.
- Determine when information is no longer needed and assist in secure disposal.

EXAM TIP Remember that the responsibility for information security is not something you can delegate to an information owner. The owner is accountable to information security policies, procedures, and operating security controls effectively. You as an HCISPP may be tested on your constant responsibility to ensure that the information owner is adhering to their duties and assess risk that the information protection is in control.

You may have heard that risk assessments and risk management planning are annual requirements. That would be incorrect. HIPAA, for example, requires risk assessments conducted "continuously to identify when updates are needed."[15] In some organizations, a complete assessment could be done annually or biannually. In others, the timing may be more often based on how things change in the environment with added policies, new systems, and interconnections, particularly with external entities. In all cases, expect risk management processes to be ongoing and not single events with specific start and stop dates.

Tools, Resources, and Techniques

The use of tools, resources, and techniques to conduct and document risk assessments and risk treatment decisions helps in a variety of ways. You may have heard the expression, "Not documented equals not done." Auditors and regulators across the globe will require proof of compliance for risk management activities. Admittedly, the existence of a reasonably simple set of file folders with up-to-date risk assessments, policies, and corrective actions plans would probably suffice. There are, however, several tools available that can assist. Based on complex regulatory requirements, these tools also serve to guide completeness in terms of what auditors and regulators may inspect.

The use of a tool can make assessing and managing risk easier. You must keep in mind that tools for risk management are only beneficial if the underlying methodology is sound. For example, US healthcare organizations would prefer tools that follow a process or methodology such as NIST SP 800-30 Rev. 1, *Guide for Conducting Risk Assessments*, depicted in Figure 6-7, which includes these steps:[16]

1. *Prepare for the assessment.* Be thoughtful and comprehensive in determining the requirements, approaches, scope, assumptions, constraints, and models. During this phase, you will identify and categorize threats, likelihood, and impact information that will support the assessment.

2. *Conduct the assessment.* As shown in Figure 6-7, this step comprises several key tasks. These tasks are at the heart of determining and evaluating the components that constitute the risk equation (for example, risk = likelihood × impact):

    a. *Identify threat sources and events.* Describe the hazards or dangers, including capability, intent, and targeting characteristics, for adversarial threats and a range of effects for nonadversarial threats.

    b. *Identify vulnerabilities and predisposing conditions.* Evaluate the weaknesses and exposures that influence likelihood that a negative event will happen.

    c. *Determine the likelihood of occurrence.* Using vulnerability information and best-available data about attackers and the possibility that a threat would happen, estimate the probability of an occurrence.

    d. *Determine the magnitude of impact.* Specify the severity and effects based on the mitigations and controls in place in response to an attack against the confidentiality, integrity, or availability of critical and sensitive information assets.

    e. *Determine risk.* Factor in current mitigating controls and other risk treatments, analysis, or calculations to assess the likelihood and impact of a risk. Again, risk equals likelihood measures multiplied by impact measures.

3. *Communicate results.* Document and share the risk assessment report. Complete risk prioritization and evaluation of additional countermeasures and risk treatment. The results will support the overall risk management process.

4. *Maintain the assessment.* Update residual risks in a risk register or other repository for archiving risk methodologies and decisions used by the organization. Keep the risk assessment current by having a continuous risk management policy and adhering to it.

ONC-OCR HIPAA Security Toolkit Application

This tool is offered by the Office of the National Coordinator for Health Information Technology (ONC), in collaboration with the HHS Office for Civil Rights (OCR).[17] It was designed by a committee of industry volunteers and experts to help organizations assess

Figure 6-7
NIST risk
assessment steps

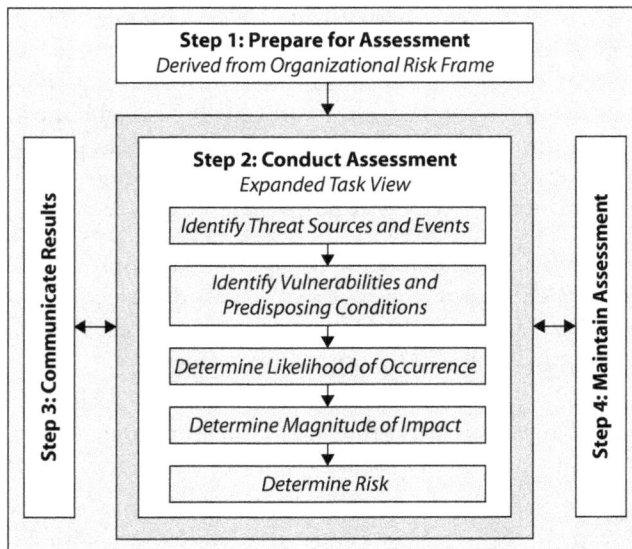

their compliance to the HIPAA Security Rule. The survey asks hundreds of questions, and each question provides the types of documents or actions that would count as evidence of compliance. An organization can choose to upload the documents into the tool for archiving and quick future retrieval, or it can simply provide a link or note about the file location. The tool is extensive, and healthcare organizations of significant size and mission may utilize the entire database. Smaller organizations can tailor the survey according to their environment. The Security Risk Assessment (SRA) Toolkit resides on a personal computer or shared network drive as an application. It is not web based or networked to a central ONC or NIST database. It is not dependent on a specific hardware or software platform: Windows, Red Hat Linux, and macOS are all supported. The tool can be used and reused.

HIMSS Risk Assessment Toolkit

Primarily for HIPAA compliance in the United States, the Health Information Management Systems Society (HIMSS) has published a risk assessment (RA) toolkit to help providers conduct a full risk assessment. It incorporates many of the popular risk management frameworks and is intentioned for smaller sized healthcare provider organizations with limited resources for privacy and security activities. The toolkit includes a set of templates, whitepapers, analyses, best practices, and other reference materials that can help you comply with the guiding regulations in managing and securing PHI. It can also help you establish a comprehensive risk management program that would start with the risk assessment. This tool is created and maintained by HIMSS member volunteers and is intentionally vendor-agnostic.

The Data Security and Protection Toolkit

In the United Kingdom, the DSP Toolkit from the National Health Service (NHS) integrates the legal requirements and guidance into an information governance application. This tool enables organizations under the purview of the DSP requirements to perform self-assessments of their compliance. Using the toolkit, healthcare organizations in the United Kingdom can demonstrate that they properly maintain the confidentiality and security of personal information.[18] The toolkit helps them control variance and partial compliance, and remediation activities can be documented, tracked, and communicated. This effectively supports UK healthcare organizations' information governance compliance through continuous improvements. According to the UK NHS, using the DSP toolkit helps healthcare organizations evaluate themselves against regulatory standards and demonstrate their trustworthiness to their patients.

Desired Outcomes

Conducting risk assessments and implementing a good risk management program requires budget, time, and expertise. The results that come from assessments and analyses are valuable. The protection of healthcare information is without question the principle desired outcome of a risk management program. Several other desired outcomes or additional benefits maximize the usefulness of the risk management process. Information that is used to formulate a risk assessment will help the organization maintain a full accounting of its assets. Understanding the threats the organization faces along with the likelihood of occurrence can assist in business resiliency, which includes disaster recovery and business continuity planning. In fact, risk management information should be used to help business and clinical leaders develop a risk strategy. For initiatives that use cloud service providers or contemplate increased data sharing initiatives with external parties for healthcare improvements, knowing the risks and how such strategic imperatives may be helped or hindered by can save the organization time, money, and energy.

Role of Internal and External Audit and Assessment

Within the organization, the use of auditors who are competent in information technology and security is an imperative to providing assurance to the executive leadership and the board of directors. In the three lines of defense security model, introduced in Chapter 2, you should recognize the internal audit function as a third-line function. Information owners are the first line, and you, as a security professional, are second line. The auditors perform assessments to review proper implementation and operation of security controls. The internal audit function can strengthen an information security and privacy governance. In US healthcare organizations, an internal auditor typically reports directly to the audit committee of the board. The auditor is nonetheless an employee of the healthcare organization. The direct reporting to the board ensures objectivity in the auditor's observations and opinions. The oversight that is provided may identify inefficiencies, poorly designed controls, and ineffective processes.

The role of oversight is just one valuable contribution of the auditor role; the same auditor can also serve the organization in more of a consultant role. This distinction does not change the reporting relationship to the board. The expertise and perspective of an auditor can be extremely helpful to management. When acting in the consultant role, an auditor can participate in projects, contribute to meetings, and otherwise give advice and suggest changes to improve the healthcare organization. The auditor should not blur the lines between consulting and oversight roles, however. When acting as a consultant, she should not use information gained in working internal issues to formulate an internal audit finding or observation. As an example of the consultant role, an internal audit can help your organization conduct a risk assessment. However, the auditor cannot identify, assess, evaluate, and respond to risk. Those are your responsibilities along with organization management. Some of the other tasks in which internal audit cannot participate are determining risk tolerances, making risk treatment decisions, and accepting accountability for risk management processes.

An effective organizational audit process includes a combination of external and internal audit teams in a comprehensive oversight program. External auditors would not act in a consultant role or as advocates for any management actions to manage risk. Information security risk is a complex and extensive profession with many specialized competencies. It is often necessary to get specific expertise from an external auditor to augment internal audit review. A good example of this is penetration testing using external suppliers who specialize in ethical hacking and conducting simulated attacks on the organization.

Another consideration for using external auditors is that over time, internal auditors can increase risk resulting from gaps in control assessments. This is potentially because of cumulative expectations from previous audits or because of shortcuts taken based on perceived understanding of organizational constructs. In short, internal auditors may develop bias, positive and negative, in overseeing the same program over many years. Although internal audit is not responsible for the information security risk assessments, external auditors can be used successfully to conduct a risk assessment, and that assessment and related auditor work papers that the external auditor agrees to share can be used to inform an internal audit. This may facilitate less costly and inefficient internal audits. In fact, the integration of external audits of information risk can permit internal auditors to focus review in areas where the external audit expressed findings, identified control weaknesses, or made observations.

If an organization does not consider using internal auditors and outsources the audit function, there are significant drawbacks. Using only external audits can be highly costly and inefficient because of the auditors' unfamiliarity with the organization. Information gathering and coordination of resources can be a problem. An outsider's view can potentially lead to misunderstandings when internal processes or management risk decisions are inaccurately judged or estimated. In reviewing security control effectiveness, the data is often persuasive but not conclusive.

Auditor professional judgement that provides meaning to results based on sampling or relatively subjective observations is always a factor with both internal and external audits. Internal auditors may provide a more applicable perspective in evaluation of control effectiveness. When used together, external and internal auditors reduce duplication of effort, strengthen the weak points, and reduce gaps to achieve the greatest level of assurance.

Identify Control Assessment Procedures Using Organization Risk Frameworks

You have a variety of choices when selecting a risk assessment procedure as part of a risk management process. Considerations include constraints on time and resources, along with the organization's mission and size. Fortunately, leading examples of risk frameworks have several points in common, which makes them useful candidates because they can be customized to fit within your constraints. Additionally, you can use ISO/IEC 27014, *Information technology – Security techniques – Governance of information security*, as a guide, which offers some other common attributes:

- **Consistent** Control of specifications and how they are measured must remain constant to build trust and value for control owners and executive leadership.

- **Measurable** The risk management system must be able to demonstrate baseline and progress toward risk reduction and information security maturity objectives.

- **Standardized** The measures used in the framework must be suitable for comparison across the organization. In fact, where data can be shared externally, measures that can be compared against other organizations using the same framework are helpful.

- **Comprehensive** Starting with a minimum requirement to satisfy legal and regulatory security requirements, the framework should be able to scale to variables such as organizational size, mission, and any additional security controls the organization considers necessary for its clinical or business functions.

- **Modular** Organizations change, and the information security environment is also dynamic. A good risk assessment framework can be tailored and adapted to these realities and still be relevant and rigorous.

According to Tenable's whitepaper "Trends in Security Framework Adoption Survey," a security framework is used by 84 percent of surveyed organizations in the United States. In fact, 44 percent of the respondents to the Tenable survey said they use multiple frameworks at the same time.[19]

One example is a companion special publication to NIST SP 800-53 Rev. 4, *Security and Privacy Controls for Federal Information Systems and Organizations*. NIST SP 800-53A, *Assessing Security and Privacy Controls in Federal Information Systems and Organizations: Building Effective Assessment Plans*, offers an approach to implementation of the NIST framework of security controls.[20] Within this implementation guidance is information about the security assessment process. The experts that collaborated to publish SP 800-53A considered the assessment of security controls to be the most critical step in risk management. Testing the operation of controls helps assure the organization that the security controls are enough to maintain the appropriate levels of security.

You may encounter some conditions that prevent proper assessment. Be on the watch for these:

- Lack of leadership expectation for risk assessments
- Insufficient oversight of the risk management program

- Security assessors who are inadequately trained and experienced to do the tests
- Operational pressures to accelerate testing or limit scope

Another example that is used routinely as a framework is the Center for Internet Security (CIS) Critical Security Controls. According to the Tenable survey, this model is used by 32 percent of organizations surveyed. This framework is less focused on risk than other examples, but it is very effective in measuring security maturity. It consists of three groups, totaling 20 actions, that have been shown to reduce the risk of the most common and likely cyber-attacks. The CIS controls are a global standard and were designed by international experts who volunteered to contribute. These individuals represented cyber-experts, consultants, academics, and auditors. The results are demonstrated controls that lead to effective control practices. They incorporate regulatory and compliance requirements applicable to hardware, software, applications, and emerging technologies such as the Internet of Medical Things (IoMT). Here are the three groups with the 20 total control titles (from https://www.cisecurity.org/controls/cis-controls-list/):

Basic CIS Controls

1. Inventory and Control of Hardware Assets
2. Inventory and Control of Software Assets
3. Continuous Vulnerability Management
4. Controlled Use of Administrative Privileges
5. Secure Configuration for Hardware and Software on Mobile Devices, Laptops, Workstations, and Servers
6. Maintenance, Monitoring, and Analysis of Audit Logs

Foundational CIS Controls

7. E-mail and Web Browser Protections
8. Malware Defenses
9. Limitation and Control of Network Ports, Protocols, and Services
10. Data Recovery Capabilities
11. Secure Configuration for Network Devices, such as Firewalls, Routers, and Switches
12. Boundary Defense
13. Data Protection
14. Controlled Access Based on the Need to Know
15. Wireless Access Control
16. Account Monitoring and Control

Organizational CIS Controls

17. Implement a Security Awareness and Training Program

18. Application Software Security

19. Incident Response and Management

20. Penetration Tests and Red Team Exercises

A third risk assessment framework you will need to appreciate is ISO/IEC 27001, *Information security management*. As we have introduced in Chapter 4, this ISO standard is part of the ISO/IEC 27000 family of information security standards. It is popular in the United States as well as internationally, as the Tenable survey reports that 35 percent of organizations report using it. ISO/IEC is the companion implementation standard for ISO/IEC 27002, *Information technology – Security techniques – Code of practice for information security controls*, which describes the best approaches.

The implementation standard is made up of 114 controls and 10 management system clauses and results in a comprehensive and thorough risk management framework. ISO/IEC 27001 is clear on the value and significance in an effective risk management process. At the center of the risk management process is the risk assessment.

With respect to aligning internal audit with the risk assessment approaches, another option you may consider integrating into the risk management frameworks are the Committee of Sponsoring Organizations of the Treadway Commission (COSO) standards. COSO was developed by private sector companies in the United States as a response to corporate fraud. In 2019, COSO published "COSO Internal Control – Integrated Framework: An Implementation Guide for the Healthcare Provider Industry."[21] In these standards, the implementation process is described as five phases:

1. **Planning and scoping**   Before the assessment begins, orientation for senior leaders is needed to gain buy-in. Timelines and priorities have to be established. The extent of the assessment must also be determined to complete the planning phase.

2. **Assessment and documentation**   In this phase, gather information and review the control structures in place, including fraud prevention, because of its prevalence in adverse impacts to the healthcare system. Recording results and findings are also part of this portion of the work. At this point, gaps and weaknesses begin to reveal risks.

3. **Remediation planning and implementation**   In this phase, countermeasures to the assessment findings are designed and steps toward mitigation are started. It is important to gain the support of information owners and security control owners no later than at this point of the assessment.

4. **Design, testing, and reporting of controls**   Once remediation efforts are completed, the assessment continues to review effectiveness of the control improvements. Communication of observations and data analysis of the evidence collected is presented to management and the governing board of directors.

5 components	17 principles
Control environment	1. Demonstrates commitment to integrity and ethical values
	2. Exercises oversight responsibility
	3. Establishes structure, authority, and responsibility
	4. Demonstrates commitment to competence
	5. Enforces accountability.
Risk assessment	6. Specifies suitable objectives
	7. Identifies and analyzes risk
	8. Assesses fraud risk
	9. Identifies and analyzes significant change
Control activities	10. Selects and develops control activities
	11. Selects and develops general controls over technology
	12. Deploys control activities through policies and procedures
Information and communication	13. Uses relevant information
	14. Communicates internally
	15. Communicates externally
Monitoring activities	16. Conducts ongoing and/or separate evaluations
	17. Evaluates and communicates deficiencies

Figure 6-8 Components of COSO Risk Assessment Framework[22]

5. Optimization of effectiveness of internal control Like other frameworks, COSO insists that risk assessment be a continuous process. Continual improvement and refinement of security controls is phase 5 of the COSO healthcare framework, but it really just creates the cycle to inform the first phase of planning and scoping to begin again.

In practice, the COSO framework is applicable as an audit approach, but it is relevant to assessing security controls. As such, it can be relevant to communicate risk to management and the board of directors, as well as to inform improvements in the overall information security system. The framework consists of five components and 17 control principles that measure efficient and effective control operation, timely open and accurate communication of results, and compliance with legal and regulatory obligations. Figure 6-8 illustrates the components and control principles.

Participate in Risk Assessment According to Your Role

The qualifications for candidates seeking the HCISSP certification require a discussion in this area that covers a variety of roles that conduct the risk assessment as well as those that support and benefit from it in terms of facilitating risk treatment decisions. We defined and described many of these positions in Chapter 1, and other sections referenced general functions most of these professionals perform. We will not repeat that information here, but instead provide relevant additional information related to supporting risk assessments:

- **Board of directors/regulators**   A healthcare system with a board of directors typically also has an audit committee that participates in the risk assessment process by establishing the information security risk tolerance level using input from organization management. In such healthcare organizations, the board and audit committee should receive regular updates concerning risk management topics, including internal and external risk assessments. In healthcare systems that have boards and those that are not commercial entities or are fully controlled as extension of government organizations, regulators participate in risk assessment by establishing risk assessment requirements. If a healthcare organization fails to meet those recommendations, the government can levy fines and penalties.

- **Executive management**   Senior management of the organization develops the risk tolerance levels based on risk factors such as operational, clinical, and financial concerns. Senior management has the ultimate responsibility of ensuring that the organization conducts risk assessments and communicates honest and accurate results to the executive management, the board, regulators, and personnel throughout the organization as required. The executive management accepts risk on behalf of the organization, and risk assessment input is crucial to that role. To enhance the executive management to be successful in understanding and making risk treatment decisions, another responsibility is extremely important: management must select and support information security leadership and be active in information governance.

- **Chief information officer (CIO)**   As a member of executive management, the CIO will be principally responsible for much of the technology, interconnections, and data protection risks. Enforcing adherence with risk mitigations and keeping residual risks minimized is within the CIO purview as the senior leader of information technology assets.

- **Chief information security officer (CISO)**   The CISO leads the team that conducts information security assessments or works with internal and external audits on other information security risk assessments. The CISO is responsible for interpreting outcomes of the assessments and taking action. Those actions may be related to updates to policy and procedures, investment in new security technologies, and remediation of vulnerabilities. The CISO may not have direct responsibility for addressing the vulnerabilities, but the role is accountable to leading efforts of those who are and providing oversight to make sure the work is done. The CISO communicates risk assessment information to executive management, the board of directors, and often regulators.

- **Privacy officer**   The privacy officer, particularly if the position is an officer of the corporation such as the chief privacy officer, will be integral to many information security risk assessments. One example is in organizations that use the Health Information Trust Alliance (HITRUST) CSF as a measurement tool.

The HITRUST CSF includes an assessment against the effectiveness and maturity of various privacy controls. Otherwise, the privacy officer can provide a wealth of knowledge on security and privacy concerns that impact the operation of controls, such as data transfer obligations and data breach notification, to name a few. Privacy officers are also versed in legal and regulatory concerns that impact proper operation of security controls and could affect calculations of the consequences that result in risk estimation.

- **Security control owners/information owners/data stewards**   These roles include information security personnel, system administrators, network engineers, and representatives from business and clinical departments. Many security controls are dependent on proper operation and daily oversight by professionals in these roles. Information owners are responsible for designing and maintaining controls for data collection, transfer, and storage, for example. Clinical representatives, likewise, often administer the access and authorization policies and procedures for systems and data in their areas, assuring that the acceptable use adheres to organizational guidelines and regulatory requirements. Information security personnel, including the CISO, are not always the owners of security controls. Every security framework includes a shared responsibility expectation between information security personnel, IT professionals, business managers, and clinical representatives who work together to operate security controls effectively and efficiently. However, the oversight of the risk management program and the conduct of the risk assessment process remain the responsibilities of the information security leadership.

- **Information technology auditors**   As we mentioned in the previous section, internal and external auditors play key roles in providing objective oversight and assurance to the organization, regulators, and the governing board. Their expertise and third line of defense function help to identify gaps where controls are not working effectively or efficiently. In some cases, internal auditors can serve as consultants to advise and champion the design of mitigating actions to improve the operation of security controls.

- **Business resiliency professionals**   These professionals include business continuity planners and disaster recovery specialists. Security control frameworks include sections on controls that measure the ability of the organization to respond to and recover from incidents and events should they occur. Business resiliency is concerned with natural as well as manmade disasters. The objectives are to keep business and clinical functions running with minimal disruption. During a risk assessment process, business resiliency professionals will participate by providing evidence to demonstrate that policies and plans are in place for each appropriate business or clinical area, not just in IT. They will also be able to demonstrate that sufficient exercises and tests were conducted to assure the organizational leadership that in a crisis the organization can respond and recover.

- **Physical security personnel** The responsibilities and functions that entail physical security extend beyond information risk management. However, the integration of proper physical security and information security has many examples. Each security control framework has controls that require or recommend processes and technologies. Personnel assigned to facility management or maintenance are often the security control owners of physical security controls. Some controls are intended to limit building access to personnel through badging systems and security guards. Other controls call for installation of surveillance solutions and use of facility alarm systems, as examples. These controls assist information security professionals and information owners in preventing, deterring, and alerting against unauthorized access and use of information assets located in areas not open to the public, such as data centers, operating rooms, and medical supply storage areas.

This list is not comprehensive, as other categories of personnel in an organization can own a security control or participate in the risk assessment process. For example, we didn't mention human resources representatives, who will likely own controls concerned with personnel security areas such as employee background checks, discipline and sanction policies, and organizational training requirements. That is not a reflection on how important these people are in managing effective controls and assessing risks in those areas. Conducting a risk assessment in an organization will involve many subject matter experts from a variety of IT, business, and clinical departments.

Information Gathering

Information gathering for a risk assessment is dependent on the risk model you select to use. You must first determine the risk factors that will be assessed along with how they are associated with one another. Earlier in this chapter, we defined some common risk factors that are used in risk models: threat, vulnerability, impact, and likelihood. You may find it useful to define subcategories of risk factors. For example, a threat can be segmented into threat sources and threat events. Information gathering is facilitated by making these determinations before conducting the risk assessment, because the methods and evaluation of the information collected relies on how useful or relevant it is for assessing the chosen risk attributes and measuring risk.

The process for gathering information will include one or more approaches. Typically, a combination of several methods works best to get the most accurate and complete assessment of control effectiveness and efficiency. Here are some examples of information gathering from NIST:[23]

- **Questionnaires** A survey of questions can be used to help control owners and respondents manage the time required to participate. The approach can also reduce any constraints meeting face-to-face may cause because of scheduling and travel. Questionnaires can be used to follow-up or provide the agenda for subsequent onsite meetings.

- **Onsite interviews**   These allow for direct observation of the operation of security controls in the business and clinical environments. This is especially true when reviewing physical controls. The interviews may involve individual and group meetings to explore responses from earlier surveys or to ask questions for the first time.

- **Document reviews**   A thorough information-gathering process will include at least a valid sampling of policies, procedures, and system output documentation. System outputs will include screen shots and audit logs. An assessor may want to review artifacts from previous audits and budgets, for example, to provide context for current and planned security controls.

- **Use of automated scanning tools**   Vulnerability management and asset management scans can provide evidence of system security controls operating effectively. These tools and others are very good sources of evidence.

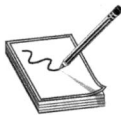

NOTE   Information gathering is an activity that starts before the assessment begins, but it can continue throughout each phase of the process.

Risk Assessment Estimated Timeline

When a risk is identified, the priorities of mitigating the risk or otherwise providing countermeasures to address it become necessary. There will never be enough time or budget to address every risk immediately. You must have a system to determine priority and then estimate resources required and timelines for completion of risk reduction. Figure 6-9 illustrates a simple matrix that you could use to help prioritize risk. The matrix also provides a categorization (extreme risk, high risk, moderate risk, and low risk) that can be used to provide a qualitative estimation of time to reduce the risk. In this case, the timeline could be immediate for an extreme risk with an imminent likelihood and catastrophic consequence. A rare risk with minor impact may be deemed acceptable with no timeline required. For a risk likelihood that is considered neutral (or about a 50 percent chance it could happen) with an impact expected to be minor, a timeline of periodic monitoring would be sufficient.

Gap Analysis

To give meaning to security control assessment, analysis of the difference between the current state of the control effectiveness and the desired or future state is necessary. That scrutiny is called a *gap analysis*. The gap analysis is not a separate activity, but part of the entire risk assessment process and the risk management program. The target of the assessment, which could be the security program in total, a specific system, or a process such as business continuity, provides a source for the initial measurements. You will need to compare a *benchmark*, a standard or best practice, against those measurements.

	Impact				
Likelihood	**Insignificant**	**Minor**	**Moderate**	**Major**	**Catastrophic**
	1	2	3	4	5
Imminent (A)	H	H	E	E	E
Likely (B)	M	H	H	E	E
Neutral (C)	L	M	H	E	E
Unlikely (D)	L	L	M	H	E
Rare (E)	L	L	M	H	H
E	Extreme: The risk requires immediate response; avoid, transfer, or mitigate				
H	High risk: Appropriate risk treatment is necessary before assuming risk				
M	Moderate risk: Management of risk with periodic monitoring sufficient				
L	Low risk: Level of risk is considered acceptable				

Figure 6-9   Risk matrix for establishing risk mitigation timelines

Information security and information risk management were introduced in Chapter 4 and will be covered again in this chapter.

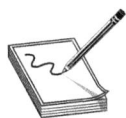

> **NOTE**   Refer to ISO/IEC 27002, NIST SP 800-53 Rev. 4, or HITRUST CSF as examples of healthcare information security and information risk management benchmarks.

When you understand the variance between the current and desired states using the benchmark, you will want to communicate the results with senior leadership, at which point they will expect you to have recommendations, including costs, for mitigation actions and corrective action plans. As you do that work, keep in mind that communication of the findings and the next steps to improvement is important, because you will increase your chances of success by getting management support and commitment at the onset.

> **CAUTION**   A gap analysis will be most useful if the assessment is objective. Information control owners will be essential to implementing improvements. However, internal personnel can find it difficult to help expose areas of weakness for fear of negative consequences. To gain trust, you should avoid blame and individual attribution. Your focus should be on system-level or process improvement, which involve teams and groups.

Mitigating Actions

Risk is ever-changing and always present. We know that as an HCISPP, your role will be important in helping your organization manage risk through a variety of risk-reduction activities. One risk-reduction approach involves mitigating actions. *Mitigation* is defined as reducing or lessening the effect of an action as measured in seriousness or severity. In terms of information risk, mitigating actions would serve to lessen the likelihood of occurrence, the severity of impact, and the seriousness of vulnerabilities, independently or in combination. An example of a mitigating action is to lessen the threat of account credential theft by implementing multifactor authentication for remote computing access as a security control. Security awareness and training for employees also serves as a risk reduction action, as employees are less likely to fall for an e-mail phishing attack and more likely to report a security incident when they appreciate information security risks and can identify issues. Another mitigating action involves diversification. In information risk, diversity is achieved through multiple copies of critical data stored in multiple locations, online and offsite, with at least one copy not accessible through the computer network to mitigate attacks such as ransomware or natural disasters.

Risk Avoidance

When a risk exceeds the risk tolerance established by the organization, the proper risk mitigation is to avoid it. Risk avoidance may be a difficult business or clinical decision. When considering exposing the organization to undue risks, the benefits may not outweigh those risks. Think of a potential third-party supplier relationship to share PHI, for example. As information risk assessment is done against that new relationship, you find that the vendor does not uphold the information security practices that your organization requires. In fact, the vendor will not sign contractual language to obligate them to protect the information to your standards, particularly where those standards are associated with regulatory requirements. In that case, avoidance of the risk is the best option. Avoidance of risk can manifest as cancelled projects, decommissioned systems, and destruction of data that is no longer needed.

Risk Transfer

Shifting risk to another entity or organization based on information security activities is another risk treatment action. This can be accomplished through several approaches. Two of the most prevalent methods are through cybersecurity insurance and contracts or other legal agreements.

CAUTION Be careful with risk transfer. In most cases, you can shift legal and financial responsibilities for the risks, but the reputational risk or loss of revenue that results from an incident or breach may still happen. For example, a business associate loses PHI from your patient population. Those patients may lose trust in your organization and seek care elsewhere, even though your organization was not at fault. Risk transfer decisions should not overstate the extent to which they reduce risk.

Cybersecurity insurance is an indemnification approach in which the organization pays premiums to guard against unplanned costs in the event of an information security incident. To get the lowest premiums and the best coverage, insurance underwriters will conduct a risk assessment against your organization to estimate the risks they are accepting to insure your organization. The costs the policy will cover may include the following:

- Notification of affected individuals after a data breach
- Fraud protections with credit monitoring and assistance to restore identity
- Investigation and forensic costs
- Restoration of computing environment

Cybersecurity insurance can provide a safeguard against excessive unplanned costs during and after a natural disaster or a successful cyber-attack. However, the use of cybersecurity insurance cannot be considered a security control that actually reduces risks, unless the use of the insurance motivates improved investment in the overall information security program to reduce cybersecurity insurance premiums and permit the organization to obtain the best policies.

Another approach to risk transfer is through contracts and other legal agreements. In the United States, this contract is a business associate agreement. Third-party suppliers, vendors, and partners with which you share information must be aware of their obligations. They must provide at least as much protection for the healthcare information they handle on your behalf as you do. Risk transfer has to be explicit, and these documented expectations and agreements are essential. Continual review of adherence to the agreements is also necessary to make sure the risk levels are not changed over time. This is a good example of business and clinical department representatives serving as the owners of the security control, because they likely "own" the relationship with the third party. You, as an HCISPP, will be responsible to provide oversight for adherence with the information risk transfer mechanism, such as the business associate agreement.

Risk Acceptance

Most importantly, do not mistake risk acceptance with risk disregard. Acceptance results only after proper risk assessment and consideration of other risk treatment actions. After mitigations are considered, transfer options are reviewed, and a compelling business or clinical reason makes avoidance infeasible, risk acceptance may be the best risk treatment action. Restated, risk acceptance is possible when risk treatments reduce the risks below the established risk tolerance levels or the benefits of exposing the organization to the risks outweigh the potential for adverse outcomes such as a data breach.

There will always be a security risk involved in collecting, using, transferring, storing, and disposing of PII and PHI. The delivery of healthcare services today is an interconnected, data-driven, and advanced IT systems industry. With public health and research pursuits added, the information risks are often global and shared between organizations in multiple national and regulatory jurisdictions. Before you accept risks, it should be obvious that a significant amount of assessment and communications must happen.

EXAM TIP Risk acceptance cannot be the correct risk treatment option, or exam answer, until after a risk assessment is conducted and other treatment options are considered.

Communications and Reporting

Once the risk assessment is completed, the corrective action plan is developed, and the cost–benefit analysis documents the recommended approaches to risk, the next order of business is to communicate the findings. This implies that communication is episodic and involves a sequence of steps; however, this is not the case. Effectively, various types and levels of communication must occur throughout the risk management program. Certainly, once there are findings, they must be communicated. There are no right answers on how and when the results of risk assessments are provided. In some ways, the role of information security and privacy is in marketing and sales, at least internally. To be effective or to have any chance of compliance, the information risk management program has to be understood by employees, championed by senior management, and funded adequately. Funding is probably the most difficult and lacking aspect of information protection in the healthcare industry.

Some of the more established ways risk management plans are communicated throughout the organization are through established committees, as discussed in Chapter 2. The information management council, the configuration control board, and any other cross-functional group meetings are great opportunities to devote an agenda item highlighting key findings or to provide ad hoc training on topics. In some of these groups, it is necessary (and advantageous) to introduce upcoming hardware and software initiatives. Once these are in place, providing the group updates on the return on investment is important. Consider, for instance, installing a new intrusion detection system. Once it is in place, the end-user community as well as senior leadership would be interested in seeing some data on how many threats have been averted over time. Knowing that these threats probably were happening prior to the new intrusion detection system and that any one of them could result in a data breach can be helpful in establishing future risk management decisions. If done correctly, this type of internal communication can help gain organizational trust and support for adequately funding future information protection initiatives.

Communication also happens at the board of directors level. The CISO or an executive management proxy delivers details on risk assessments on a periodic basis. Here are some examples:

- Enterprise risk assessments done by internal and external experts, such as those required by HIPAA
- Penetration testing conducted by external subject matter experts
- Audits from regulatory agencies
- Results of assurance assessments such as those required for ISO/IEC 27001 certification
- Business resiliency tests and exercise outcomes

Communication to the board of directors should remain at a strategic or program level. The objective to communication at this level is to instill confidence in management and gain support for thorough and convincing plans to improve where necessary. Because the board oversees management's operating models and performance considering risk tolerance levels, their awareness and advocacy are important in the risk management program.

Understand Risk Response

A central process in risk management is to correct weaknesses or close any vulnerability gaps once they are identified. The corrective action plan is a formal, organized management tool that identifies these discrepancies. Importantly, the plan describes the actions needed to mitigate identified risks. These actions will relate to prescribed actions from sources such as NIST and ISO. Another key aspect of a corrective action plan is assigning responsibility for implementing the mitigation to an individual. Once that is accomplished, management-level accountability can be applied by way of monitoring the plan for desired outcomes.

As described earlier, even the best corrective action plan may still result in residual or accepted risk. The corrective action plan enables management to identify this reality clearly and document the risk assessment that resulted in a decision to accept the risk and why; in the event variables change, the risk can be readdressed. If variables change (if impact is greater than originally presumed, for example), the prescribed mitigation activity may become feasible.

The corrective action plan is useful beyond helping to address vulnerabilities and manage risk. It can assist information protection efforts in including trending and analysis. The components of a corrective action plan imply its use to support business cases as a cost–benefit tool. Probably most important to information security and privacy, the corrective action plan maintains organizational knowledge and helps communication.

All of the following aspects improve a healthcare organization's information protection program:[24]

- **Trending and analysis** When the corrective plan is managed and updated in concert with an annual risk assessment, it is a terrific historical data source. Management can use the data to measure the cost and effectiveness of controls put in place to mitigate vulnerabilities. Subjective decisions based on the likelihood of an exploit happening or a potential impact can be refined based on actual occurrences.

- **Supporting business cases** Done correctly, corrective action plans contain financial information that can be monitored. Future investment in information protection can be justified (or rejected) by comparing them against successes and failures. Proving return on investment in information protection is often elusive.

Properly managing a corrective action plan is a huge benefit in easing return on investment concerns by management. A corrective action plan can actually support accepting a risk. In these cases, the corrective action plan serves as documentation of the decision processes that were conducted and rationale for making the decision to accept the risk. If conditions change, such as increased risks, the corrective action plan can be adjusted to implement other risk treatment options.

- **Maintaining institutional knowledge** In an organization with a mature information protection program, institutional knowledge is a valued element. Otherwise, the program must rely on an individual or the competency of the current workforce, and a change in workforce results in a change in institutional knowledge. Having a library of corrective action plans and the analysis that goes with each ensures that the organization can maintain an information protection program even if there is turnover in the workforce.

- **Facilitating effective communication** The importance of communicating the corrective action plan to senior leadership cannot be understated. Using the corrective action plan tool and its related information capabilities satisfies the responsibility that information protection personnel have in creating information protection awareness, communicating to senior leadership, and documenting outcomes for compliance efforts.

Use Controls to Remediate Risk

Every healthcare organization faces information risk. The ability to deal confidently with risk is related to the proper implementation and maintenance of a security control environment. When we refer to the NIST cybersecurity framework, we note that control frameworks can be categorized according the control function, such as identify, protect, detect, respond, and recover. Another view of risk remediation controls is commonly used to categorize them. The categories are related to phases or timing of the control use. Phase controls can be administrative, technical, and physical. Let's revisit the prevent, detect, and correct control phases in Table 6-1.

Your understanding how to select controls based on effectiveness during a certain phase or based on timing considerations will improve your risk mitigation activities.

Prevent	Detect	Correct
Security awareness training	Security incident and event monitoring (SIEM)	Operating system/application upgrade
Firewall	Intrusion detection system	Fire suppression systems
Door locks	Antimalware	Patch management of software vulnerabilities
Security guards	Motion detectors	Sanction policies for security violations
Data loss prevention system	Vulnerability management scanning	Incident response plans

Table 6-1 Sample Table of Security Control Phases

Preventative, detective, and corrective security controls are present in the standards with which you are familiar. NIST SP 800-53 Rev. 4, for example, identifies more than 160 controls. Recall that based on the security categorization of the information asset, the number will change. As a refresher, a high security categorization may require that significantly more controls be implemented than a moderate categorization, and in turn a low security categorization requires even fewer. ISO/IEC 27001 lists more than 130 controls in different areas, but this is not an exhaustive list. You can implement additional controls according to the requirements of your organization. Using the control frameworks as a catalog of security controls, focusing on the phase of controls (prevent, detect, correct) can bolster your risk remediation efforts.

Administrative Controls

Policies and procedures are the basis of administrative controls. These controls are intended to inform the healthcare organization workforce on what protected healthcare information is, what to do to protect it, and what to do when there is a problem. Examples of administrative controls are contracts and legal agreements that tell third parties what to expect and what obligations they have accepted. Laws and regulations are another form of administrative control. Administrative controls such as the following can be effective in any security control phases:

- **Administrative preventative controls** These include security awareness programs, risk management policies, and disaster recovery plans. Business associate agreements are administrative preventative controls as well.

- **Administrative detective controls** Examples include asset inventory procedures and vulnerability management scan reconciliation.

- **Administrative corrective controls** Incident response plans and employee sanction policies are effective in response and recovery risk mitigation phases.

Physical Controls

Physical controls can be effective in each phase. Controls can be as simple as wall or door locks or more sophisticated technical solutions for physical security such as surveillance systems with facial recognition. Security guards and emergency responders may also be an important component of physical security. Here are some examples of physical security controls per phase:

- **Physical preventive controls** These are probably obvious because of the deterrence they provide, but secure buildings, fences, locking cages for network equipment racks, and security guards are just a few examples.

- **Physical detective controls** Risk mitigation comes from the use of surveillance systems, smoke and fire alarms, and motion detectors.

- **Physical corrective controls** When an incident happens, some physical controls can be effective responses. For example, a fire suppression system can mitigate loss of property and information assets.

Technical Controls

The use of software and hardware systems and applications to prevent, detect, and correct risks are technical security controls. Technologies or tools have improved risk mitigation as solutions such as firewalls, data loss prevention systems, intrusion detection systems, and SIEMs have automated scanning and alerting processes. The ability to manage vast amounts of data from audit logs and maintain a view of the computing environment would be impossible security tasks without technical security control solutions. In each phase of security controls, technical risk mitigation is evident:

- **Technical preventive controls** These are used to block or prohibit an unwanted action. Firewalls and intrusion prevention systems are common devices used to mitigate the risks of unauthorized access to network resources.

- **Technical detective controls** SIEM technologies, for example, continually ingest threat intelligence from external sources and correlate that information against large stores of data gathered from internal computing asset logs. These solutions identify and alert against potential infiltration to the network and exfiltration of data.

- **Technical corrective controls** An example of this type of control is patch management. As vulnerabilities are discovered, technology is used to create an application package of updates. Through centrally managed patch distribution technology, the updates reach a majority of information assets. For the portion of computing assets that cannot be centrally managed, patches are applied through manual update of the software.

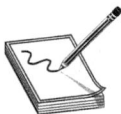

NOTE A security control can be effective across multiple phases. For example, a security guard can be a preventative control as well as a detective and corrective security control. An antimalware application can mitigate risk across all the phases of security controls and can block, identify, or quarantine any malicious code.

Participate in Continuous Monitoring

By now, you understand that risk assessment and, by extension, risk management is a continuous process, not a one-time evaluation at a specified time. Your role in that continual process will take several forms. On a daily basis, you will be reviewing metrics and indicators from SIEMs, threat intelligence from internal and external sources, and reports from security tools and audit logs. Within the organization, you may participate or lead committees and governance groups to integrate monitoring of information risks with major concerns such as organizational risks, fraud, and data use. Depending on your role in the organization, you may also provide continuous monitoring and reporting for strategic planning for risk treatment actions and risk mitigation projects within the information security program. These monitoring activities are reserved for executive management and board-level communications.

Starting at an operational level, you will be expected to monitor risk to the environment. Numerous information security tools can assist you in mitigating risk. You can, for example, use endpoint protection and detection capabilities such as antimalware and advanced persistent threat software. At the network level, you can employ tactics such as firewalls and intrusion detection systems Data loss prevention (DLP) technologies can help prevent and detect unauthorized access and transfer of sensitive data. Add to this the use of SIEM that ingests threat intelligence to stay current on threats that can be detected in your environment, and you begin to see a full spectrum of tools and techniques that you will use to monitor and then report changing risk levels within the organization.

You should also consult a few risk mitigation guidelines as you develop risk mitigation strategies. Two leading examples are the MITRE ATT$K techniques and the CIS controls and CIS controls implementation groups.[25,26] Both are open standards that you can use to examine specific threats and the corresponding tools or techniques that these groups recommend. For example, the MITRE ATT$K matrix suggests a risk mitigation to deal with the drive-by compromise in which an attacker attempts access by normal web browsing but then tries to do an injection of malware: MITRE advises keeping software up-to-date and prohibiting pop-up ads as two of several mitigations. Likewise, the CIS controls implementation group offers guidance for running automated vulnerability scanning as a mitigation to identify vulnerabilities, remediate them, and minimize the window of opportunity for attackers. These are just samples of the information available to assist information security personnel in participating in continuous risk monitoring.

Because the risks faced by organizations change almost daily, an HCISPP must also stay current on threat intelligence. An individual organization is likely not able to fund, gather, and analyze the vast amounts of data that exists in this area. Searching the dark web or researching adversarial actors probably exceeds the capabilities and time available for healthcare organization staff. Therefore, a mixture of open source (no-cost) threat intelligence sources and participation or membership with professional, industry-based groups that provide threat intelligence and information sharing among member organizations is an imperative. Examples of open source groups include the SANS Internet Storm Center, the Department of Homeland Security's (DHS) National Cybersecurity and Communications Integration Center (NCCIC), and the US Computer Emergency Readiness Team (US-CERT). The National Health ISAC (H-ISAC) and the HITRUST C3 are examples of membership services. Using these sources to monitor continuously changes in risks external to your organization may alter your projections for likelihood and impact.

It is not enough to simply monitor risk within the information security department. You must communicate the changes to keep the board of directors and the rest of the organization current. Drawing from what you learned in Chapter 2, the information governance function within the healthcare organization should be informed of changes in threats and vulnerabilities and how they alter impact and likelihood measures. Periodic updates to the audit committee of the board and the entire board of directors should contain top information security risks that may result in regulatory action, significant financial loss, or reputational damage such as data breach or disruption of services. Appropriate topics for these groups are risks with third-party suppliers, longstanding open audit findings, and select risk mitigation activities that improve security maturity levels. The exact content will depend on your organization, the risks your organization face, and the focus areas of senior management and the board members.

Within the organization, risk is continuously monitored through participation and updates to internal information governance committees and groups that information security leads or serves as a member. We introduced examples in Chapter 2—including the risk management steering committee that looks at organizational risks of financial, operational, and information security concerns. There should also be an information management steering committee with purview over various collection, use, transfer, storage, and disposal issues for information assets in the organization. Although these groups and committees may have different names depending on the organization, the information governance functions of managing risk and overseeing information use should have such governance groups in place with authority codified in policy and procedures. It is applicable for these groups to have a regular report of existing, accepted risks; progress on risk mitigations; and current appraisal on any changes to the threat environment that will alter priorities or previous risk treatment decisions.

Chapter Review

In this chapter, we introduced the process of examining information risk in a healthcare organization. We examined some terminology and activities within the risk management process, such as the risk equation Risk = Likelihood × Impact. All healthcare organizations face risk, and risk cannot be completely eliminated. Risk treatment decisions such as avoidance, mitigation, transfer, and acceptance are necessary, and the HCISPP is central to the decision process. Where risk must be accepted, actions can be taken to minimize the likelihood of risk occurring or reduce the impact if it does. Sometimes, the elements of risk are so incompatible with the business of healthcare that the risk must be avoided (in other words, actions cannot be taken). This chapter addressed activities related to participating in risk management activities, starting with the risk assessment. We also introduced development of remediation actions plans using leading security frameworks and security controls.

The chapter also addressed risk communications as it applies across organizations, including keeping team members informed of identified risks, monitoring risks, and responding to risks. Additionally, the chapter covered the process for performing exception handling, reporting to management and organizational functional areas, and measuring risks based on established metrics.

The chapter also included how to estimate timelines or timeframes for conducting the risk assessment and how often they should occur, as well as how to conduct a gap analysis and develop corrective action plans and plan of action and milestones for identified risks or other weaknesses. As a healthcare information security and privacy professional, you can expect to participate in efforts to remediate gaps, including selecting and implementing the types of security controls and safeguards and controls related to time.

Healthcare organizations are mandated to go through a risk management process. Some frameworks were introduced in this chapter with scenarios for how they might apply in your organization. The most salient point about information risk in healthcare is that it can lead to patient harm in addition to other enterprise risks such as financial, operational, and reputational risks. Healthcare-savvy information protection programs will understand and factor in patient care and patient safety in risk decisions. With proper communication of these issues and the findings of the risk management process, information protection can integrate and enable healthcare business strategy, clinical practices, and third-party relationships.

Questions

1. Which of the following National Institute of Standards and Technology (NIST) special publications details the risk management process?

    A. NIST SP 800-53 Rev. 4

    B. NIST SP 800-30 Rev. 1

    C. NIST SP 800-37 Rev. 2

    D. NIST SP 800-60 Vol. 1 Rev. 1

2. To find a qualitative measure for the likelihood of a denial-of-service attack, which would be a recommended source?

    A. Expert opinions from threat intelligence sources

    B. Value of information assets expected to be taken offline due to the attack

    C. Historical financial records of department services downtime

    D. Lost revenue from diverted patients from other organizations in previous attacks

3. Which of these is a variable in considering the risk of a decision?

    A. Controls

    B. Cost

    C. Impact

    D. Frequency

4. At a high level, NIST 800-39 builds a risk management framework around which of these activities of a risk management program?

    A. Framing, assessing, responding, monitoring

    B. Framing, controlling, responding, monitoring

    C. Framing, assessing, restoring, monitoring

    D. Framing, assessing, responding, motivating

5. Which risk management framework specifically tailors its approach to healthcare?

    A. ISO/IEC 27001

    B. HITRUST

    C. NIST RMF

    D. Common Criteria

6. If you must perform an action that increases risk, you may choose to do what to approach the residual risk by implementing one or more administrative, physical, and technical controls?

   A. Avoid

   B. Transfer

   C. Mitigate

   D. Accept

7. A security guard who is present at the front desk of your hospital is an example of what type of phase security control?

   A. Preventative

   B. Detective

   C. Corrective

   D. All of the above

8. You have implemented an intrusion detection system for the local area network. You begin to collect data to show the number of attacks detected and prevented. You present the information and trends to the information management committee. You recommend hiring a new security engineer based on the workloads and requirements. This scenario is an example of what proper use of corrective action plans?

   A. Facilitating effective communication

   B. Trending and analysis

   C. Supporting business cases

   D. Maintaining institutional knowledge

9. Because medical devices have special configuration considerations, the information security officer decides to implement a compensating control to ensure that the company is mitigating against virus infiltration via an enclave, or virtual private network architecture. Which of these suggest a valid reason for implementing the compensating control?

   A. The architecture solution meets or exceeds the original intent of the prescribed control of protecting against virus infiltration.

   B. Medical devices are regulated by an external agency and cannot be administered by healthcare organizations.

   C. Physicians must approve any changes to medical devices because medical devices often provide diagnostic and treatment support, so patient safety is at issue.

   D. Antivirus software is not applicable to systems that do not provide office automation services.

10. At the completion of a risk assessment and development of a corrective action plan, which would be a logical next step in the risk management program?

   A. Budgeting for future information security upgrades

   B. Filing results with regulatory agencies

   C. Creating a risk management archive

   D. Communicating results to the organization

Answers

1. C. NIST's Risk Management Framework is detailed in SP 800-37 Rev. 2, *Risk Management Framework for Information Systems and Organizations: A System Life Cycle Approach for Security and Privacy*. A, NIST SP 800-53 Rev. 4, *Security and Privacy Controls for Federal Information Systems and Organizations*, can be used to establish security controls to use in the risk assessment. B, NIST SP 800-30 Rev. 1, *Guide for Conducting Risk Assessments*, is one part of the entire risk management process only. D, NIST 800-60 Vol. 1 Rev. 1, *Guide for Mapping Types of Information and Information Systems to Security Categories*, also offers guidelines for a portion of the entire risk management process.

2. A. Of the choices, only gathering expert opinions from threat intelligence sources would result in a subjective qualitative measure such as high, medium, or low. B would be a measure in money and perhaps an additional amount for time and energy needed for replacement and would not address probability of the attack. C is also an objective measure of money and therefore quantitative. D is another example that would not address probability of attacks and would result in a financial indicator that does not satisfy the question.

3. C. The impact of the exploit of a vulnerability is one of the variables that must be considered in making risk-based decisions. Impact is the expected outcome if the scenario happens. It can be measured in subjective (loss of reputation) and objective (dollars for fines) terms. A is incorrect because controls are the safeguards that may be put in place to reduce risk. B is not the best answer because cost is a consideration of compensating controls. Those controls that make sense compared to how much they cost to implement against what value they provide are selected. D is incorrect because frequency may be a variable related to likelihood, which is also a variable, but it is not a variable by itself.

4. A. Framing, assessing, responding, and monitoring are the prescribed high-level activities identified in NIST SP 800-39. The other options contain words that are not applicable to the list found in the publication. B includes controlling, which is not correct; however, choosing controls to put in place is part of a risk management program, yet not at a high level. C includes restoring, which is not applicable. D, motivating, is incorrect; although communicating the risk management program and findings of the risk assessment is crucial to motivating the organization, NIST 800-39 does not point to motivation in this regard.

5. B. The HITRUST Common Security Framework is the only representative in this group that applies specifically to healthcare organizations. A is incorrect because ISO/IEC 27001 is an information risk management framework, but it is applicable across any industry that handles sensitive information. C, the NIST RMF, also has applicability across multiple industries, especially US federal government systems. D is incorrect because the Common Criteria is an assessment or accreditation program that assigns a level of assurance to common hardware and software security products and is not specific to healthcare.

6. C. According to the definitions of these valid actions taken to address residual risk in an organization, mitigate is the only option in which you implement one or more controls to minimize the likelihood and negative impact of a risk. A is incorrect because avoiding a process or action that has risk is specifically ruled out by the question, as you must perform the action that increases the risk. B is incorrect because transferring the risk means contracting or outsourcing liability. D is incorrect because accepting the risk can happen when the impact of the risk is not severe enough to preclude the organization from taking the chance.

7. D. All of the choices are correct. A security guard can be an effective preventative security control because of his or her presence. The guard mitigates the risk of an intruder. Also, a security guard can act as a detective security control as he or she walks around the data center on periodic rounds or monitors a surveillance camera. Finally, a security guard can be a corrective security control when he or she extinguishes a fire or apprehends an intruder.

8. C. The data is being used to support the business case for hiring a new person. Collecting data to demonstrate objectively that the intended impact is happening for the control that is put in place is a great example of supporting a business case for the cost of implementing and maintaining the intrusion detection system with a new hire. A is incorrect because facilitating effective communication is only part of the use of this report of a corrective action plan that includes implementing a new technical detection solution. B is incorrect because the intrusion detection system was just implemented, and trending and analysis information is probably not mature enough. D is incorrect because maintaining institutional knowledge does not apply to this scenario. Over time, the data will be beneficial for measuring the effectiveness of the corrective action plan.

9. A. Although not the prescribed control from a set of standards, a compensating control with equal rigor meets or exceeds the original requirement. B, C, and D are incorrect; all point to common reasons why some healthcare organizations and medical device manufacturers believe medical devices cannot be secured the same way as office automation computers and networking equipment. Some of the reasons are based in fact. For instance, medical devices are regulated by the US Food and Drug Administration (FDA), but the FDA does allow software configuration for security enhancement as long as the changes are coordinated and approved by the medical device manufacturer, making B incorrect. C is incorrect because although medical devices are often used for diagnostic and treatment purposes, physicians do not necessarily have a role in approving modifications. However, all clinical personnel should receive communication about such changes and provide concurrence when feasible. D is not the most relevant answer because antivirus software is almost always applicable to medical device software; most medical devices use common OSs and applications to operate. That said, exception lists and other additional configuration efforts need to be made based on types of file extensions and traffic that medical devices process to ensure legitimate files are not quarantined or blocked inadvertently.

10. **D.** A good risk management program is good only if it is communicated throughout the organization from senior leadership down. Awareness must be built into clinical practices and business processes to ensure that corrective actions succeed and that future events are prevented to the extent possible. Though getting information security acquisition into future budgets is important, A is incorrect because it may not cover all findings because some corrective actions may be no cost or nontechnical to fix. B is incorrect because there may not be any requirement to send results to a regulatory agency. C is incorrect because a good risk management program is not static, so simply filing the result away in an archive until the next assessment is not recommended.

References

1. Williams, J. 2020. "OWASP Risk Rating Methodology." https://owasp.org/www-community/OWASP_Risk_Rating_Methodology.

2. NIST. 2004. *Federal Information Processing Standards: Standards for Security Categorization of Federal Information and Information Systems*, FIST PUB 199. https://nvlpubs.nist.gov/nistpubs/FIPS/NIST.FIPS.199.pdf.

3. Stine, K., R. Kissel, W. Barker, J. Fahlsing, and J. Gulick. 2008. *Guide for Mapping Types of Information and Information Systems to Security Categories*, NIST Special Publication 800-60 Vol. 1 Rev. 1. https://csrc.nist.gov/publications/detail/sp/800-60/vol-1-rev-1/final.

4. Barrett, M., J. Marron, V. Y. Pillitteri, J. Boyens, S. Quinn, G. Witte, and L. Feldman. 2020. *Approaches for Federal Agencies to Use the Cybersecurity Framework*, NISTIR 8170. https://nvlpubs.nist.gov/nistpubs/ir/2020/NIST.IR.8170.pdf.

5. NIST. 2011. *Managing Information Security Risk: Organization, Mission, and Information System View*, Special Publication 800-39. https://nvlpubs.nist.gov/nistpubs/Legacy/SP/nistspecialpublication800-39.pdf.

6. NIST. *Managing Information Security Risk: Organization, Mission, and Information System View*.

7. NIST. 2018. *Risk Management Framework for Information Systems and Organizations: A System Life Cycle Approach for Security and Privacy*, Special Publication 800-37 Rev. 2. https://nvlpubs.nist.gov/nistpubs/SpecialPublications/NIST.SP.800-37r2.pdf.

8. Adapted from M. Scholl, et al. *An Introductory Resource Guide for Implementing the Health Insurance Portability and Accountability Act (HIPAA) Security Rule*, NIST Special Publication 800-66 Rev. 1. https://nvlpubs.nist.gov/nistpubs/Legacy/SP/nistspecialpublication800-66r1.pdf.

9. HealthPocket. 2019. "What's the difference between Medicare and Medicaid?" https://www.healthpocket.com/medicare/medicare-vs-medicaid#.XrAm5G5Fw2x.

10. Centers for Medicare & Medicaid Services Information Security and Privacy Group (CMS). 2018. *Risk Management Handbook (RMH)*, Ver. 1.1, Chapter 14: "Risk Assessment (RA)." https://www.cms.gov/Research-Statistics-Data-and-Systems/CMS-Information-Technology/InformationSecurity/Downloads/RMH-Chapter-14-Risk-Assessment.pdf.

11. CMS. 2019. "Information Security and Privacy Library." https://www.cms.gov/Research-Statistics-Data-and-Systems/CMS-Information-Technology/InformationSecurity/Information-Security-Library.

12. NIST. 2012. *Guide for Conducting Risk Assessments*, Special Publication 800-30 Rev. 1. https://nvlpubs.nist.gov/nistpubs/Legacy/SP/nistspecialpublication800-30r1.pdf.

13. NIST. 2020. "National Vulnerability Database: Vulnerability Metrics." https://nvd.nist.gov/vuln-metrics/cvss.

14. First.org. 2019. *Common Vulnerability Scoring System version 3.1 User Guide*, CVSS Rev. 1. https://www.first.org/cvss/v3-1/cvss-v31-user-guide_r1.pdf.

15. US Department of Health and Human Services, Office for Civil Rights. 2019. "Guidance on Risk Analysis." https://www.hhs.gov/hipaa/for-professionals/security/guidance/guidance-risk-analysis/index.html.

16. NIST. *Guide for Conducting Risk Assessments*.

17. HealthIT.gov. 2019. "Security Risk Assessment Tool." https://www.healthit.gov/topic/privacy-security-and-hipaa/security-risk-assessment-tool.

18. National Health Service (NHS). 2020. "Data Security and Protection Toolkit." https://www.dsptoolkit.nhs.uk.

19. Tenable. 2016. "Survey Report: Trends in Security Framework Adoption." Available for download at https://www.tenable.com/whitepapers/trends-in-security-framework-adoption.

20. NIST. 2014. *Assessing Security and Privacy Controls in Federal Information Systems and Organizations: Building Effective Assessment Plans*, Special Publication 800-53A Rev. 4. https://nvlpubs.nist.gov/nistpubs/SpecialPublications/NIST.SP.800-53Ar4.pdf.

21. Schandl, A., and Foster, P. 2019. "Committee of Sponsoring Organizations of the Treadway Commission (COSO): An Implementation Guide for the Healthcare Provider Industry." https://www.coso.org/Documents/COSO-CROWE-COSO-Internal-Control-Integrated-Framework.pdf.

22. Committee of Sponsoring Organizations of the Treadway Commission (COSO). 2013. "Internal Control – Integrated Framework: Executive Summary." https://www.coso.org/Documents/990025P-Executive-Summary-final-may20 .pdf?source=post_page.

23. NIST. *Guide for Conducting Risk Assessments*.

24. CMS. 2015. *Risk Management Handbook*, Volume III, Standard 6.2: "Plan of Action and Milestones Process Guide." https://www.cms.gov/Research-Statistics-Data-and-Systems/CMS-Information-Technology/InformationSecurity/Downloads/RMH_VIII_6-2_Plan_of_Action_and_Milestones_Process_Guide .pdf.

25. MITRE ATT&CK. 2020. "ATT&CK Matrix for Enterprise." https://attack .mitre.org.

26. The Center for Internet Security (CIS) Controls V7.1 Implementation Groups are available for download at https://www.cisecurity.org/controls/cis-controls-implementation-groups.

CHAPTER 7

Third-Party Risk Management

This chapter covers Domain 7, "Third-Party Risk Management," of the HCISPP certification. After you read and study this chapter, you should be able to:

- Inventory third parties that handle sensitive information for the organization
- Design and conduct third-party risk assessments when required
- Respond to information privacy and security events caused by external suppliers
- Integrate privacy and security requirements in establishing third-party arrangements
- Understand the role in third-party risk mitigation activities
- Establish and enforce secure external information disclosures such as breach notifications

The healthcare organization cannot possibly provide all products and services required to deliver patient care and sustain business operations. Numerous third parties are essential to augmenting and supporting a healthcare organization's activities. For example, medical coding and billing are commonly accomplished by an external organization under contract to the healthcare organization. In the United States, third parties, or business associates, can be contracted to handle protected health information (PHI) on behalf of the healthcare organization. With the data flow for sensitive health information extending beyond the healthcare organization to third parties, new vulnerabilities are present. Add to this the growing mandate from regulators and payers alike to share more data, even among competitors. For a healthcare organization to have a firm information protection program in place, it must know its third parties and conduct periodic reviews to determine how well third parties handle PHI. This chapter illustrates why information risk management for third parties is important in the context of scenarios common to healthcare operations.

Managing risk when using third parties is subject to legal restrictions in countries with privacy and security regulations, but it also follows the leading privacy and security frameworks. According to the Generally Accepted Privacy Principles (GAPP), a healthcare organization "may outsource a part of its business process and, with it, some responsibility for privacy; however, the [healthcare] organization cannot outsource its ultimate responsibility for privacy for its business processes. Complexity increases when the entity that performs the outsourced service is in a different country and may be subject to different privacy laws or perhaps no privacy requirements at all."[1] In all circumstances, the organization that outsources a business process will need to ensure that it manages its privacy responsibilities appropriately. The healthcare organization (prior to sharing sensitive personal information with a third party) must share its expectations, policies, or other specific requirements for handling protected health information. In return, the third party must provide written agreement to adhere to these requirements.

If you have a friend or colleague who works in a healthcare organization in a department called Vendor Management, or something similar, ask him or her about third-party management. Many healthcare organizations must manage several hundred to perhaps a thousand third parties. In short, managing the organization's contractual agreements is daunting, and so are the information and privacy concerns with the relationships that include handling PHI. These concerns are within the realm of your responsibilities and are covered in this chapter.

Understand the Definition of Third Parties in the Healthcare Context

Healthcare organizations are typically large employers in a community. Doctors, nurses, administrative personnel, and maintenance workers alike live and raise families in the same community in which they work. Even with the sizeable workforce the healthcare organization employs, it probably requires many external partners to supply, provide, or support the organization with products and services. Within the United States, this business agreement is established through a business associate agreement (BAA), which contracts with a third party to handle PHI on behalf of the healthcare organization (the "Covered Entity," as defined in HIPAA). In other countries, the same type of arrangement should be outlined in contractual agreements with terms and conditions that outline the expectations for proper information use.

Knowing what a third-party organization is and the significance of the relationship is important for several reasons:

- Assessment of third parties is a preventive security control to help reduce risks.

- Data shows that 23 percent of data breaches happen because of a third-party action to some extent.[2]

- Healthcare organizations may suffer reputational and financial loss, even if the third party causes the data breach.

- Studies indicate that business associate data breaches tend to involve more affected individuals.[3]

In Chapter 1, you learned that the reason the term "third party" is used to define the relationship is because the first two parties are the patient and the healthcare organization. Third parties are organizations that provide services in support of the first two parties.

EXAM TIP Exam questions concerning third parties are most likely referring to services such as medical coding, billing, and transcription services as examples, not business agreements between covered entities such as hospitals and health insurers. Sometimes health insurers are referred to as third parties based on the role they play with healthcare delivery organizations and patients as a third party paying for services delivered.

Maintain a List of Third-Party Organizations

The process of managing the risk of third-party relationships begins with having an accurate and comprehensive inventory of the third-party organizations the healthcare organization uses. It is vital that you create and maintain an up-to-date inventory of third-party vendors, suppliers, and contractors with which your organization has business and clinical agreements. Due diligence requires initial review of the terms and conditions of any agreement as well as assessment of the privacy and security practices of the third party. The healthcare organization has an obligation to make sure the third-party organizations they work with have privacy and security controls in place. With that information, you can establish and maintain a database or inventory of the third parties that handle sensitive information.

Within the inventory, you should categorize the third parties according to the levels of risk they present for the healthcare organization. Depending on your organization, you may use categories such as criticality of the relationship, which would consider the size or value of the engagement; the volume and types of PHI the third party handles; and the cost of replacement of the vendor considering competition or proprietary capabilities. Criticality also depends on the location of the third party. The third party could work within the healthcare organization or at another location, including in a foreign country. Some of the impacts of criticality categorization are listed here:

- Frequency of risk assessment of the third-party relationship
- Types of documents required by the third party to demonstrate good security controls (such as SOC 2 reports, ISO certifications, or external penetration testing results)
- Transfer of risk through additional contractual terms and conditions such as increased limits of liability or proof of cybersecurity insurance by the third party

Your inventory of third-party risk management must also consider third parties that use other third parties. This is complicated and hard to determine sometimes, so maintaining the inventory can help. As part of the assessment process, you will ask the third party to disclose any of these downstream business relationships. HIPAA defines the downstream third parties as *subcontractors* to the business associates.[4] Obligations included in the BAA along with any additional terms and conditions in contracts should flow through to the subcontractors.

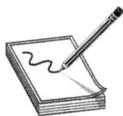

> **NOTE** Downstream subcontractors to business associates are also considered business associates and subject to HIPAA in the United States.

Third-Party Role and Relationship with the Organization

We covered third parties in healthcare in Chapter 1. In this chapter, we focus specifically on the risks the relationships present as well as your role in assessing and mitigating those risks. Third-party business and clinical relationships expand the capabilities of the healthcare organization and reduce costs—at least those are the objectives. When the objectives are not realized because of an information security event or a data breach, the benefits are quickly eroded. The HIPAA Privacy Rule identifies the reality that healthcare organizations cannot provide all healthcare services and actions autonomously. The Privacy Rule establishes provisions for healthcare organizations to share protected healthcare information with third parties, aka business associates, if there were assurances that the business associate would also protect the healthcare information. The Privacy Rule also stipulates the strict conditions for the information use. The business associate can use the information only in support of the healthcare organization, not for any other use, especially uses in support of the business associate's other activities, such as marketing.[5]

Third-party staff may or may not actually perform the work outside of the healthcare organization. Some third-party employees work right beside the employees of the organization, sometimes doing the same work. For example, because many healthcare organizations have implemented electronic health records (EHRs), the work required to connect any existing data systems, engineer the local area network, and prepare physical environments to house the equipment often require additional staffing. Healthcare organizations need to procure the services of contracted staff to help the current workforce accomplish EHR implementation in a timely, cost-effective manner. Some of these services are provided by consultants working onsite, and some are handled remotely by experts who can provision services or transfer data as required.

A sizeable number and/or variety of third parties can support the healthcare organization through a contract or financial agreement while not actually employed by the healthcare organization. Several types of third parties require more explanation, because their relationships with healthcare organizations create impactful scenarios. Within these scenarios, some interesting concerns arise that those who protect healthcare information must appreciate.

A third-party company in a European Union (EU) healthcare setting can provide services or products for a data controller. Under the EU Data Protection Directive (DPD), this is an allowable relationship as long as a Safe Harbor treaty is in place (for data flow outside of the European Union) or a model contract is in place with already approved clauses from the data authority.[6] In the United States, the relationship is focused on the healthcare sector and formalized using a BAA.

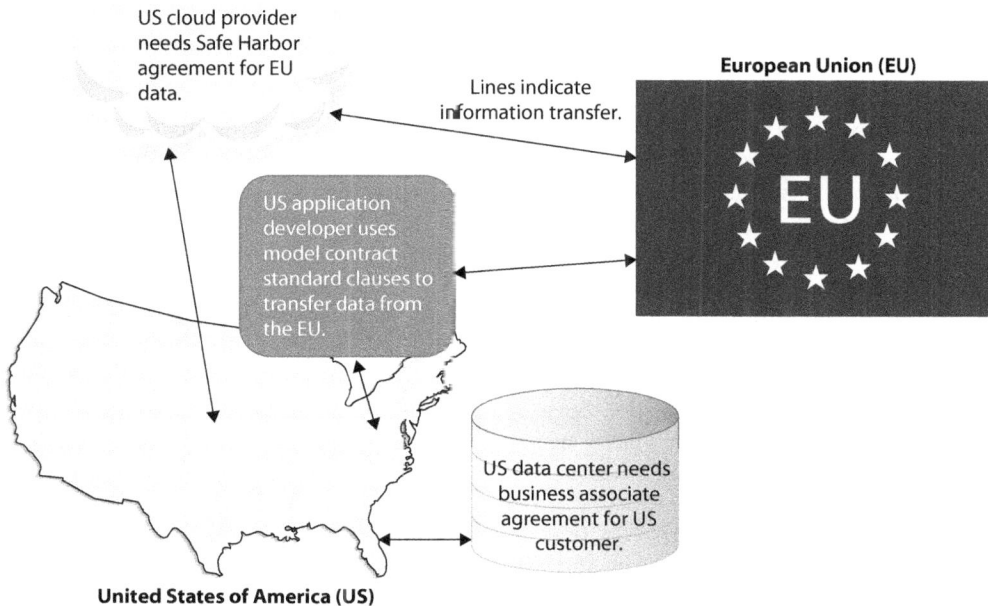

US cloud provider needs Safe Harbor agreement for EU data.

Lines indicate information transfer.

European Union (EU)

US application developer uses model contract standard clauses to transfer data from the EU.

US data center needs business associate agreement for US customer.

United States of America (US)

Figure 7-1   Third parties in healthcare providing international support

Our review of this information here is important, because the relationship between the third party and the healthcare organization may be unusual from the third party's perspective. If, for example, the third party provides similar services to other industries or handles nonpersonal information, the requirements of regulatory guidance such as HIPAA and the EU DPD can be challenging to meet. Figure 7-1 shows how transferring information within US borders is controlled via BAAs. Transferring data across US and EU borders requires another type of administrative agreement, previously covered by Safe Harbor and model contract standard clauses and now Privacy Shield provisions.

Outsourcing

Outsourcing services, functions, and products is widely used in most organizations. Internationally, forecasts say outsourcing of healthcare information technology will exceed $61 billion in revenue in the United States by 2023.[7] Outsourcing enables healthcare organizations to focus more on their core mission, to reduce costs, and to increase access to highly skilled staff. While the outsourced model extends beyond information technology, a majority of healthcare information privacy and security concerns with third parties resides in the outsourcing of information technology processes.

The model for outsourcing consists of completely transitioning responsibility for the performance of key objectives to a third party. That does not, however, mean the healthcare organization can transition responsibility for privacy and security concerns to the third party. In some cases, the outsourcing is so extensive that the only employee of the healthcare organization who has any contact with the third party is a management staff member. A single healthcare organization employee may be responsible for managing the information risk relative to sharing protected health information. In other cases, the third party is directed by a healthcare organization employee who has the relative qualifications to accomplish the same tasks, but the third party is in place to augment that capability. A great example is a chief information officer who manages the contract and the third-party personnel who provide the entire information technology function for the healthcare organizations. Another example is a patient administration director who oversees all the patient billing functions and accomplishes the process by using a third-party vendor.

The other variance in the total outsourced model is whether the vendor works onsite or offsite. Using the patient billing scenario, it's likely that the billers work from a location other than that of the healthcare organization. In fact, it is increasingly probable that they work from home. Another information security–related example is the managed security service provider (MSSP) that is hired to provide outsourced monitoring and management of security devices and systems, such as firewalls and intrusion prevention appliances. Revisiting the outsourced information technology example, help desk personnel and network administrators better serve the organization when they are onsite staff. This would facilitate attendance at information governance meetings, which would be appropriate from time to time. Some tasks require the information technology staff to be present rather than remotely accessing the local area network or end-user device.

Staff Augmentation

In addition to totally outsourced services, healthcare organizations can contract for support in a more tailored fashion. The reason staff augmentation is mentioned here is because in some cases, contract employees are viewed more as the healthcare organization's workforce members. They receive all the same training as staff, and access to information systems is administered along with employed staff. The covered entity (the healthcare organization) may be liable for employees' actions as well as those of any contract staff supplied by a business associate. Like the rest of the covered entity's workforce, the covered entity is responsible for the business associate's adherence with many of the security and privacy controls that are components of the covered entity's information security program. In other words, the contractor takes day-to-day direction from the healthcare organization rather than from his or her company.

Entry security badging, network access, use of a company-owned computer, and receipt of periodic security awareness communications are all examples of how a contract staff member uses the same security and privacy controls used by employees of the organization. Staff augmentation could comprise a consultant hired to help a healthcare organization implement a clinical application, possibly in the emergency department.

The contracted employee may accomplish tasks based on the direct supervision of the shift supervisor. Terrific examples of these types of arrangements are contracted nursing personnel and temporary employees.

An important distinction and implication between an outsourced third-party arrangement and a staff augmentation contract is in how a data breach may be viewed from a regulator's point of view. A data breach caused by a contract staff member, who is considered a workforce member under US law, may be a liability for the healthcare organization, not the third-party company. To illustrate this, consider another example: a nursing agency that supplies a nurse temporarily to a hospital may not by liable under HIPAA if that nurse causes a data breach; instead, the healthcare organization itself may be deemed liable for the breach. These complicated distinctions require legal review and interpretation. The intent of introducing them here is to emphasize the importance of managing (and assessing) the risk introduced by third parties and how third-party support is delivered.

EXAM TIP Pay attention to exam questions that introduce a distinction between onsite contractor support, such as staff augmentation, versus offshoring and services rendered at another location managed by a third party. Liability and responsibility can change depending on the workplace location.

Outside Legal Counsel

Many healthcare organizations employ lawyers with and without specific healthcare background or experience as part of their internal staff. But even when organizations have employed legal representation, they may choose to retain (on a contract) the services of legal counsel not employed by the organization; these are called outside legal counsel. These legal professionals and firms perform many different types of services, from reviewing contract language and the content of compliance programs (such as the information risk management program), to reviewing other administrative controls the healthcare organization wants to make sure it is properly managing. Outside legal counsel may also help the organization defend itself in malpractice claims, defend against data breach cases (in the United States), perform forensic investigations, and otherwise represent the healthcare organization in litigation. In the context of managing outside counsel as a third party to the healthcare organization, the same types of risk management review must be done for any outside counsel that handles PHI as for any other third party performing similar data use services. (And a good outside legal counsel will advise their customers to do as much!)

Third-Party Risk in the Cloud

Beginning with one of the emerging third-party relationships in healthcare, the cloud provider example enables you to examine several important considerations. Think about a cloud service provider that supports a healthcare customer as well as customers in retail, banking, or education. If the transfer of data includes collecting, storing, or transmitting protected health information, the cloud provider must meet HIPAA compliance standards in the United States. It must also be able to provide documentation of its independent audit report. This is in addition to any requirements the cloud provider may or may not have with its other customers.

The move to cloud services for healthcare organizations is happening internationally. There are good reasons for this, such as unprecedented pressures to reduce costs, improve health outcomes, and respond to regulatory changes, to name a few concerns. Cloud solutions promise to help healthcare organizations implement complex health information technology (IHIT) systems at a fraction of the cost. NIST SP 800-144, *Guidelines on Security and Privacy in Public Cloud Computing*, provides a terrific synopsis of the upsides and downsides of cloud computing from a privacy/security perspective.[8] Benefits include improved staff specialization and resource availability, while Internet-facing systems and multinet hosting arrangements introduce new vulnerabilities (for some customers).

Table 7-1 describes common examples of cloud computing service delivery models to help illustrate the variety of products and services available in *cloud computing*. Table 7-2 describes the formats that cloud computing can take. In sum, cloud computing offers convenience, rapid innovation, and lower total cost of ownership.

With an understanding of the types of cloud offerings, you can look at some scenarios in which healthcare organizations may face challenges using them. This means that information privacy and security issues arise when you consider a third party and a type of cloud to use, and as you evaluate that relationship over time.

Cloud Service Delivery Model	Description
Software as a Service (SaaS)	The service provider offers an application for use by the customer. EHRs that are offered over the Web or patient portals are good examples of SaaS applications. To access the service, the healthcare organization and the end user do nothing more than access the application via a web browser. The hardware and software resources required are the responsibility of the service provider.
Platform as a Service (PaaS)	This model enables a healthcare organization to use service provider resources to run a specific application on a shared software platform in the cloud. The service provider may offer access to a MySQL or Oracle database (shared resource) that is used by the healthcare organization's front-end application (not shared with others).
Infrastructure as a Service (IaaS)	When the healthcare organization requires more computing capability, it may opt for a cloud IaaS. On demand, the healthcare organization can acquire more bandwidth, storage, or even physical hardware access. The healthcare organization would not have to increase staff or physical space onsite to acquire the additional capabilities. And it can scale back down when the capabilities are no longer needed.

Table 7-1   Cloud Computing Models

Cloud Architecture (Format)	Characteristics
Private	A private cloud devotes resources to a single customer. It can be a form of intranet with a configuration of servers located behind the customer's firewall. However, a type of private cloud that follows the intent of cloud services is the virtual private cloud, where customer assets are logically provisioned or configured within the service provider's overall cloud offering. Thus, the customer gains all of the dedicated resource aspects with some of the cost reduction. The private cloud in any form is the most expensive type of cloud.
Public	Public clouds offer the most flexibility and scalability. They maximize cost effectiveness and can rapidly respond to customer demand. A public cloud supports multiple customers across any industry, geographic boundary, and type of data involved. For the most part, all resources, processing, and bandwidth are shared among all customers.
Community	A community cloud combines public and private clouds. The customers sharing resources are defined and segmented according to predefined criteria. A healthcare-specific example consists of multiple hospitals and provider organizations that collectively make up an integrated delivery network on a community cloud.
Hybrid	A hybrid cloud is actually an integration of some or all of the other cloud types. Instead of having only a community cloud or a private cloud, the healthcare organization may have a public cloud for the patient portal, a private cloud for the EHR, and a community cloud for a health information exchange with its affiliated providers and third parties.

Table 7-2   Cloud Computing Formats

TIP   Cloud providers and data centers (private clouds) are extremely important third parties in healthcare. With this understanding, you can begin to apply the same principles to cloud applications such as an EHR, billing operations, or health information exchanges.

Although it's true that cloud providers introduce levels of risk to healthcare organizations in terms of information privacy and security, as described in Chapter 5, the risk can be worth it because cloud computing does offer measurable benefits. Most healthcare organizations do not have or desire to have in house the capabilities that cloud providers can quickly provide (such as large storage facilities, processing power, resource provisioning, and network redundancy). Although healthcare organizations need to understand the cloud computing process to assess risks, many cloud providers do not fully understand the unique privacy and security pressures for healthcare. This lack of understanding can be a source of information risk. The healthcare organization needs to ensure the cloud provider can meet applicable regulatory standards. If it cannot, the organization must continue to evaluate cloud providers until it finds one that can comply and deliver all the benefits and standards required.

> **CAUTION** Today in the United States, cloud providers are specifically subject to HIPAA as BAs. In the past, cloud providers often did not enter into BAAs. Their position was that, as cloud providers, they did not access the data and therefore were not subject to HIPAA. The recent passage of the Omnibus HIPAA Final Rule in 2013 clarified the definition of business associate with specific regard to naming cloud providers and data centers as business associates, whether the cloud provider agrees to sign a BAA or not.

In sum, healthcare organizations must carefully consider the issues and evaluate potential cloud solutions before leaping into binding agreements. Healthcare organizations that do not heed this advice will encounter problems when regulators remind them that compliance cannot be outsourced to a third party—in this case, to the cloud. What your cloud provider does or does not do will be your responsibility in terms of privacy and security of sensitive information.

Third-Party Risk in Data Disposition

In the information management lifecycle, destroying or disposing of data is the final step. It is also one of the most vulnerable processes.[9] When data is no longer needed, it often receives less protection because the organization tends to relax control. In many cases, the data disposition, destruction, or disposal process is conducted by an outsourced company that specializes in this function. Some examples include paper shredding, electronic media erasure, and hardware recycling.

Whether the data is in a paper or an electronic format, a healthcare organization needs to ensure that the PHI it marks for disposition is safeguarded all the way through the final steps of making it unreadable and indecipherable. Otherwise, theft and unauthorized disclosure can occur as PHI is taken from loading docks, where medical records await pickup from the data disposition company, for example. As many personal computers are donated to community organizations and schools, a data disposition company may have authority to make the donation, but any sensitive information must be completely removed from the hard drives. A healthcare organization must conduct third-party risk assessment and auditing oversight to make sure its sensitive data is not disclosed under these types of scenarios. A certification of destruction from the third party would be required when data is disposed.

Third-Party Risk in Nonmedical Devices

A special category of third party has evolved as printers, faxes, and scanners have become commonplace in healthcare environments. If an organization is not careful, these devices can be sources of a data breach. Because these devices copy, e-mail, and transmit data by changing paper documents into electronic images, they often store data on local storage media. A third-party company contracted to maintain and service these devices may not know the nature of the data the hard drives contain. But if it is PHI, that data may leave the healthcare organization as the devices move to be serviced or replaced. Similar to the data disposition companies, nonmedical device repair and supply companies must be under contractual obligation to protect the healthcare information that may be present on these devices. This means proper destruction, disposal, and reuse provisions must be in place. It also means the healthcare organization has risk management responsibilities with respect to the third party that manages nonmedical devices that includes auditing compliance with the use of PHI.

Health Information Use: Processing, Storage, Transmission

Your role includes helping to establish and monitor the technology and procedures used for processing, storage, and transmission of any PHI that a third party may handle for your organization. In some cases, the responsibility will entail designing interconnections and implementing new security controls. In other scenarios, you may need to review and evaluate already existing safeguards implemented by the third party.

In all cases, the third-party entity will receive terms and conditions in contracts or legally binding documents. In addition to ensuring that your organization and third parties adhere to all applicable regulatory requirements, you will be responsible for informing and enforcing the requirements to the organization as well as the third party. For example, the authorization for access to data and systems must be limited based on your organization's requirements.

CAUTION The guiding principle for a third-party arrangement to handle PHI for your organization (or if you work in an organization that handles PHI for a healthcare organization) is that the safeguards that the healthcare organization must satisfy are extended through contract and law to the third party.

To emphasize the important concepts here with a practical example, we'll add another common third-party relationship. Using HIPAA as a regulatory guide, a covered entity is required to enter into a BAA with a cloud service provider. It does not matter what type of service model the covered entity uses, because the principles remain the same. The cloud service provider is a business associate and is subject to HIPAA regulations, just like the covered entity.[10]

Additional contractual obligations can be made where the cloud service provider must ensure services in a service level agreement, often supplemental to BAA terms and conditions, to include the following:[11]

- Availability of data and systems.

- Business resiliency and support of contingency operations.

- Performance of backup sufficient to restore and recover successfully from disasters.

- Terms for data disposal or return to customer after the agreement ends or when the data is no longer needed. In HIPAA and GDPR, for example, the requirement for adequate information protection by the third party extends beyond the contract life if the third party has to maintain the data for a valid reason.

- Expectations for third-party security responsibilities.
- Limited use and authorized disclosure provisions as well as retention guidelines.

If you are working for the covered entity, the considerations outlined here are expected to be part of your ongoing risk assessments and risk management program. In international healthcare organizations, the practice of assessing risk and outlining the expectations of the third party to adhere to at least the same regulatory and organizational policies you, as the customer, does is nonetheless imperative.

International Regulations for Data Transfer to Third Parties

Related to international trade implications, the variations in regulatory standards pose concern for healthcare organizations transferring information to third parties internationally. US healthcare organizations are subject to HIPAA even if PHI is stored by a third party (including cloud providers) in another country that may not have the same data geographic restrictions, auditing, and breach notification requirements. According to the EU DPD, and later in GDPR, international concerns for auditing and monitoring are similar, in that data controllers must request the logging of processing operations performed by the provider.

In the United States, HIPAA codifies the requirements a bit more in that the healthcare organization must ensure that third parties adhere to security controls for authentication, error reporting, breach notification, and accounting of disclosures. The healthcare organization must ensure that any international third party follows applicable regulations if a breach of data occurs. The HIPAA requirement for patient notification in certain circumstances, for example, is not relaxed simply because a healthcare organization stores data outside of HIPAA jurisdiction.

CAUTION It bears emphasis that a significant obstacle to using offshore third parties, or companies that provide products and services outside of the host country, is that jurisdictional differences may make enforcement of law and contractual obligations difficult.

Canadian and EU healthcare organizations have additional privacy concerns even beyond the need for Safe Harbor or model contract language. These governments and their domestic healthcare organizations in particular have expressed concern with cloud providers that collect, store, and transfer information to and from the United States. The US Patriot Act makes it undesirable—and even illegal—for Canadian and EU healthcare organizations to use US-based cloud service providers, because US law allows authorities to look at their PHI in certain circumstances. The 2001 US Patriot Act was fortified by the 2018 Clarifying Lawful Overseas Use of Data (CLOUD) Act. With respect to the current GDPR, EU citizens' data stored in US cloud provider computers is subject to US government access on demand.[12] That said, remember that under all leading privacy and security regulations, access to PHI has provisions for legal authorities to access with additional patient consent. For instance, the United Kingdom's Regulatory of Investigatory Powers Act, much like the US Patriot Act, mandates similar levels of government access.[13]

Unauthorized Disclosure of Data Transferred to Third Parties

This may seem obvious, but third parties have a significant impact on healthcare organizations because they cause a high percentage of data loss and data breach. Even with robust risk management from the healthcare organization, unauthorized disclose still happens. With proper contracts and legal agreements in place, financial liability can be properly applied to the third party. But from a reputational perspective, the healthcare organization is still affected negatively. For instance, a patient billing company receives files and has access to databases of healthcare information. If the third-party offices are burglarized and computer equipment is stolen, the third party may have to pay the fines and penalties for a breach. But patient notification will be done by the healthcare organization. Patients will probably not make the distinction between responsible parties.

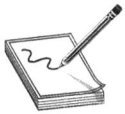

NOTE A database of third-party unauthorized disclosures in the United States is publicly available at www.privacyrights.org. If nothing else, examining the database presents a clear picture of the frequency and magnitude of the impact that third-party unauthorized disclosure has on healthcare organizations.

Apply Management Standards and Practices for Engaging Third Parties

NIST refers to the management of third-party risk as "Cyber Supply Chain Risk Management" (C-SCRM).[14] The process is similar to overall risk management lifecycles that include identifying, assessing, and mitigating information risks. In this case, risk management is tailored to address risks incurred by outsourcing and contractual relationships that support the healthcare organization. A simple way to start this discussion is to remember that building security controls into the relationships at all phases of the third-party arrangement or supply chain lifecycle is much better than trying to address issues after the contract or agreement is in place. Some general phases in the lifecycle include the following, which are depicted in Figure 7-2:

1. **Planning** Understand the business requirements and help design the data use specifications with any information transfer needs.

2. **Selection** Perform due diligence initial risk assessment activities during evaluation of third parties.

   - Make sure the third party has an information protection program aligned with privacy and security regulations (HIPAA, EU DPD, ISO, PCI, and so on).
   - Make the effort to review any objective assessments by qualified auditors (SOC2 HITRUST, ISO 27001 and so on).
   - Check reference accounts to understand past performance for the third party.
   - Visit the third party's facilities.

Figure 7-2
General phases
in third-party risk
management
lifecycle

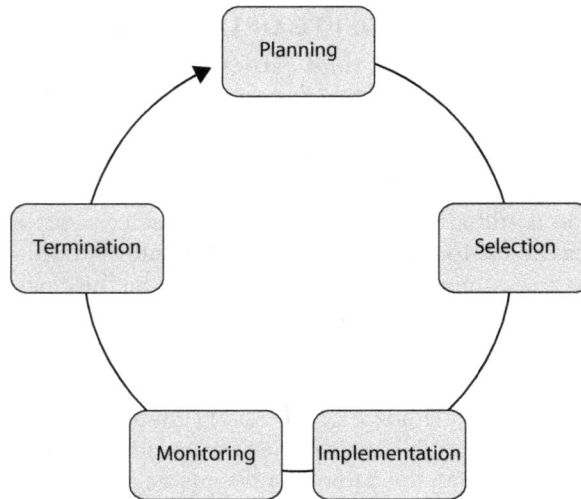

3. **Implementation**   Select connection controls or a trust model for the interconnection, including secure data transfer technical controls such as encryption plus identity and authentication management.

4. **Monitoring**   Assess compliance with the contract terms that will consist of periodic risk assessments, reviews of service level agreements, and performance satisfaction ratings. As part of the contract, a right to review and audit should be present.

5. **Termination**   As third-party relationships end, security and privacy concerns must be included in the decommissioning of systems and disposition of any data that the third party no longer has authorization to access or store.

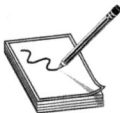

NOTE   During the process of considering alternatives and making a choice between third parties in US healthcare organizations, you can use language developed from the US Department of Health and Human Services (HHS) to determine each third party's ability to comply with a BAA. A template, available at https://www.hhs.gov/hipaa/for-professionals/covered-entities/sample-business-associate-agreement-provisions/index.html, can be used or it can be customized for your organization (provided the resultant document is compliant with minimum HHS requirements). Once a third party is selected, the document is signed by both parties.

Relationship Management

In addition to risk management frameworks that help healthcare organizations oversee third parties that handle PHI, several other types of documents and agreements are necessary. These help the healthcare organization communicate requirements, evaluate performance, and hold all parties accountable for compliance. Without the use of one or more of these administrative controls, healthcare organizations have little reason to expect a third party will apply appropriate safeguards or be responsive enough, particularly if a healthcare organization's expectations exceed those of the third party's customers from other industries. We outlined some examples of the major types of relationship management tools in Chapter 3, including SLAs, contracts, and interconnection security agreements.

We have introduced and explained several leading risk management frameworks that healthcare organizations can use to evaluate and manage internal risk. These same tools can be used to evaluate and manage third-party vendors. The same risk assessment and remediation work should be done for each external vendor with respect to their processes, policies, and controls in place to protect your information. We will not repeat the information here concerning the leading risk management tools such as the NIST RMF, HITRUST CSF, or the ISO 27000 family of standards, but keep in mind that these tools can all be applied to third parties that handle PHI for your organization.

One leading risk management framework that is presented as a vendor risk-specific framework is the Office of the Comptroller of the Currency (OCC) in the US Department of the Treasury.[15,16] We mention this because the framework is used by many leading assessment organizations internationally, such as the Santa Fe Group's Shared Assessments. Shared Assessments was established in 2005 and is present in more than 115 countries worldwide (mostly in the financial industry).[17] It specializes in assessing third-party vendors that handle sensitive information. You can see some similarities in its lifecycle risk management model compared to those already discussed. A couple of differences are in contract negotiations (SLAs, for example) and in the termination phases. The OCC lifecycle (see Figure 7-3) also integrates some overarching concepts that fit into the other risk management frameworks we have covered. Here are some examples:

- **Oversight and accountability** Of course, someone from the healthcare organization must be responsible for the contract. They should be accountable for results and be integrated into the information governance structure of the healthcare organization.

- **Documentation and reporting** As part of the information governance structure, the accountable person must be able to communicate relevant details, events, and performance measurements. All of this must be documented and the documents retained.

- **Independent reviews** In addition to periodic assessments and audits, both onsite and remotely through vendor self-assessment, an objective independent assessment is a best-practice idea as well. Remember that a solid risk management component is to access and review all objective audits of the third party that they already maintain. For example, give credit for FISMA ratings, ISO certifications, SOC 2 assessments, and HITRUST audit results.

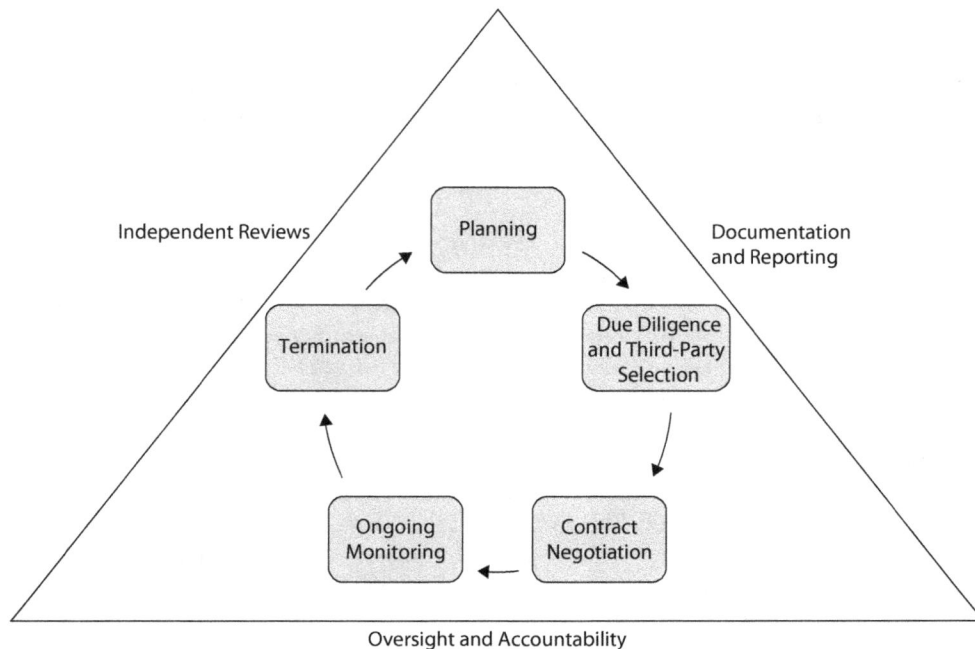

Figure 7-3 OCC risk management lifecycle

Determine When a Third-Party Assessment Is Required

Each organization will need to determine when and how it wants to assess its third parties. Of course, some regulatory pressures may influence the frequency. We have established that an initial assessment is essential. After that, most third-party relationship frameworks indicate that an annual frequency for review is sound practice. In any event, organizational standards for vendor management will set the expectations, which will factor criticality of the service, sensitivity of the data, or level of risk to the healthcare organization because of the third-party relationship. The conduct of the assessment can vary as well. The organization may choose to allow a self-assessment reported to the healthcare organization via a questionnaire or an interview through a remote assessment, or the healthcare organization may insist on an onsite audit. In all cases, updating and provisioning of a current copy of any information risk–related assessment documents such as the SOC 2, ISO 27001, or an external firm's penetration test reports would also be necessary.

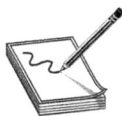

NOTE As of September 2013, HIPAA, through an amendment with the Omnibus Final Rule, has formalized and clarified the responsibility of healthcare organizations to conduct security reviews of their third-party subcontractors and vendors that handle protected health information.

Organizational Standards

The proper approach for managing third-party information risk is to start with an enterprise-inclusive perspective. This means that although information protection experts may lead or design the processes, it takes many stakeholders from within the organization to establish a strong third-party information risk program. Personnel from clinical and business functions, along with corporate departments such as finance and procurement, must join together to create a program that builds in risk management rather than bolting it on after a third party has been selected (or worse, after the contract is signed). Add to this multidisciplinary team legal and vendor management functions, and you can meet the objectives of good risk management in this area. This team, which can include people from areas not specifically mentioned and based on specific third-party relationships, will contribute to development of the request for proposals, contract terms and conditions, and business and clinical objectives for the relationship.

Here are some specific components of the organizational standards:

- *Be practical.* Overly complicated processes may be seen as an impediment, and some stakeholders may be motivated to circumvent the process or parts of it.

- *Be consistent.* Exceptions should not become the rule. If there is a perception of favoritism or excessive waivers for certain business or clinical areas, this may become another justification for working around the standards.

- *Streamline use of third parties.* Many organizations have large portfolios of vendors. Where one vendor can satisfy multiple stakeholders' requirements, the costs of risk assessments and oversight can be reduced. Overall risk can be reduced where high performing vendors are used for multiple requirements too.

- *Set good standards.* Choose those standards that are aligned with industry frameworks such as the NIST Cybersecurity Framework that includes supply chain management and ISO 27001 third-party and processor controls. This helps the organization meet or exceed regulatory requirements too.

- *Follow the third-party risk management lifecycle.* Remember that the process begins with planning, goes through termination, and begins again with a replacement solution. Information protection has a role in every phase of the lifecycle.

This approach describes how an organization can establish processes that align to internal policies. However, the emphasis is not on fitting a third-party relationship selection into an information protection constraint. It is the opposite. By involving multiple stakeholders in the organization and conducting due diligence, understanding the risks incurred, performing ongoing monitoring, and being ready for unintended incidents, the business and clinical stakeholders can obtain the products and services they need. At the same time, the risk to the healthcare organization can be reduced to a tolerable level.

Triggers of a Third-Party Assessment

Throughout this chapter, we covered several routine times when a third-party assessment would be required or beneficial. In addition to regularly scheduled events initially and annually, sometimes an out-of-cycle assessment may be needed. Keeping in mind considerations for the costs of additional assessments, criticality of the third party, and the sensitivity of the information that is exchanged, the following are some events that can trigger a third-party assessment:

- Failure to perform to the contract or SLA
- A data breach relative to another organization
- New personnel in key positions
- Information outage and unsatisfactory disaster recovery
- Leadership inquiry or interest item
- Possible recompete for a new provider

These triggers are facilitated by ensuring that a right to audit is included in contractual terms and conditions. The BAA should include this condition for US healthcare organizations.

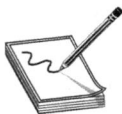

NOTE The usefulness of a right to audit for US healthcare organizations is demonstrated by a provision in the HIPAA Omnibus Rule, which authorizes the HHS to perform audits on business associates.

Support Third-Party Assessments and Audits

A primary role of a healthcare information privacy and security professional is to help organize and conduct the required assessments and audits of third parties. The overall consideration for a third-party audit will be whether the activity will be conducted. Based on factors such as how much risk the third party introduces or how familiar the third party is to the organization, one of the following assessment approaches may be useful:

- **Self-assessment** The vendor responds to a survey provided by the healthcare organization.
- **Onsite** The healthcare organization's employee observes and interviews the vendor onsite.
- **Remote** With or without a self-assessment, the third-party vendor is reviewed using relevant third-party material such as past performance attestations, marketing material, any legal proceedings against the third party, and other considerations.
- **Hybrid** This uses a combination of onsite and offsite approaches.

These approaches can be useful for the initial assessment in the planning or selection phase and in the annual or periodic assessment process. If a third-party vendor triggers an out-of-cycle assessment because of a potential data loss incident, a different approach from these assessments can certainly be chosen. That said, because the SLA or contract is a risk transference vehicle, it can help determine the appropriate type of assessment approach.

The next step may be your biggest obstacle in participating in the third-party risk assessment process. Even though the third party is not part of the healthcare organization, no special considerations apply to reduce standards that apply internally to the organization. The third party must have all the controls in place that are required by contract and by law. For instance, if there are information security and privacy training requirements, it is not acceptable to excuse the vendor from them. Sometimes healthcare organizations are tempted to give credit to the vendor for training provided by the healthcare organization. Unfortunately, under most circumstances, that does not meet requirements.

Remember, for example, that a component of the required training deals with the third-party organization's policies and procedures, not those of the healthcare organization. Another example is not having access to the third party's facilities. If within the contractor SLA the negotiated terms and conditions permit access by the healthcare organization to visit the third party's onsite premises and conduct an inspection, that should be part of the audit. Relaxing that standard because of reluctance of the third party to support the inspection adds undue risk to the healthcare organization.

When faced with third-party vendors that do not comply with assessment and audit requirements, your role in the organization will be to document findings and communicate them to more senior leadership. This is an incredibly important role. Properly organizing these types of assessments (using the correct approach, using valid assessment tools, following contracts, and communicating all findings) is a linchpin to reducing the risk of third-party data breaches. Once again, you know that the results of several industry surveys demonstrate that third parties commonly cause data breaches. The underlying causes tend to be the lack of oversight we have just described and desire to avoid.

Information Asset Protection Controls

During the risk assessment process, the effort will be to understand the security and privacy controls the third party uses. This can come from assessment documents or audits that detail the frameworks or control sets. You may also choose to use a survey to ask about the frameworks or to obtain answers about specific controls. Regardless of your chosen approach, particularly the survey, you should be aware that vendors are asked to fill out a lot of questionnaires. If you use a standard questionnaire, the vendor may have already completed it for another customer.

Here are some valid and popular risk assessment tools:

- **Center for Internet Security (CIS) Critical Security Controls** This tool is effective because it seeks information from the third party based on security controls that mitigate the most common or prevalent attacks. The selection of the Top 20 controls is based on historical data and firsthand knowledge of security experts concerning what security controls reduce the most risk. The Critical Security Controls are drawn from the leading industry resources, including the NIST Cybersecurity Framework, NIST SP 800-53, ISO 27000 series, and regulations such as PCI-DSS, HIPAA, and FISMA.

- **Consensus Assessments Initiative Questionnaire (CAIQ)**   The Cloud Security Alliance (CSA) developed the CAIQ to assess the information protection controls specific to cloud service providers and third parties that host data centers.

- **ISO 27001 Questionnaire**   A precursor to ISO 27001 certification, organizations may have completed the questionnaire based on the ISO 27001 body of controls, yet did not seek certification. This completed questionnaire would be sufficient to document a robust information protection program provided the responses were satisfactory.

- **NIST SP 800-171 Rev. 2**   This publication is applicable because NIST SP 800-171 Rev. 2, *Protecting Controlled Unclassified Information in Nonfederal Systems and Organizations*, is a standard for government agencies to use a commercial third-party entity as a supplier of information services. Used with NIST SP 800-171A, *Assessing Security Requirements for Controlled Unclassified Information*, the guidance extends requirements such as NIST SP 800-53 Rev. 4, *Security Controls*, to nongovernmental agencies in a manner that translates to the commercial sector while maintaining confidentiality, integrity, and availability to sufficient standards for the government agency.

- **Standardized Information Gathering (SIG) Questionnaire**   An industry consortium of accounting firms, corporations, and information technology firms make up the Shared Assessments group, which authored the SIG questionnaire to provide a standardized, repeatable, and reusable assessment document that appraises 18 different risk domains.

- **Payment Card Industry Data Security Standards (PCI DSS) Questionnaire**   In organizations that handle credit cards or are considering establishing a third-party relationship for such services, the PCI DSS questionnaire can help gather data about security controls relevant to the PCI standards.

Healthcare information is a valuable commodity. With the reliance on third parties to handle PHI on behalf of the healthcare organization and the fact that so many data breaches result from third-party mishaps, their proper assessment is vital. The use of one or more assessment tools may make it a little easier for the third party to comply. However, in reality, the industry-tested and validated questionnaire can assist you with the daunting task of initial assessment, ongoing monitoring, and periodic reassessment, because it is probably ready when you need it.

Compliance with Information Asset Protection Controls

The healthcare organization needs to assess whether or not the third party is adhering to information asset controls. As we have described earlier, the healthcare organization may choose to use a questionnaire to survey the third party to assess compliance. Questionnaires have a drawback, however, in that they may lack objectivity because third parties themselves are filling them out. Because the healthcare organization must conduct due diligence to assess compliance with information protection, a questionnaire may be insufficient based on the criticality of the vendor, the sensitivity of the information, and the value of the engagement.

A complementary approach is to use external audits or results of assessments of the third party. These results can increase confidence in the information protection programs of the third parties. Here are some examples of external assessments and audits you may look for and accept in addition to or in place of a questionnaire:

- **Service Organization Controls (SOC) report**   This series of assessments designed by the American Institute of Certified Public Accountants (AICPA) is meant to demonstrate the effectiveness of security controls. A SOC 2 is most likely the type of SOC report you will see, because it provides a view of security control effectiveness over a period of time. It can be used to address privacy, security, availability, processing integrity, and confidentiality individually or in combinations that can include all components. There are other versions of SOC—SOC 1 and SOC 3. The SOC 1 involves primarily financial controls and evaluates control functionality at a particular point in time. The SOC 3 is the same assessment as the SOC 2 with the same components, but the report is suited for a general audience.

- **ISO certification**   Some companies want to demonstrate trustworthiness to signal that their commitment to information protection exceeds the satisfaction of the ISO 27001 assessment tool mentioned earlier. These organizations seek certification by external certification bodies under the ISO information security certification process.

- **Health Information Trust Alliance (HITRUST)**   Within US healthcare organizations, including business associates, HITRUST Common Security Framework (CSF) certification has grown in recognition and credibility. The CSF is aligned with the top information security frameworks and standards created by NIST, ISO, and HIPAA. HITRUST also incorporates relevant Centers for Medicaid and Medicare Services (CMS), PCI DSS, and several US state information security and privacy laws, for example. As more healthcare organizations use and require the CSF certification, the tool is useful as a benchmark in the industry. The CSF can be used to self-assess, and through certification, an external assessment can be made by a qualified assessor.

Some organizations maintain a need to conduct a self-designed questionnaire in light of the examples of standard tools. There are reasonable concerns with using the tools or accepting completed questionnaires that appear to be generic responses. In such cases, a combination of self-created questionnaires and acceptance of precompleted assessments from external entities can be an acceptable compromise. The key consideration is that the healthcare organization achieves the objective of gaining confidence that the third party is capable of compliance with information protection requirements.

Communication of Results

During the risk assessment process, you may find issues. There are two distinct lines of communication you will use to communicate these results. First, the stakeholders in the activity will need to be informed of security control findings, lack of assessment material, or unacceptable contractual language. These gaps may indicate increased risks, and in some cases, the findings may prevent or prohibit the organization from entering into a third-party relationship with the supplier or vendor. That may be unpopular, but it's better to know early in the planning phase before selection.

The other communication requirement is with the third party itself. As you uncover issues, it is best to share concerns with the third party. The intention is to gain clarity if there are questions and to determine if remediation is possible to facilitate selection of the third party for contracted services. It is frustrating when a third party disagrees with your findings. However, if you base your requirements on industry validated assessment tools such as those described in this chapter, you can be confident in your assessments. That resolve leads us to the topic of remediation efforts in which you, as an HCISPP, will participate.

Participate in Third-Party Remediation Efforts

At times, you may be required to participate in third-party remediation efforts, such as remediation efforts that result from the risk assessment process. When you find issues and communicate them with the third party, the remediation process begins, and you will be required to track the items to completion. The third party may need assistance in designing proper controls or finding solutions to close controls gaps. As an HCISPP, you may be able to provide recommendations based on your subject matter expertise; there may be debate, however, as to whether the recommendations equate to free consulting services. The remediation of findings ultimately benefits your organization, in that a third-party relationship is established with sufficient information protection controls in place. As we have mentioned, this reduces risk and lowers potential for negative financial, operational, reputational, and clinical impacts.

Another opportunity for third-party remediation activities is after a cybersecurity event or a data breach occurs. These events are characterized by a higher sense of urgency and priority. Your role in these events will be aligned with contractual and legal obligations. Starting with a third party's requirement to notify your organization of a breach, remediation begins immediately. Coordination to contain the crisis and notification of your patient population should be part of the process. Assuming that the event prompts an out-of-cycle risk assessment to determine root cause and discover any security control ineffectiveness, your role will begin to resemble the routine remediation procedures we described in the preceding paragraph. Tracking and closing security control findings will be required. However, in contrast with routine risk assessment and control remediation, with remediation efforts post breach or after a cyber-attack, the pressures to remediate the issue to the satisfaction of your organization and external regulatory agencies add pressure, scrutiny, and importance.

In some cases, an official remediation order from the government, legal authorities, or regulators will dictate the actions and pace of change the third party must satisfy. Your role may be to participate in assuring that your organization is informed of progress. Of course, that is assuming that after a breach or cyber-attack, your organization did not cancel the contract and end the relationship with the third party. In that case, you may be called upon to assess and recommend continuing the relationship or ending it through the use of a contract termination clause (that you may have helped negotiate, by the way).

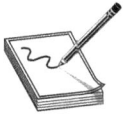

> **NOTE** Documentation is a point of emphasis. As the relationship with a third-party supplier is a contractual agreement, proper documentation and recordkeeping of risk assessments, communications between the organizations to present findings, and remediation efforts are part of what is needed to support additional negotiations, resolve disputes, and make decisions for business and clinical stakeholders.

Respond to Notifications of Security/Privacy Events

For incidents caused by third parties, the HCISPP will be expected to lead or participate in the healthcare organization's response, communication, and remediation activities. A large percentage of incidents are caused by improper handling of PHI by a third party. According to the Ponemon Institute (a privacy and information management research firm), in its 2015 "Fifth Annual Benchmark Study on Privacy and Security of Healthcare Data," third-party organizations accounted for 39 percent of all breach cases.[18] These remain the most costly form of data breaches because of additional investigation and consulting fees. The prevalence of third parties causing data breaches has been noted around the globe. Keep in mind that the healthcare organization's incident response team may activate and oversee the overall incident investigation. Based on contractual obligations and legal requirements, the third party will have significant responsibility and should bear the costs of the investigation (and notifications, if required). Figure 7-4 depicts the coordination with third parties that the incident response team may need to oversee.

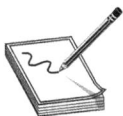

> **NOTE** The exact numbers of data breaches and information security incidents vary between years of measurement, data sources, and survey respondents. The key point is that third parties account for approximately 25 to 40 percent of information protection issues that impact the healthcare organization.

Internal Processes for Incident Response

If the third party suspects a data incident is underway that has originated in its organization, as it complies with contractual obligations and legal requirements, it must ensure that initial reports are sent to the healthcare organization in the prescribed timeframes. These reports may incite the healthcare organization to activate its incident response team. Additional responsibilities the healthcare information security and privacy professional can expect to perform are as follows:

- Coordinating with the third party during the investigation
- Corroborating any findings of the third party against the healthcare organization's environment

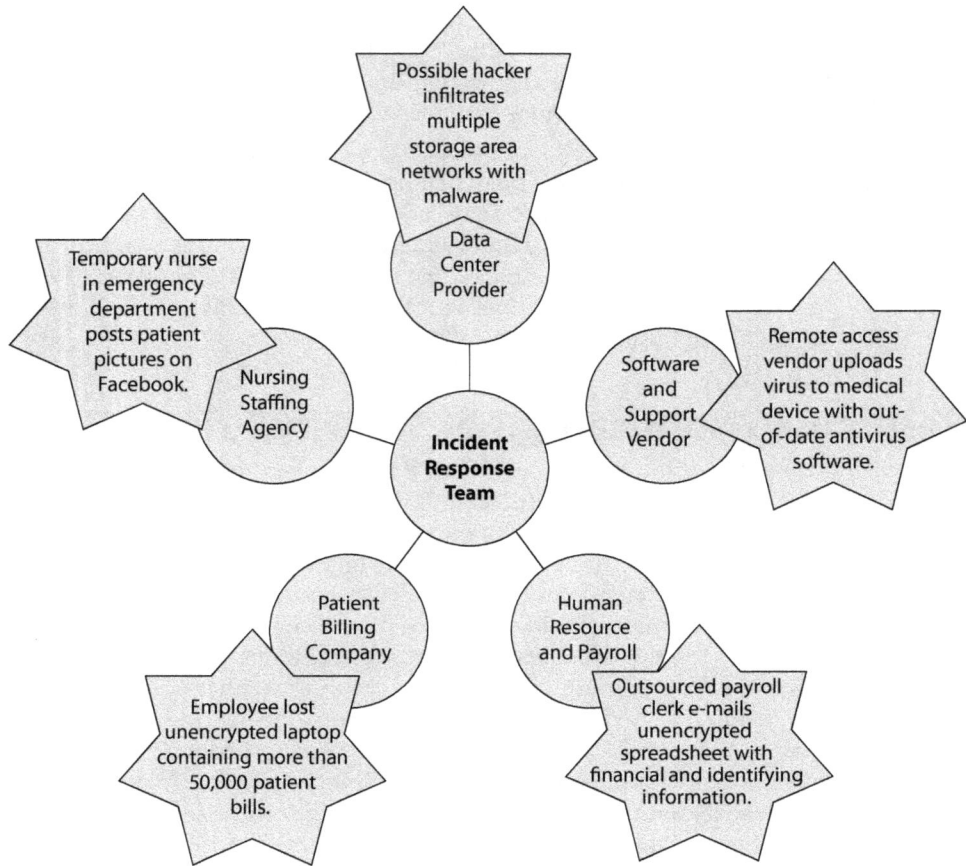

Figure 7-4 Incident response team and third parties

- Identifying, in the case of malware, infiltration of the healthcare organization, which may also be evident as attackers target multiple hosts
- Escalating the incident within internal reporting processes (senior leadership, vendor management, and so on)
- Assisting the third party with all communications to be made in community updates and notification activities to the media, regulators, and affected individuals
- Leading the notification responsibilities or delegating the actions to the third party
- Ensuring that third-party actions adhere to contractual obligations and legal requirements
- Making sure notifications are made in the prescribed manner
- Minimizing disruptions in services

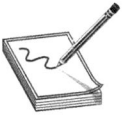

NOTE During incident investigations and data breach notification timeframes, healthcare organizations should implement controls to manage the flow of information through their spokesperson. Normally, one central point of contact is established for any external requests for information. All other employees, including members of the incident response team, are highly discouraged from providing comments to the media or details about the incident to patients. The guidance is to refer these requests to the central point of contact. When there is a toll-free number for patients to call, that number is provided. Having these central contact points readily available (on a web site or broadcast in the media) is not only required, but it is helpful in controlling rumors; it also helps to prevent the spread of incorrect information and helps prevent the investigation from being compromised.

As with an incident that originates inside the healthcare organization, the third party will progress to the containment, eradication, and recovery phases. The healthcare organization will closely monitor the progress. Whether the incident response team is activated or a third party determines whether the evidence indicates a data breach, communication with the healthcare organization must continue. Other pertinent responsibilities in monitoring the third-party progress may include the following:

- Assisting with digital forensics to preserve evidence
- Continuing to coordinate any media press releases and notices to regulators and affected individuals once the incident is determined to be a data breach
- Vulnerability scanning to ensure proper eradication and recovery if there are interconnections of systems between the third party and the healthcare organization
- Documenting costs to the healthcare organization as they apply to any downtime, assisting in managing the third-party activities, and checking performance against service level agreements

When the incident occurs, the third party should follow a process that is similar to that of the healthcare organization. Lessons learned and additional training on previous events should be incorporated into the organization's risk assessments and information security programs. Doing this may help to prevent the next problem and reduce incidents by third-party organizations.

Following are some responsibilities to consider in the post-incident phase:

- Including previous incidents in the next risk assessment done by the healthcare organization
- Updating any contractual documents and service level agreements
- Providing any financial data relative to investigation, oversight, and downtime to internal management for possible reimbursement from the third party
- Incorporating third-party incidents into healthcare organization training and awareness as well as incident response team training scenarios

As much as possible, an incident response plan must integrate procedures that handle events originating at a third-party supplier with a holistic perspective. Consider the third party as an extension of your organization. The incident response plan that integrates internal stakeholders inside of business continuity plans, disaster recovery, or organizational crisis management teams is not just for internal events. It is common to activate internal response teams to manage the organization through an event that happens to a third-party supplier.

Relationship Between Organization and Third-Party Incident Response

There is an old proverb that we can paraphrase: "The best time to plant a tree is 20 years ago. The second-best time is today." Drawing from the proverb, the relationship between the organization and third-party incident response must be established and tested before the need for the incident response occurs. A plan is needed that assigns clear roles and responsibilities for key personnel who are leading the incident response for each organization. The plan should be part of the overall negotiation and review before a contract is signed. If that did not happen in your organization when the third-party contract was signed, plant the "tree" today: Develop the plan and a schedule to test the plan with your current critical third-party suppliers before you need to respond to an incident. It is chaotic and ineffective to develop procedures and assign roles and responsibilities during a cyber event or data breach.

Make sure that you actually review the current plans for incident response that the third party uses. You need to understand who is responsible for certain actions and when those actions may occur. For example, a security manager may be the responsible party to notify you when the third party suspects a potential or actual data breach. A senior manager in the third-party organization may have the role of escalating communications to regulators or other external entities, including the public media. You should ensure that your and the third-party's plans align with regard to the timing of incident responses and input from your organization. Imagine a third party announcing a data breach to the local news station before you have had the chance to activate your organization's incident response team and escalate communication!

Breach Recognition, Notification, and Initial Response

A third party is probably not going to notify you of a security issue until they are sure that a data breach has occurred. They may be contractually obligated and otherwise legally obligated to notify your organization, but the reality is that they are probably going to do some initial investigation and containment before they notify you. Breach recognition requires some certainty. Making notifications and sharing information only to determine there was no unauthorized access or data loss may sound like good news, but after the process has started for initial response, frustration increases, costs are incurred, and credibility is diminished. In sum, make sure a breach has actually occurred before you announce it.

In the European Union under GDPR, Article 33, the notification rules stipulate that data controllers must notify the data protection authority within 72 hours. The same section mandates that data processors, third parties to the data controller, must make notification to the data controller immediately upon determination of a data breach.[19] If doing that is infeasible, some exceptions exist, but the reasons for delay must be disclosed. The imperative to notify individuals is less stringent. The data controller is permitted to determine whether the data breach is likely to affect the privacy of the individual adversely. If the breach has adverse impact, Article 33 directs the data controller to notify the affected individual "as soon as possible." The data authorities intend to keep individual notifications to those with adverse impact versus over-notifying individuals and creating notification fatigue.

HIPAA poses similar timeframes and guidelines for initial notification of data breaches. The law adds complexity around the size of the data exposure. If it involves more than 500 records, the healthcare organization must notify the HHS OCR within 60 days, or sooner. Notification of affected individuals must also fit within that timeframe. When less than 500 records are involved, the notification starts with the affected individuals within the 60-day timeframe. For volumes of data breaches under 500, each one is reportable to the OCR, but only on an annual basis at the beginning of the calendar year. For any amount of records, a third party or business associate must notify the covered entity healthcare organization within 60 days.[20]

EXAM TIP Understand that the 60-day timeline for business associates, covered entities, and other notification requirements for HIPAA are not sequential. The intention is to accomplish all notifications in 60 days unless there are exceptions and reasonable delays. Don't fall for a question that indicates a notification event could take 120 or 180 days when you add up the timelines. The law's intent is for practical and prompt notification.

As we move into the next section, we will explore notification more thoroughly. It is important to consider and determine who will actually do the notification. This happens at or before contract signature in the best case. Going back to the point made in the first paragraph of this section, you must be certain that a data breach has occurred before the required notifications occur. In addition, determining who is responsible for making notifications depends on who is being notified—external regulatory agencies, the media, or affected individuals. The fact is that notification may be the responsibility of a third party other than your organization. Many cybersecurity insurance policies include provisions for these services and they are prenegotiated. The costs of making notifications will also need to be understood and written into the contracts, particularly when those services are not covered in cybersecurity insurance policies or when no policy exists.

Respond to Third-Party Requests Regarding Privacy/Security Events

Responsibilities may be limited to internal activities culminating with notification of senior management. Regardless of the limitations, your understanding of how the healthcare organization leadership must interact with external agencies during and after an incident will be valuable. What follows is an overview of how that interaction should happen and under what conditions.

Law Enforcement

Once an incident is determined to be a crime, senior leadership will notify law enforcement. In the United States, this includes authorities such as the Federal Bureau of Investigation (FBI) and Secret Service as well as local and state agencies. Internationally, relevant law enforcement agencies will have jurisdiction and should be notified. Law enforcement can assist in the investigation and advise the organization on evidence collection. Law enforcement also can help determine when additional notification actions may take place, such as delaying notification if it would interfere with an ongoing investigation.

EU Data Authorities

The notification responsibilities in the European Union relate to electronic information and are founded in telecommunication industry regulations. This is changing as notification has been integrated into Europe's overall privacy doctrine. Currently, when a data breach occurs, the data controller (healthcare organization) is mandated to notify the appropriate EU nation's supervisory data authority of the personal data breach. When it is determined that the breach presents a high risk to the affected individual, the data controller is required to make personal notifications.

Affected Individuals

In the United States, healthcare organizations must notify individuals (of any number) once the incident has been evaluated and there has been sufficient risk of disclosure. The organization determines the risk of disclosure through a specific risk assessment process, described later in this chapter in the section "Risk Assessment Activities." If the risk analysis confirms that the incident is in fact a data breach, healthcare organizations in the United States are mandated to notify affected individuals. Even the form of the notice is prescribed. The individual notice must be made within 60 days and must be in written form, delivered by first-class mail or, alternatively, by e-mail if the affected individual has agreed to receive such notices electronically. When the contact information is out of date or incorrect for 10 or more people, the healthcare organization must take alternative measures. It can post the notice on the organization's web site or engage the media to broadcast the information.

The notice in any format must include the following elements:

- A description of the breach
- Types of information that were involved
- What affected individuals can do to reduce chances of additional harm
- Recommendation to obtain a credit report, monitor bank accounts, and so on
- A brief description of what the healthcare organization is doing to investigate the breach, mitigate the harm, and prevent further breaches
- Contact information for the covered entity, including a toll-free number for individuals to call to determine whether they were affected by the breach

In the European Union, as the proposed notification rules gain acceptance, the imperative will be to notify the supervisory authorities within 24 hours. The imperative to notify individuals is less stringent, however. The data controller is permitted to determine whether the data breach is likely to affect the privacy of the individual adversely. If the breach has adverse impact, the data controller may notify the affected individual. The data authorities intend to limit individual notifications to those with adverse impact versus over-notifying individuals and creating notification fatigue.

Media

The media plays a role in broadcasting the nature and extent of the breach. It will also help notify individuals and the community about actions they can take to protect themselves. In the United States, healthcare organizations are required to notify the media (newspapers, television stations, and so on) when the breach impacts 500 residents of a state or jurisdiction. The media press release must be issued within 60 days of breach discovery. The content of the media notification will be the same as the elements included in the notification to affected individuals.

Public Relations

While the incident is ongoing, the healthcare organization will continue to interact with the media and the community. Typically, one person serves as the spokesperson for the healthcare organization in front of the media. This helps ensure continuity and reliability of messaging and proper dissemination. Public relations personnel will create press releases to update the media and community continually. These updates may be placed in local newspapers, periodicals, and social media outlets. The public relations personnel may oversee the content that is placed on any web site created and dedicated to communicating data breach issues with affected individuals and other interested parties. In some cases, the lessons learned from the data breach can be shared with other healthcare organizations. Public relations personnel may contribute to this process to help develop the message for others to present or deliver it firsthand at professional organizations' meetings, seminars, and other educational events.

Health Information Exchanges

In some circumstances, a data breach by a healthcare organization may result in the need to notify other external stakeholders. For instance, if a healthcare organization participates in a health information exchange (HIE), the healthcare organization may need to notify the exchange or other member institutions. HIEs exchange identifiable patient information for clinical care purposes. Because of the organizational relationships resulting from HIEs, healthcare organizations may incur new notification responsibilities.

Organizational Breach Notification Rules

Remember that under HIPAA, the risk of disclosure threshold is important to determine whether the data incident is a breach under the law (impermissible use). According to the US HHS, "a breach is, generally, an impermissible use or disclosure under the Privacy Rule that compromises the security or privacy of the protected health information."[21]

Unless the healthcare organization can show through a risk of disclosure assessment that the PHI has a low probability of compromise or further disclosure, the disclosure is considered a data breach. The components of that type of risk assessment are as follows:

- The identifying elements that may constitute PHI and the potential elements that can be used to reidentify the information
- The person who handled the information through unauthorized disclosure or access
- A determination of whether the information was retained and viewed by the person
- An evaluation of mitigations resulting from exposure of the PHI

In the analysis, the organization may determine that notification actions are not required. In addition to the risk assessment determination, three disclosure scenarios would also serve as exceptions to the Breach Notification Rule in HIPAA:

- A person working for a covered entity or business associate inadvertently obtains or views PHI. Although the access is unauthorized, it is accidental and the person acted within the authority of the covered entity or business associate.
- An inadvertent disclosure occurred between two people authorized to access PHI in general, but not the information exchanged at that particular time. For example, a physician sends an e-mail to another physician with patient information. The sending physician misaddressed the e-mail. The receiving physician normally has authorization to view PHI, but not specifically for this patient or in this case. The information cannot be disclosed by the parties beyond that exchange.
- The unauthorized recipient would not have been able to read or maintain the PHI.

This definition describes organizational breach notification considerations based on US healthcare organizations. Of course, healthcare organizations around the globe have similar procedures and requirements. The following section will examine some examples.

International Breach Notification

By now, you should be convinced of the importance of notification of affected individuals, regulators, and the media to help preserve the privacy and security of PHI even after the data has been breached. After a data breach in the United States, the notification effort is intended to minimize damage and harm. This is true in other countries as well, where the external reporting requirements vary, but have the same general intention to minimize the harm to affected individuals. Here are some of the notification procedures:

- **Canada** According to PIPEDA, the external notification of the affected individuals and the privacy commissioner is mandatory for organizations subject to the law. In select provinces, such as Alberta and Ontario, rules are in place to make external notification mandatory as well.[22]
- **People's Republic of China** China's Cybersecurity Law (2017) requires that in the event of a suspected or actual data breach of personal information, an organization must mitigate the impacts and notify affected individuals.

The government requires timely notification to the proper agency. However, the regulation and relevant specification guidance for implementation does not dictate an actual timeline for notification.

- **Israel**   The enactment of the Privacy Protection Regulations (Data Security), 5777-2017, in 2018 interestingly does not require organizations to notify affected individuals unless the regulatory authority, called a Database Register, specifically determines notification is necessary. The determination is based on a categorization of databases that hold sensitive information as either a high or an intermediate level of security. If the data breach involves these categories of databases, it is designated as a serious security incident. The Database Register will also confer with the head of the Israel National Cyber Authority to decide whether notification is warranted because of the potential harm to the data subject.

Organizational Information Dissemination Policies and Standards

You should keep in mind several guidelines when you are participating in a data breach response and notification action. We have covered external communication, but internal communication is also important. A data breach may involve a relatively small portion of the organization in containment, investigation, remediation, and notification, but you can be certain that many more people in the organization are aware of the event. Unfortunately, these people do not always have the best view or the most accurate information. What they share with one another and outside the organization can detract from your official notification processes.

Here are some suggestions for creating internal communication to help keep staff members informed:

- *Employees should receive practical and frequent communication.* Rumors and gossip will happen relatively quickly. Start communication as soon as possible to counteract this.

- *Honest communication that is authentic is best.* Employees can be a terrific source of public relations advocates for the organization during this setback. Give them information they can share with friends, family, and the general public at home and online where possible.

- *Stay connected with employees.* Maintain regular communications, with accurate and official updates.

- *Authorize managers at all levels to share approved communications.* The sense of order that leaders can instill will be beneficial in an otherwise chaotic event.

- *Allow for feedback from employees.* In particular, employees who serve customers or patients can provide valuable information that helps improve notification expectations.

As the incident response team follows the established procedures and the external notifications are underway, internal communications done correctly will help the organization reduce the impact of a data breach. Brand and reputational impacts can also be lessened. Of course, even with internal communications, the information that you share should be appropriate for public disclosure—absent specific attack information or exposed vulnerabilities, for example. Focus on providing information to help employees answer the types of questions they may be asked.

In addition to details provided in public notifications, you may want to ensure that employees know the following:

- The steps the organization is taking to recover
- Assurance of continued business operations and safe patient care
- Actions affected individuals can take and who to contact
- A point of contact for employees to ask additional questions
- Instructions for employees that include to whom media inquiries are referred

CAUTION Keeping employees informed should not be confused with permitting employees to act as official spokespeople for external notifications regarding the breach. The intent is to reduce incorrect information sharing and uncertainty within the organization, which can add to the negative impact of a data breach outside the organization.

Risk Assessment Activities

The risk assessment process stipulated by the HIPAA Breach Notification Rule is meant to assist healthcare organizations comply with the reporting requirements. The process also helps determine the qualitative risk of disclosure in terms of high, medium, or low. Where the risk of disclosure is low enough, external notifications are not required. We know that this risk assessment process begins with a determination of whether or not PHI was disclosed as part of the incident. It is possible that the attacker accessed systems or databases that did not have PHI. This underscores the importance of knowing where your organization has PHI stored. Without that clarity, you cannot rule out PHI disclosure if data of any type was potentially accessed.

The risk assessment continues on to determine the magnitude or scope of the breach. The number of records, the files accessed, e-mail transfer to a third party, data exfiltration, or ransomware encryption are considerations of how extensive the impacts might be. The amount of time the attacker had unauthorized access to the information is also something that factors into the risk assessment. It is not uncommon for unauthorized access to continue undetected for months. Once the scope is understood, the damages must be estimated. If the adversary actually viewed the data or used it in some way, such as offering it for sale or attempting to gain medical care fraudulently, the extent of the data breach increases the assessment of risk level.

To complete the risk assessment process, consider the mitigations to the risk. Even after you've understood aspects such as what data was breached, by whom, its scope, and any actual use of the data, factor in any mitigating actions the organization has taken. A lost laptop with three gigabytes of PHI is mitigated by proving the laptop had acceptable encryption of the data at rest. Another example is where a determination can be made that the disclosure was incidental and by accident; in this case, ensure that the data was not used and was disposed of promptly and properly to stop further disclosure.

Chain of Custody Principles

In a data breach investigation, especially one in which an external adversary conducts an attack that lasts several months and accesses multiple systems, the investigation will result in a large volume of evidence. Your understanding of the principles that govern chain of custody will prevent that evidence from becoming unusable.

Evidence is needed to help with the risk assessment for notification as well as to ensure that recovery actions are successful. Keep in mind that recovery and restoration to normal operations should not be rushed in case the access for the attacker has not been completely removed from the environment. The other value of evidence and the reason chain of custody must be maintained is because the data from the investigation are required and essential for any legal proceedings after the data breach, including regulatory inquiries and class action lawsuits. Chain of custody principles ensure that the proper documentation and processes are in place for gathering, using, and storing evidence to prevent any contamination of evidence or tampering with evidence to preserve legal validity.

In data breach remediation that involves a third party, the healthcare organization should ensure that the chain of custody is preserved in the investigation even if the third party is in charge of the evidence collection and handling. If the healthcare organization has special expertise in staff with forensics experience or even secure storage capabilities, the third party can extend the chain of custody to the healthcare organization. By adhering to chain of custody principles to properly document and prevent changes to the integrity of the evidence, the healthcare organization can support the investigation if third parties lack sufficient resources.

Promote Awareness of Third-Party Requirements

Entering into a contract with a third party to handle PHI for your organization does not make the third party a data controller under GDPR or absolve a covered entity of its responsibilities under HIPAA. It is important to make sure business stakeholders, clinical managers, and information protection professionals know this, especially in the context of data breach response. As the data breach risk assessment process unfolds, your organization must cooperate as much as possible with the third party in the determination of whether or not a breach has happened, who must be notified, what information was lost or at risk, and what containment and recovery actions must occur.

Other stakeholders in the processes of managing third-party relationships need to participate by holding third parties accountable. Your organization will rely on its information governance process, vendor management, legal counsel, and the individual business or clinical leaders who manage the relationship. As part of supporting awareness of third-party activities before, during, and after a data breach, you can emphasize the roles and responsibilities that are outside of information privacy and security departments.

Again, the responsibility of the data collectors or covered entities does not stop when the contract is signed. The third parties definitely have defined responsibilities during these crises, but the stakeholders do as well, and they need to be aware, trained, and practiced in how to execute those responsibilities when needed.

Information Flow Mapping and Scope

Third-party risk management centers on understanding the flow and scope of information that transfers between the organizations. Regulators and legal frameworks identify the concerns of data subjects or patients depending on where you work. Assuring that reasonable and adequate controls are in place for information transfer and sharing is required. Also, the regulations require the healthcare organizations that collect the data to know where the data is, where it goes, to whom, and under what conditions. Under Article 30 of the GDPR, for example, organizations must have a thorough information processing accounting, which can be provided to data supervisory authorities on demand.[23]

The components of an information flow and scope for third-party data sharing, in general terms, provides clarity in the following areas:

- Describing the entire information lifecycle
- Considering intended and potential unforeseen uses
- Incorporating the information mapping and sharing implications into training
- Planning for any potential scope increases for information use

An information map can help the organization manage a data breach response, whether or not a third party handles the information. The number of affected individuals depends on the organization's knowledge of what data exists and where. Otherwise, organizations have to over-notify in an abundance of caution, adding to expense and reputation damage. Here are some considerations for developing an information map:

- Document the sources of information collected and data elements such as name, Social Security number, diagnoses, procedures, biometrics, and so on.
- Detail how the information is collected via paper forms, online, medical device reporting, and so on.
- Specify accountable information collectors and maintainers.
- Identify the media and locations used for storing the information, such as paper documents, digital files, and databases, as well as storage within the organization in leased data centers or with a cloud service provider.
- Record who has access to the data and to what extent.
- Map the transfer and sharing activities for the information.
- Catalog any technical interconnections between organizations.

By adhering to a strict process of knowing how data comes into your organization and third party organizations, you can be assured of a comprehensive awareness of information flow and the scope of data for which you and your third parties are responsible. This can minimize the impacts of data breaches, notification actions, and ultimately costs and long-lasting damages to your organization. It seems obvious, but this practice also protects your patients and customers by limiting their exposure to the identity theft, worry, and financial burdens they can face when your organization suffers cyber incidents resulting in unauthorized access and data loss.

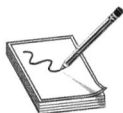

> **NOTE** Although Social Security numbers are PII and mentioned as part of the information mapping process, increasingly healthcare organizations are refraining from collecting those data elements and using them as identifiers. However, where they are collected, they must be included in the information flow and mapping procedures to protect them.

Data Sensitivity and Classification

Referring back to our topics on asset management and information lifecycle, we can apply the same concepts to third-party management. As we conduct information flow mapping and scope, we categorize the sensitivity and classification of the information that is shared. This will inform the frequency and rigor of third-party risk assessments and the risk analysis that needs to be conducted during investigations of a data breach. Understanding the particular data elements that may have been exposed during an attack supports notification. Affected individuals may respond differently when data elements that are exposed are limited to name and address, versus unauthorized access to PHI and Social Security numbers. The criticality of data elements varies.

NIST's guidance on cyber supply chain risk management includes a focus on critical systems for the commercial sector. Although the guidance is not specific to data, you can draw inferences from the material because a measure of criticality of a third party concerns what types of information they handle and how much. NIST recommends third-party risk management that identifies the systems or components that are most vulnerable and will cause the greatest organizational impact if compromised.[24] It follows that in healthcare systems that collect, transfer, use, and store PHI would be tiered based on levels of criticality. The data itself would be assigned a level of sensitivity and classification. Refer to the "Data Classification" section in Chapter 1 to review specific levels you may want to use. Having this information written into third-party risk management plans and incident response processes will help your organization respond to a cyber event or data breach that starts with your third party. If notification actions are required as a result, your organization will be able to accomplish the communications properly.

Privacy and Security Requirements

As mentioned, privacy deals with the information we need to protect, and security deals with how we protect the information. This concept is relevant in third-party risk and incident response as well. Stakeholders in the healthcare organization who manage or sponsor the relationship with an external third party need to realize which privacy and security requirements the healthcare organization must adhere to, and these requirements should be extended to the third party. Following are some privacy requirements in third-party risk that the stakeholders should comprehend:

- Determining whether the data shared with the third party constitutes personal or health information subject to privacy law (such as HIPAA, GDPR, PIPEDA)
- Ensuring that confidentiality is protected for customers through adequate privacy practices and accessible notices of privacy practices
- Adhering to prevailing regulation for the jurisdiction per region, nation, and US state level, for example, with emphasis on breach notification requirements

These are just a few requirements with privacy implications. These requirements are more than just concerns with meeting legal standards. In the event of a data breach, meeting privacy requirements will facilitate breach notification, ranging from a determination of no breach to notification of affected individuals, regulators, and the media, all in consultation with legal counsel. Along with these privacy requirements, stakeholders in your organization must understand many other security concerns, such as the following:

- Technical controls that are in place to limit access to authorized personnel only
- Physical safeguards such as cipher-locked rooms and environmental controls to protect computing equipment
- Administrative requirements including mandatory HIPAA or information security training for all employees at the third-party organization

While you as an HCISPP understand the need to assess privacy and security requirements for third parties, stakeholders can add value. Because they interact with the third party more often than you may, they can be a first line of defense in managing the risk, especially when stakeholders understand the privacy and security requirements.

Risks Associated with Third Parties

There is a shared responsibility between the business and clinical sponsors of the third-party relationship and the privacy and security personnel in the organization to manage the risks associated with third parties. We know that responsibility for information protection remains with the healthcare organization in that due diligence in risk management must be accomplished. Contracting with a third party does not remove the healthcare organization's responsibility for security. Stakeholders need to understand the implications to risk that the contractual work involves. When there are changes to the work, the stakeholders are in the perfect position to inform privacy and security personnel. In some cases, due diligence would require a new risk assessment. As an example, contracting with a laboratory company to collect samples and health information, provide tests, and report back to the referring physicians requires an initial assessment and subsequent periodic assessments. However, outside of that routine, you may need to conduct a new risk assessment if the electronic health record software in the laboratory changes from an on-premises–managed solution to a hosted cloud service model (such as SaaS). Business and clinical stakeholders should know to report this type of a change within the healthcare organization.

Chapter Review

You now have a more holistic approach to managing the risk of third parties in healthcare. The value of these relationships will continue to grow as technology advances, pressures to control costs continue to mount, and access to specialized personnel becomes more difficult. The healthcare organization will find it advantageous to outsource many of its services and products and share access to PHI. Without exception, however, the responsibility for healthcare organizations and data collectors to maintain the privacy and security of this information cannot be outsourced with the information sharing. Therefore, understanding how to manage third-party risk appropriately is a central competency of the healthcare information privacy and security professional. This process includes making an accurate and comprehensive inventory of third-party suppliers with which your organization works. As an HCISPP, you will be required to support due diligence through conducting risk assessments of third parties when needed. Your responsibilities will extend to the actions taken when third-party relationships result in a cyber incident or a data breach. Each organization must be aware of and take mandatory actions, including breach notification, and you will participate in these.

Building a culture within a healthcare organization that values managing this risk is no easy task. It starts with incorporating front-line business and clinical representatives who sponsor the third-party relationships. It is a shared responsibility to manage third-party risk between information protection professionals and the stakeholders in the healthcare organization. You are expected to build awareness in the organization through training and internal communication programs. If all of this is done well, perhaps the only data breaches a healthcare organization may experience will be simulated events during testing of the incident response plans.

Questions

1. To manage third-party information risk properly, a healthcare organization should:

   A. Inventory all third parties that handle protected healthcare information

   B. Assign an objective clinical staff member to review all service level agreements

   C. Use the same vendor for all services that require the handling of protected health information

   D. Ensure that patient consent is obtained to share information with third parties

2. An EU healthcare organization discovers a database server interconnected to the public Internet behind a firewall that has been accessed by an internal unauthorized person who was caught before he could copy or transfer the data. The healthcare organization would be required to notify:

   A. Affected individuals

   B. Data authorities

   C. Data controllers

   D. European Commission

3. When you conduct an initial risk assessment of a potential third party, which of the following would be part of the documents you would collect and review?

   A. SOC 2 assessment, external penetration test summary, ISO 27001 certification

   B. Balance sheet, credit ratings, PCI DSS reports

   C. HITRUST certification, human resources policies, Notice of Privacy Practices

   D. External risk assessment results, vulnerability scanning logs, previous data breach disclosures

4. As an HCISPP, your pertinent responsibilities in monitoring the third-party progress may include:

   A. Corroborating any media reports of the third-party data loss

   B. Leading the investigation and remediation as a subject matter expert

   C. Scanning and review any interconnections between the organizations

   D. Identifying affected individuals from your organization to provide advance notice

5. A prominent healthcare insurance company works with a health savings company under a signed business associate agreement. Customers deposit portions of their salary in the health savings account to be used for certain authorized medical expenses. Records of the transactions, billing information, and some health information are maintained by the business associate. Last week, the health savings company notified you that they had experienced a data breach seven weeks prior. They have had a qualified cybersecurity forensics team collect data, and they are sure it is an actual data breach. Now they are involving you as part of the notification requirements of the business associate agreement. Of the following options, which is the most appropriate next action your organization takes?

   A. Terminate the contract for cause so no more customers are harmed.

   B. Conduct an independent penetration test to verify the findings.

   C. Perform an out-of-cycle risk assessment to establish corrective action plans.

   D. Notify regulators within the next week, if possible.

6. Outsourcing health data management to third parties is:

   A. Not regulated by law in the United States, but is regulated in Canada

   B. Illegal in the United States and European Union but not in Canada

   C. Covered in leading privacy and security frameworks

   D. Helpful in reducing information risk to the healthcare organization

7. The international trade impact of having a Safe Harbor agreement in place is:

   A. A US cloud provider could contract with an EU healthcare organization

   B. Data authorities would provide model contract standard clauses

   C. The US government could have access to EU data controller health data

   D. A US healthcare organization could use an EU utilization review firm

8. A service level agreement or a business associate agreement are contractual obligations that help an organization manage risk through:

   A. Transfer

   B. Avoidance

   C. Tolerance

   D. Treatment

9. In monitoring third parties, healthcare organizations should:

   A. Ensure outside counsel does inspections

   B. Include them in information governance groups

   C. Conduct annual and periodic audits as needed

   D. Assign a board member to interview them

10. One of the most cost-effective ways to promote organizational awareness of privacy and security concerns with information management by third parties is:

    A. Investing in a software-only data loss prevention application

    B. Conducting audits of third parties with clinical leadership personnel

    C. Publishing service level agreements on an organization's intranet

    D. Providing training upon hire and annually

Answers

1. **A.** The first step the healthcare organization should take is to inventory all third parties that handle health information and what services they provide. B is incorrect because involving a clinical staff member has benefit but is not an applicable step in the process. C is incorrect because it is highly improbable and likely cost-prohibitive to use the same vendor for all required services. D is incorrect because patient consent is not necessarily needed for transferring health information to a third party that is supporting healthcare operations.

2. **B.** The GDPR specifically requires notification to the supervisory data authorities. A is incorrect because the scenario does not describe a high risk of disclosure where one person accesses a database but does not cause further disclosure or criminal use of the information. This assessment of risk can preclude notifications to affected individuals. C is incorrect because data controllers are entities that actually make the notifications to the data authorities. D is incorrect because the European Commission may ultimately receive the notification, but the GDPR requirement is to notify supervisory data authorities.

3. **A.** Of the choices, only SOC 2 assessment, external penetration test summary, and ISO 27001 certification are all useful documentation to help you conduct a reliable third-party assessment prior to engaging in a business relationship. B is incorrect because only PCI DSS reports would help assess information risk. However, the financial position of a third party may be a consideration in terms of their ability to invest in privacy and security as well as recover from a data breach, including paying for notifications and breach recovery activities. C is incorrect, because although HITRUST certifications are relevant, the other listed documentation would not be adequate to assess risk properly, even though the information may be eventually needed to conduct due diligence. D is incorrect because the reliability and independence of these reports may not exist. Even the data breach disclosures may be under-reported if you consider the requirement to update regulators annually in the United States.

4. **C.** When a third party notifies your organization of an actual or a potential data breach, the only correct action listed is to scan and review the interconnections to investigate any potential exploitation of your organization as well. A is incorrect because you would probably not be a spokesperson for the organization, and you would not comment on an ongoing investigation of a third-party organization. B is incorrect because although you may assist in the investigation, the third party would lead the investigation. D is incorrect because notification would happen at a coordinated time by the proper organizational representatives, and advanced notification would be highly inappropriate.

5. **D.** Your organization may be tempted to do all of these actions, but regulator notification is the most applicable. To keep notification to regulators within the HIPAA-required 60 days, at least a notification of a potential data breach is appropriate. A is incorrect, although terminating the contract may occur later as your organization assesses the value of the third-party service in light of the data breach. B is incorrect because an external firm has provided confirmation of a data breach. C is incorrect; although it is relevant, this would not occur before your organization satisfies legally required notifications. A risk assessment may even wait until a decision is made to keep the contract in place versus terminate for cause.

6. **C.** The provisions for allowing information sharing with third parties is included in regulatory guidance internationally and in privacy and security principles. A is incorrect because both the United States and Canada regulate the third-party use

of health information. B is incorrect because the use of third parties to support healthcare in the European Union, United States, and Canada is entirely legal, as is proper health information sharing. D is incorrect because information risk is inherently increased by introducing information sharing with an external, third-party organization. This is the main point of this chapter.

7. A. Safe Harbor enables EU health organizations to transfer sensitive data to US companies that satisfy the requirements. B is incorrect because model contracts are used in place of Safe Harbor agreements. C is incorrect because this agreement applies to US companies only, not governments. D is incorrect because it is irrelevant; the Safe Harbor agreement is an EU requirement. The US healthcare organization would be subject to HIPAA, but the EU utilization review firm would not be, so the third-party contract would probably not happen. This has nothing to do with Safe Harbor.

8. A. Service level agreements and business associate agreements help to manage risk through transferring the risk to a third party. B is incorrect because the action does not make the risk disappear; the organization still faces some risk from the third party. C is incorrect because risk tolerance may inform the decisions the organization makes to engage with third parties, but contractual agreements likely do not change risk tolerance levels set at the management and board levels. D is not the best choice, because it is too general. Risk transfer is one action related to overall risk treatment, as is risk avoidance or not contracting with a third party.

9. C. Healthcare organizations are required to conduct annual or periodic audits of third parties that handle their PHI. A, B, and D are incorrect in terms of feasibility and cost. A, outside counsel, is an expensive option, and unless there is a high risk and the healthcare organization wants a more formal interpretation, outside counsel is probably not involved with third-party risk monitoring. B is incorrect because, although it may be wise to include third parties in some activities of information risk management within the healthcare organization, having them as regular members of any internal boards and committees is not practical. D is incorrect because there is little chance a board member would interview an individual third-party organization as a risk assessment measure. However, it may be possible to have a board member meet with a collection of third-party vendors as part of an "industry day meeting."

10. D. Although often overlooked, staff training on managing third-party risk (along with protecting healthcare information in general) is a cost-effective way to promote awareness of privacy and security concerns. A is incorrect. Although this may be less costly than hardware technology purchases, there is no expectation of the application's effectiveness. B is incorrect because using clinical personnel to augment auditing while not providing patient care would not be cost efficient; it would be costly. C is incorrect because publishing service level agreements on the intranet provides no context or explanation to the average user of those services and does not increase organizational awareness.

References

1. American Institute of Certified Public Accountants (AICPA) and Canadian Institute of Chartered Accountants (CICA). 2009. "Generally Accepted Privacy Principles." https://www.cpacanada.ca/-/media/site/operational/ms-member-services/docs/00250-generally-accepted-privacy-principles.pdf?la=en&hash=284 D936484F7D77307F80A9951E015D551B62DBC.

2. HIPAA Journal. 2020. "2019 Healthcare Data Breach Report." https://www .hipaajournal.com/2019-healthcare-data-breach-report.

3. Dolezel, D., and A. McLeod. 2019. "Cyber-Analytics: Identifying Discriminants of Data Breaches." Perspectives in Health Information Management. https:// www.ncbi.nlm.nih.gov/pmc/articles/PMC6669366.

4. US Department of Health and Human Services (HHS). 2013. "Business Associate Contracts: Sample Business Associate Agreement Provisions." HHS.gov. https:// www.hhs.gov/hipaa/for-professionals/covered-entities/sample-business-associate-agreement-provisions/index.html.

5. HHS. 2019. "Business Associates." HHS.gov. https://www.hhs.gov/hipaa/for-professionals/privacy/guidance/business-associates/index.html.

6. Information Commissioner's Office (ICO). 2004. "Model Contract Clauses: International transfers of personal data." https://ico.org.uk/media/1571/model_ contract_clauses_international_transfers_of_personal_data.pdf.

7. CISION PR Newswire. 2016. "Healthcare IT Outsourcing Market to Account for US$61.28 Billion in Revenue by 2023, Shaped by Focus on Improved Healthcare Administration: Transparency Market Research." https://www.prnewswire.com/ news-releases/healthcare-it-outsourcing-market-to-account-for-us6128-billion-in-revenue-by-2023-shaped-by-focus-on-improved-healthcare-administration-transparency-market-research-571974461.html.

8. Jansen, W., and T. Grance. 2011. *Guidelines on Security and Privacy in Public Cloud Computing*, NIST Special Publication 800-144. https://csrc.nist.gov/ publications/detail/sp/800-144/final.

9. Swire, P., and K. Ahmad. 2012. *Foundations of Information Privacy and Data Protection: A Survey of Global Concepts, Laws and Practices*. Portsmouth, NH: International Association of Privacy Professionals.

10. HHS. 2017. "Guidance on HIPAA and Cloud Computing." HHS.gov. https:// www.hhs.gov/hipaa/for-professionals/special-topics/cloud-computing/index.html.

11. Badger, M., T. Grace, R. Patt-Corner, and J. Voas. 2012. *Cloud Computing Synopsis and Recommendations*, NIST SP 800-146. Download available from http://www.nist.gov/manuscript-publication-search.cfm?pub_id=911075.

12. Huffman, B., C. O'Donoghue, A. Splittgerber, and M. Eichenberger. 2018. "Potential conflict and harmony between GDPR and the CLOUD Act." ReedSmith Client Alerts. https://www.reedsmith.com/en/perspectives/2018/06/ potential-conflict-and-harmony-between-gdpr-and-the-cloud-act.

13. UK government. 2016. "Investigatory Powers Act 2016." legislation.gov.uk. http://www.legislation.gov.uk/ukpga/2016/25/contents.

14. See "Cyber Supply Chain Risk Management," https://csrc.nist.gov/Projects/cyber-supply-chain-risk-management, and *Supply Chain Risk Management Practices for Federal Information Systems and Organizations*, NIST SP 800-161, https://nvlpubs.nist.gov/nistpubs/SpecialPublications/NIST.SP.800-161.pdf.

15. Office of the Comptroller of the Currency (OCC), US Department of Treasury. 2013. "Third-Party Relationships: Risk Management Guidance," OCC Bulletin 2013-29. https://www.occ.gov/news-issuances/bulletins/2013/bulletin-2013-29.html.

16. OCC. 2017. "Third-Party Relationships: Supplemental Examination Procedures," OCC Bulletin 2017-7. https://www.occ.gov/news-issuances/bulletins/2017/bulletin-2017-7.html.

17. Santa Fe Group Shared Assessments. 2020. "Vendor Risk Management Maturity Model." https://sharedassessments.org/vrmmm.

18. Ponemon Institute. 2015. "Fifth Annual Benchmark Study on Privacy and Security of Healthcare Data." https://iapp.org/media/pdf/resource_center/Ponemon_Privacy_Security_Healthcare_Data.pdf.

19. The General Data Protection Regulation (GDPR). 2018. "Notification of a personal data breach to the supervisory authority," Article 33 GDPR. Intersoft Consulting. https://gdpr-info.eu/art-33-gdpr.

20. HHS. 2013. "Breach Notification Rule." HHS.gov. https://www.hhs.gov/hipaa/for-professionals/breach-notification/index.html.

21. HHS. 2013. "Breach Notification Rule." HHS.gov. https://www.hhs.gov/hipaa/for-professionals/breach-notification/index.html.

22. Office of the Privacy Commissioner of Canada. 2018. "What you need to know about mandatory reporting of breaches of security safeguards." https://www.priv.gc.ca/en/privacy-topics/business-privacy/safeguards-and-breaches/privacy-breaches/respond-to-a-privacy-breach-at-your-business/gd_pb_201810.

23. GDPR. 2018. "Records of processing activities," Article 30 GDPR. Intersoft Consulting, https://gdpr-info.eu/art-30-gdpr.

24. NIST Computer Security Resource Center. 2020. "Cyber Supply Chain Risk Management." https://csrc.nist.gov/Projects/cyber-supply-chain-risk-management.

About the Online Content

This book comes complete with TotalTester Online customizable practice exam software with 250 practice exam questions.

System Requirements

The current and previous major versions of the following desktop browsers are recommended and supported: Chrome, Microsoft Edge, Firefox, and Safari. These browsers update frequently, and sometimes an update may cause compatibility issues with the TotalTester Online or other content hosted on the Training Hub. If you run into a problem using one of these browsers, please try using another until the problem is resolved.

Your Total Seminars Training Hub Account

To get access to the online content you will need to create an account on the Total Seminars Training Hub. Registration is free, and you will be able to track all your online content using your account. You may also opt in if you wish to receive marketing information from McGraw Hill or Total Seminars, but this is not required for you to gain access to the online content.

Privacy Notice

McGraw Hill values your privacy. Please be sure to read the Privacy Notice available during registration to see how the information you have provided will be used. You may view our Corporate Customer Privacy Policy by visiting the McGraw Hill Privacy Center. Visit the **mheducation.com** site and click **Privacy** at the bottom of the page.

Single User License Terms and Conditions

Online access to the digital content included with this book is governed by the McGraw Hill License Agreement outlined next. By using this digital content you agree to the terms of that license.

Access   To register and activate your Total Seminars Training Hub account, simply follow these easy steps.

1. Go to this URL: **hub.totalsem.com/mheclaim**

2. To register and create a new Training Hub account, enter your e-mail address, name, and password on the **Register** tab. No further information (such as credit card number) is required to create an account.

    If you already have a Total Seminars Training Hub account, enter your e-mail address and password on the **Log in** tab.

3. Enter your Product Key: `3xqt-79gh-gfwn`

4. Click to accept the user license terms.

5. For new users, click the **Register and Claim** button to create your account. For existing users, click the **Log in and Claim** button.

    You will be taken to the Training Hub and have access to the content for this book.

Duration of License   Access to your online content through the Total Seminars Training Hub will expire one year from the date the publisher declares the book out of print.

Your purchase of this McGraw Hill product, including its access code, through a retail store is subject to the refund policy of that store.

The Content is a copyrighted work of McGraw Hill, and McGraw Hill reserves all rights in and to the Content. The Work is © 2021 by McGraw Hill.

Restrictions on Transfer   The user is receiving only a limited right to use the Content for the user's own internal and personal use, dependent on purchase and continued ownership of this book. The user may not reproduce, forward, modify, create derivative works based upon, transmit, distribute, disseminate, sell, publish, or sublicense the Content or in any way commingle the Content with other third-party content without McGraw Hill's consent.

Limited Warranty   The McGraw Hill Content is provided on an "as is" basis. Neither McGraw Hill nor its licensors make any guarantees or warranties of any kind, either express or implied, including, but not limited to, implied warranties of merchantability or fitness for a particular purpose or use as to any McGraw Hill Content or the information therein or any warranties as to the accuracy, completeness, correctness, or results to be obtained from, accessing or using the McGraw Hill Content, or any material referenced in such Content or any information entered into licensee's product by users or other persons and/or any material available on or that can be accessed through the licensee's product (including via any hyperlink or otherwise) or as to non-infringement of third-party rights. Any warranties of any kind, whether express or implied, are disclaimed. Any material or data obtained through use of the McGraw Hill Content is at your own discretion and risk and user understands that it will be solely responsible for any resulting damage to its computer system or loss of data.

Neither McGraw Hill nor its licensors shall be liable to any subscriber or to any user or anyone else for any inaccuracy, delay, interruption in service, error or omission, regardless of cause, or for any damage resulting therefrom.

In no event will McGraw Hill or its licensors be liable for any indirect, special or consequential damages, including but not limited to, lost time, lost money, lost profits or good will, whether in contract, tort, strict liability or otherwise, and whether or not such damages are foreseen or unforeseen with respect to any use of the McGraw Hill Content.

TotalTester Online

TotalTester Online provides you with a simulation of the HCISPP exam. Exams can be taken in Practice Mode or Exam Mode. Practice Mode provides an assistance window with hints, references to the book, explanations of the correct and incorrect answers, and the option to check your answer as you take the test. Exam Mode provides a simulation of the actual exam. The number of questions, the types of questions, and the time allowed are intended to be an accurate representation of the exam environment. The option to customize your quiz allows you to create custom exams from selected domains or chapters, and you can further customize the number of questions and time allowed.

To take a test, follow the instructions provided in the previous section to register and activate your Total Seminars Training Hub account. When you register you will be taken to the Total Seminars Training Hub. From the Training Hub Home page, select **HCISPP® HealthCare Information Security and Privacy Practitioner All-in-One Exam Guide TotalTester** from the Study drop-down menu at the top of the page, or from the list of Your Topics on the Home page. You can then select the option to customize your quiz and begin testing yourself in Practice Mode or Exam Mode. All exams provide an overall grade and a grade broken down by domain.

Technical Support

For questions regarding the TotalTester or operation of the Training Hub, visit **www.totalsem.com** or e-mail **support@totalsem.com**.

For questions regarding book content, visit **www.mheducation.com/customerservice**.

access (1) The ability of a person, or user, to interact with information or a technology asset such as a computer network by entering the appropriate credentials; (2) a principle within privacy and security frameworks that grants data subjects rights to review, challenge, and keep copies of information that is collected about them. The term "access" is often confused with "authorization" and "authentication" because of their interrelated relationship within identity and privilege management. Each concept does have distinctions to differentiate them.

access control A type of control used to ensure that access to assets is authorized and restricted based on business and security requirements [ISO/IEC 27000]. It affects the ability for a user or other entity to do something with a computer resource, and usually refers to a technical capability such as reading, creating, modifying, or deleting a file; executing a program; or using an external connection.

access limitation A standard that requires that access to sensitive information be limited to the minimum amount necessary and only to those with a need to know based on their role in the organization and reason for the information request.

accountability
The property that ensures that the actions of an entity may be traced uniquely to the entity [ISO 7498-2].

Accountable Care Organization (ACO) A formal organizational care delivery and resourcing model that is currently applicable to Medicare patients only. Physicians, hospitals, and other relevant health service professionals are testing ACO models that merge their organizations contractually to provide a broader set of healthcare services.

accounting of disclosures A right assigned in HIPAA in which healthcare organizations must keep and be able to provide to patients and regulators a record of all information disclosed, by whom, and to whom outside of the healthcare organization.

Accreditation Association for Ambulatory Health Care (AAAHC) An organization that develops accreditation standards for patient safety, quality, value, and measurement of performance for healthcare organizations. Because its focus is in ambulatory health care, AAAHC surveys can be more efficient and meaningful with better-equipped, peer-based accreditation processes.

Accreditation Canada Formerly known as Canadian Council on Health Services Accreditation (CCHSA), this organization provides accreditation for more than 1000 client organizations, ranging from regional health authorities, to hospitals and community-based programs and services. Like the Joint Commission and the AAAHC in the United States, the Canadian surveyors and auditors are not government employees, and they do not take direction from the government.

accuracy   The quality or state of information precision that is vital to the health of the patient. Accuracy must be the rule with regard to the entire scope of a patient's medical entry and overall healthcare record. A patient—or, for that matter anyone, including care providers—who determines information within the record is in error has the right to request an amendment or change to the record or entry.

administration   The various people who manage or provide support for the provision of healthcare. At every level of the healthcare organization, from the chief executive officer to the ward clerk, administrative individuals provide appropriate levels of management and leadership. At the most senior level, administration refers to the management of internal and external forces to achieve specific goals.

American College of Radiology (ACR)   An organization founded in 1923 that is at the forefront of radiology evolution, representing nearly 40,000 radiologists, radiation oncologists, nuclear medicine physicians, and medical physicists. Its core purpose is to serve patients and society by empowering members to advance the practice, science, and professions of radiological care [https://www.acr.org].

American National Standards Institute (ANSI) Accredited Standards Committee (ASC) X12   An ANSI committee that develops protocols for HIPAA transactions as part of a larger body of work for all electronic transactions. There are more than 315 X12-based standards and a growing collection of X12 XML schemas for healthcare, insurance, government, transportation, finance, and many other industries. X12N is used for healthcare claims.

annualized loss expectancy (ALE)   A calculation of the single loss expectancy multiplied by the annual rate of occurrence, or how much an organization could estimate to lose from an asset based on the risks, threats, and vulnerabilities.

annualized rate of occurrence (ARO)   An estimate based on data showing how often a threat would be successful in exploiting a vulnerability.

anonymization   A process that removes the association between the identifying data set and the data subject [ISO/TS 25237]. Protected health information (PHI) in anonymization includes elements eliminated or manipulated with the purpose of hindering the possibility of returning to the original data set.

architecture   A general term that describes a focus on principles for information asset design and interconnectivity based on models and conceptual diagrams. It is often described as both art and science.

assessment   A process conducted by information privacy and security professional to determine levels of risk an organization may face by implementing a system, contracting with a third-party supplier, or publishing a new web site, as examples. Assessments are based on established standards or objectives to permit comparison and evaluation.

audit   An inspection and/or appraisal conducted against a "standard" with an explanation of how the activity should be performed (normally a process or procedure). The auditor works to determine whether the described process conforms to the standard and whether the operators are following the appropriate processes.

authorization   Granting of access rights and user privileges to operate information technology assets.

availability   Ensuring timely and reliable access to and use of information [NIST SP 800-53].

awareness   Possession of an informed perspective that all employees or certain groups of employees should have with regard to information privacy and security controls, responsibilities, and risks. It is achieved through initial, annual, and periodic training and communication about information protection.

bachelor of science in nursing (BSN)   A four-year academic degree in the science and principles of nursing granted by a tertiary education university or similarly accredited school. Can be combined with an RN (registered nurse) license, but BSN is not synonymous with an RN designation, which can be attained with a two-year academic degree.

biomedical technician   Personnel who maintain medical devices and are responsible for many information privacy and security controls.

body area network (BAN)   A sensor or multiple sensors located on a person's body that act as endpoint computing devices on a network. These sensors send and receive signals wirelessly to other medical devices and LANs.

breach   The compromise of information. In healthcare, a breach is usually specific to the unauthorized disclosure or loss of medical information as it is shared electronically.

breach notification   Following a breach of protected health information, healthcare organizations must inform several entities about the breach and the actions the organization is taking in response. Entities to be contacted are affected individuals, the government, and, in some cases, the media. In addition, third parties who handle PHI must notify the healthcare organization they support if a breach occurs at or by the third party.

bundled payment   A more predetermined payment model than fee-for-service, bundled healthcare delivers compensation to a healthcare provider based on expected costs for each acute care episode, not necessarily on the actual costs.

business associate (BA)   In the United States, a person or organization that performs functions or activities on behalf of, or certain services for, a covered entity that involve the use or disclosure of protected health information [US HHS].

business associate agreement (BAA)   A special type of contract, mandated by HIPAA in the United States, between a covered entity (CE) and a business associate (BA). The BAA should explicitly spell out how a BA will report and respond to a data breach, including data breaches that are caused by a business associate's subcontractors. In addition, HIPAA BAAs should require a BA to demonstrate how it will respond to an Office of Civil Rights (OCR) investigation.

business continuity   The actions an organization must be able to perform in an effort to continue its mission should an unforeseen event occur. Not all continuity operations are specific to information technology and systems.

business partner   A particular subcategory of vendor for healthcare organizations, business partners provide a product or service for the healthcare organization, but not within a transactional type of relationship. They are characterized as having a longer or recurring relationship with the healthcare organization, commonly described in a contract or formal, written obligation.

business process reengineering   Involves the radical redesign of core business processes to achieve dramatic improvements in productivity, cycle times, and quality. These improvements typically come from automation of manual processes or the implementation of a new technology.

capitation   A strict predetermined compensation model that provides a payment arrangement of a set amount for each person covered by a third-party payer. Providers agree in advance to accept a fixed amount for each person, known as a covered life, based on a specified time period, typically a year, whether or not that person seeks care.

Centers for Medicare and Medicaid Services (CMS)   An operating division of the US Department of Health and Human Services (HHS) that combines the oversight of the Medicare program, the federal portion of the Medicaid program, State Children's Health Insurance Program, Health Insurance Marketplace, and related quality assurance activities.

certified registered nurse anesthetist (CRNA)   In the United States, an advanced practice registered nurse who has acquired graduate-level education and board certification in anesthesia.

choice   A concept that covers the right a person has to withdraw earlier authorizations whenever he or she wants. The person must make the request in writing, and it goes into effect once the healthcare organization receives it. This privacy principle upholds the right of individuals to opt in or opt out of information collection and use related to them.

clearinghouse   (1) An intermediary between the healthcare provider and payer; (2) a covered entity subject to HIPAA. The clearinghouse function is not limited to changing paper-based information to digital. It also serves to streamline the claims processing and revenue collection of the provider.

clinical workflow   A general term for depicting the different procedures and examples of activities clinicians use to provide patient care. Concerning electronic data and electronic health records (EHRs), clinical workflows depict how information travels through the data framework—by whom, to whom, when, and how frequently.

cloud computing   A collection of software, platforms, and infrastructure provided as a service to consumers via the Internet from remote locations external to the consumer's organization.

coding   Translation of provider notes, exam information, and data that results from patient care and clinical operations from unstructured human language to alphanumeric data sets that are used for documenting and transacting disease description, injuries, symptoms, and conditions for additional clinical workflow and payment.

Common Criteria for Information Technology Security Evaluation   Criteria used by independent licensed testing and evaluation laboratories to assess the effectiveness of various hardware and software tools. The output or list of evaluated products can be used by healthcare information privacy and security personnel to select, purchase, and implement approved products [ISO/IEC 15408]. Usually referred to as Common Criteria.

compensating controls   The security controls employed in lieu of the recommended controls in the security control baselines described in NIST Special Publication 800-53 and CNSS Instruction 1253 that provide equivalent or comparable protection for an information system or organization. Can be used when legitimate technical or business restrictions are known and adequate risk mitigation through other security controls is in place to reach acceptable risk tolerance levels.

completeness   A part of data integrity that requires personal data to contain all relevant elements, such as a medical record that includes all visits for an individual patient. Missing records do not satisfy a completeness requirement.

confidentiality   The process of protecting information so that it is not made available or disclosed to unauthorized individuals, entities, or processes [ISO 7498-2].

configuration control board (CCB)   A formal organizational committee that makes decisions regarding whether or not proposed changes to the enterprise network should be implemented. Includes hardware, software, business and clinical systems, applications, and network architecture changes.

consent   Agreement, approval, or permission granted voluntarily by a competent person [ISO/TS 17975]. In healthcare, a patient's data should not be disclosed without the data subject's consent. HIPAA permits but does not require a covered entity to obtain consent for use or disclosure of PHI for treatment, payment, or healthcare operations.

context-based access control   A control that is not set at the user level but is based on settings within the firewall that control traffic flow based on application layer protocol session information.

continuity of operations   Similar to business continuity, the planned and actual ability to continue performance of essential functions under a broad range of circumstances.

continuous monitoring   Process used constantly to detect compliance and risk issues associated with an organization's operational environment.

control   A management, operational, or technical limitation, safeguard, or countermeasure to mitigate risk or ensure compliance with a standard. Under some standards, a control may be categorized as administrative, physical, or technical. Controls may also be classified as preventative, detective, or correction as time-based safeguards.

control variance   A range of acceptable values within any risk framework.

corrective action plan   A detailed plan of each area, such as a single Administrative Safeguard from the HIPAA Security Rule, and the actions necessary to meet compliance requirements for that one safeguard. Using the NIST Risk Management Framework language, you may want to develop a Plan of Action and Milestones as part of your corrective action plan.

covered entity   An entity subject to HIPAA and defined in the law as a health plan (insurer), health care clearinghouse, or healthcare provider (hospital).

create   The initial phase of the data lifecycle that includes the collection and intake of information. Information sources could be the patient, a provider, or any number of different medical devices and diagnostic tools.

data analytics   Employing information gained from processes that normalize, standardize, model, and turn data into usable formats to support decision-making and clinical practices.

data authority   An independent body as established by the in the General Data Protection Regulation (GDPR) in the European Union that monitors the data protection level in a member state, gives advice to the government about administrative measures and regulations, and starts legal proceedings when a data protection regulation has been violated. Also called the data protection authority and the supervisory authority in relevant guidance.

data breach   A security incident involving unauthorized access to information or data loss of personally identifiable information (PII) or PHI. *See also* breach.

data classification   A value relative to the sensitivity and criticality of information as defined by the organization. The classification level will determine what level of information protection controls will be applied to information collected, maintained, retained, used, and disposed of when no longer needed.

data controller   An entity or entities in the European Union that determine the purposes for why and how any personal data is, or is to be, processed. This entity can be a person, an organization, or a group of people who are not collectively an organization. The data controllers must ensure that information use complies with the EU Data Protection Directive (DPD).

data destruction   Various processes and methods used to permit the destruction of data and media in forms of IT storage, including shredding, degaussing, and sanitizing, based on data retention requirements. An important factor in deciding which method is appropriate is the organization's risk and mitigation policies. The overall goal is to prevent unauthorized access to sensitive information in the last stage of the data lifecycle.

data encryption Secure coding or cryptographic translation of data into a form that is unintelligible without a deciphering mechanism [NIST SP 800-47]. Data is rendered unreadable or unusable for recipients that do not possess a decryption key to change the data into clear text.

data processor In the European Union, those who process the data on behalf of the data controller but are not employees of the controller. By comparison, a business associate is an example of a data processor in the United States specific to the healthcare industry.

Data Protection Directive (DPD) Officially Directive 95/46/EC, it covers the protection of individuals in the European Union with regard to the processing of personal data and on the free movement of such data. Replaced by the General Data Protection Regulation (GDPR), effective 2018.

data retention The legal or policy-related requirements that state how long an organization must store or retain records.

data sharing agreement Often referred to as a data use agreement (DUA), an obligating document used to describe the access to and expectations for a third party's use of a healthcare organization's patient information. It will clearly indicate and limit the period of time the data sharing will occur, the systems the third party will access, and how the data will be used (and disposed of). Data sharing agreements can cover additional parameters.

data subject In the European Union, the person to whom the data refers or pertains [ISO/TS 14265].

data taxonomy The organization of elements of information into categories and classifications that are standardized to allow for common definitions and terminology and that facilitate data analytics and information exchange.

defense-in-depth Consists of coordinating various defensive controls for your systems or applications to protect the overall integrity of organizational assets. In the IT world, examples of defense-in-depth include the use of antivirus and antimalware software, firewalls, encryption, intrusion detection and prevention, and biometric authentication.

degaussing Erasing or eliminating the unwanted magnetic field on storage media such as a hard drive disk. In layman terms, degaussing erases the 0's and 1's. Because of magnetic hysteresis, it is generally not possible to reduce a magnetic field completely to 0, so degaussing typically leaves a remnant, an effect known as bias.

de-identification Removal of identifying data elements from information so that the rest of the data cannot be used to identify someone. It reduces the privacy risk associated with collecting, processing, archiving, distributing, or publishing PII and PHI [NIST SP 800-188]. Under the HIPAA Privacy Rule, de-identification occurs when data has been stripped of common identifiers by either of two methods: by the removal of 18 specific identifiers (Safe Harbor Method), or by the formal determination of an experienced statistical expert that the statistical risk of re-identification is very small.

designation of privacy officer The designation or assignment in writing from management of a person who oversees the development, implementation, maintenance of, and adherence to privacy policies and procedures. Required by most privacy regulatory requirements around the world. Privacy officers often must have specific experience or training.

diagnosis-related groups (DRGs) Foundational classifications and codes used for quality of care and reimbursement matters. The basis of the US healthcare system reimbursement, DRGs consist of codes for severity of illness, prognosis, treatment difficulty, need for intervention, and resource intensity.

digital forensics The investigation, collection, and preservation of potential digital evidence used to determine relevant circumstances after a cyberattack or data breach.

Digital Imaging and Communications in Medicine (DICOM) A standard method for transferring images and information between medical devices such as digital diagnostic imaging devices, called modalities (X-ray, ultrasound, computed tomography, and so on), to facilitate use in various vendors' electronic health records (EHRs).

disaster recovery (1) The planning and policy development that is required to respond to a natural or manmade disaster; (2) an organization's ability to resume operations after a natural or manmade disruption to information technology assets and business operations.

disclosure As a principle within privacy frameworks, data collectors should inform data subjects about who is collection and using their data.

disclosure limitation A control by which disclosure of healthcare information is limited to treatment, payment, and operations. Leading privacy frameworks generally limit disclosure but also provide specific exceptions where public safety and health considerations outweigh the need for individual privacy.

disposal The final stage of the data lifecycle. There are three common disposal options for sensitive information: overwriting, degaussing electronic media, and physical destruction as the process applies to both paper records and electronic hardware containing digital information. All options must render sensitive information useless or unreadable.

doctor of osteopathic medicine (DO) A medical professional with a doctorate degree conferred through a US medical school who focuses on osteopathic medicine. These physicians have the same credentials and privileges as physicians and surgeons with a Doctor of Medicine (MD) academic degree.

due care The amount of attention that an ordinary and reasonable person or organization would be expected to provide to avoid negative consequences.

due diligence A threshold or standard that is reached after what is considered reasonable and comprehensive review and mitigation of risk.

e-iatrogenesis (1) A phenomenon related to the concept of illness or injury actually introduced in the delivery of healthcare, such as a patient suffering a bacterial infection after being admitted to the hospital. (2) In security and privacy terms, e-iatrogenesis is the unintended consequences that result from health information technology and security interventions, such as a computer system becoming inoperable after security software updates are installed.

electronic health record (EHR) An electronic version of a patient's medical history that is maintained by the provider over time and may include all of the key administrative clinical data relevant to that person's care under a particular provider, including demographics, progress notes, problems, medications, vital signs, past medical history, immunizations, laboratory data and radiology reports [Centers for Medicare and Medicaid Services (CMS)].

emergency medical technician (EMT) A medical professional who has undergone special training to provide first response to emergency situations and to handle traumatic injuries and medical care at accident scenes.

employer-based insurance Insurance coverage offered as an employment benefit, in addition to salary and other enticements. The insurance company collects employee premiums from the employer.

environmental services The department and staff responsible for housekeeping, janitorial, laundry operations, and linen distribution in the healthcare organization.

eradication The removal of any malicious activity or artifacts left by an intrusion. The activity falls within the containment, eradication, and recovery phase of data incident response.

European Union (EU) An economic and political union of 27 member states that are located primarily in Europe. The European Union is an integrated governance of independent member states operating as one entity for cooperative and intergovernmental negotiated decisions by the member states.

event (information) Any observable occurrence in a system or network. Events can be authorized actions, such as a user sending e-mail or a server receiving a request for a web page. If the event has a negative effect, it is called an adverse event [NIST SP 800-53].

evidence Information collected in an investigation that may prove cause and extent of activity relating to an incident. Because it is used in legal proceedings, evidence must be collected and handled in a specific, controlled manner to prevent tampering or degradation.

exception handling The process of responding to the occurrences of exceptions, which involve noncompliance with computing policies and standards. Where policy requirements are clearly articulated but cannot be met, a request must be made to explain reasons for noncompliance and any mitigations that can be made instead, including compensating controls.

exposure   The estimation of the level to which a weakness could have financial, reputational, operational, or clinical consequence in the event of an adverse event.

Federal Information Security Management Act (FISMA)   A US law enacted in 2002 as Title III of the E-Government Act of 2002 (Public Law 107–347, 116 Stat. 2899). The act supported improvements and investments in information systems security as a significant component of national security in the United States as well as economic interests.

fee-for-service   A payment model in which treatment is paid for based on each exam, consultation, intervention, and so on. It offers the greatest freedom of choice for patients in selecting providers and healthcare options.

gap analysis   A step in the risk assessment process that identifies the steps specific to the organization, and in some cases the functional unit, department, system, or application necessary to resolve the risks and weaknesses identified during assessments, audits, or other forms of analysis.

General Data Protection Regulation (GDPR)   The law governing information privacy and security throughout the European Union. It replaced EU DPD in 2018.

Generally Accepted Privacy Principles (GAPP) framework   Principles designed by the American Institute of CPAs (AICPA) and the Canadian Institute of Chartered Accountants (CICA) to assist organizations in creating an effective privacy program that addresses their privacy obligations, risks, and business opportunities. Important components within these privacy principles are drawn from relevant local, national, and international privacy laws, regulations, guidelines, and leading business practices.

Good Clinical Research Practice (GCP)   A set of guidelines that provides public assurance that the rights, safety, and well-being of research subjects are protected and respected. The requirements also ensure the integrity of clinical research data.

governance (information)   A strategic approach to managing the information assets of an organization that involves oversight and the authority to examine risks versus benefit and value for the use of information. Governance establishes and monitors relevant information use policies and procedures.

governance structure   A body, such as a board of directors, that requires support from the highest levels of an organization and that must be supported by a well-defined framework for program sponsorship at all organization levels, including executive levels in the owner and program management organizations. Governance structures must provide for clear leadership and establish the requisite ethical, safety, and other cultural foundations that successful programs require.

Health and Human Services (HHS)   A cabinet-level department of the US government with the goal of protecting the health of all Americans and providing essential human services. HHS oversees regulatory aspects for healthcare delivery and payment, including compliance with HIPAA [www.hhs.gov].

Health Information and Management Systems Society (HIMSS) A not-for-profit organization dedicated to improving healthcare quality, safety, cost-effectiveness, and access, through the best use of information technology and management systems [https://www.himss.org].

health information exchange (HIE) An organization that exists to facilitate the electronic sharing of healthcare information across multiple healthcare organizations. Typically, HIE organizations are not affiliated or under the same corporate structure, but they may be. In any case, the HIE supports information transfer within a region and community.

Health Insurance Portability and Accountability Act (HIPAA) Federal legislation passed by the United States Congress and signed by President Bill Clinton in 1996. It has been known as the Kennedy–Kassebaum Act after two of its leading sponsors, then Senators Ted Kennedy and Nancy Kassebaum. It was initiated to help make healthcare operate more effectively and efficiently through administrative simplification and health insurance improvement and consists of several amendments: the Privacy Rule, the Security Rule, HITECH Act, and the Omnibus Final Rule [Public Law 104–191, 110 Stat. 1936, enacted August 21, 1996].

Health Level 7 (HL7) (1) A protocol developed to enable different information systems to exchange health data between applications using a standard; (2) the organization that builds this standard.

health maintenance organization (HMO) A healthcare organization that enrolls patients who pay a fixed amount to receive healthcare services. Patients are then eligible to receive care at lower cost from providers who have agreed to prenegotiated fees from the HMO.

health records management (HRM) An organization that handles the designated record set for a healthcare provider. An HRM organization may be engaged, for example, because the provider does not have adequate space or expertise, or it may not be able to invest in the hardware or software (data center) to manage the information.

high-deductible health plan with savings option (HDHP/SO) A high-deductible health insurance plan that enables enrollees to use tax-preferred funds (a health savings account, or HSA) to pay plan cost sharing and other out-of-pocket medical expenses. For a relatively low premium, an enrollee gets catastrophic insurance coverage. For all healthcare received up to catastrophic care, the enrollee must pay a high deductible.

impact The extent of damages expected or experienced by a threat event happening.

incident (information) An occurrence that actually or potentially jeopardizes the confidentiality, integrity, or availability of a system or the information the system processes, stores, or transmits or that constitutes a violation or imminent threat of violation of security policies, security procedures, or acceptable use policies [NIST SP 800-128].

incident response team   A designated group of personnel responsible for reacting to information security incidences or any emergency incident, such as a natural disaster or an interruption of business operations.

indemnity insurance   The model for insurance payment that is based on fee-for-service. A patient receives healthcare services, pays for it at the point of care, and then submits a claim to the insurance company for reimbursement.

information asset identification   The process used to identify any data, device, or other component of the environment that supports information-related activities. Assets generally include hardware, software, and data type information.

information asset validation   A method for determining the worth of an asset based on factors such as historical records, documented returns on investment, or replacement costs.

information lifecycle management (ILM)   A comprehensive approach to managing the flow of information from creation and initial storage to the time when it becomes obsolete and is deleted.

institutional review board (IRB)   A formal organizational committee that has been designated to approve, monitor, and review biomedical and behavioral research involving humans.

Integrating the Healthcare Enterprise (IHE)   An initiative by healthcare professionals and the healthcare industry to improve the way computer systems in healthcare share information. IHE promotes the coordinated use of established standards such as Digital Imaging and Communications in Medicine (DICOM) and HL7 to address specific clinical needs in support of optimal patient care [https://www.ihe.net].

integrity   The security and privacy concern that information and programs are changed only in a specific and authorized manner.

International Classification of Diseases (ICD)   The foremost and most widely known hierarchal medical classification system, designed to categorize diseases so that morbidity and mortality rates can be tracked and reported. The use of ICD codes—14,000 in total—are significant in the digitization of healthcare records and electronic record systems.

International Organization for Standardization (ISO)   The world's largest developer of voluntary international standards, which provides state-of-the-art specifications for products, services, and good practice and helps to make businesses more efficient and effective.

Internet of Medical Things (IoMT)   A category of medical devices and applications that are healthcare information technology (HIT) systems or that connect to HIT systems through Wi-Fi, online computer networks, and cloud platforms. IoMT leverages machine-to-machine communication to collect, store, analyze, and transfer personal health data at an unprecedented scale and depth.

interoperability   The availability of data with regard to its ability to be transferred between connected systems and applications.

Joint Commission   An independent, not-for-profit organization headquartered in the United States, with a few offices worldwide, that conducts assessments of healthcare organizations. Joint Commission accreditation is considered important to demonstrate a healthcare organization's commitment to quality and compliance with performance standards. In fact, in the United States, some reimbursement conditions are contingent on the organization having a current Joint Commission certification. Formerly known as the Joint Commission on Accreditation of Healthcare Organizations and Joint Commission on Accreditation of Hospitals.

least privilege   The concept that users of information should be granted access only to the information they need to perform their duties. Also known as the need-to-know principle. Least privilege does not mean that all users will have extremely limited functional access; some employees will have significant access if that is required for their position.

legal contracts   A legally binding agreement between entitles that generally includes four main elements: must be between two or more parties, all parties must be competent to consent, the agreement must be something of value, and the agreement must be lawful.

legal medical record   A portion of the entire medical record that should (at least) contain patient care decisions, document the care provided for purposes of reimbursement, and serve as evidence in legal proceedings about such care.

legitimate purpose   An important concept of the HIPAA Privacy Rule, which recognizes the legitimate need for public health authorities and others responsible for ensuring public health and safety to have access to protected health information to carry out their public health mission. Under HIPAA, this concept is referred to as the "legitimate business purpose," in that an organization requires the information to perform its mission. Under the EU DPA, personal data can be processed only for specified explicit and legitimate purposes and may not be processed further in a way incompatible with those purposes.

licensed practical nurse (LPN)   A nurse who completes a year-long (typically) certified educational program. Often these programs are affiliated with a teaching hospital that provides some hands-on experience for the students. After nurses complete the program, they must pass an additional licensing exam. In some states, they may be called licensed vocational nurses.

likelihood   A function of risk that is the chance an occurrence will happen to exploit vulnerability and result in some impact.

limited collection/limited data set   Under HIPAA, a set of data in which most of the PHI has been removed.

lines of defense model   A risk-management framework used to outline and clarify roles and responsibilities in three major categories, or lines of defense. When used for information privacy governance, the model guides oversight of the functions from the board of directors and reduces gaps in roles and responsibilities through layers of oversight, which is required for effective information privacy governance.

local area network (LAN)   A computer network that interconnects computers within a limited area such as a home, school, computer laboratory, or office building using network media.

logging   (1) The action of recording actions taken by a user or users of a system; (2) the recording system itself; (3) actions of system transactions (may be remote system actions).

logical access   A system that prescribes not only who or what (for example, in the case of a process) is to have access to a specific system resource but also the type of access permitted.

Logical Observation Identifiers Names and Codes (LOINC)   A widely accepted code system specially formulated for identifying laboratory and clinical observations. To be able to exchange observations and measurements electronically across multiple independent lab systems, LOINC uses a universal code system with a maximum field size of 7.

malpractice   An instance of negligence or incompetence on the part of a medical professional.

managed care   A mechanism to control cost, improve quality, and increase access that has evolved over the last 50 years. The key feature of managed care is in the integration of healthcare delivery and payment within one organization.

Manufacturer Disclosure Statement for Medical Device Security (MDS2)   A method for information gathering related to the risks associated with medical devices that are capable of being connected to an organization's networks, normally completed by the manufacturer.

master of science in nursing (MSN)   An advanced-level postgraduate degree for registered nurses in medical practices and other healthcare delivery settings. For educators and management positions, this can be an entry-level requirement. Nurses with this level of academic training often seek positions as health administrators, in health public policy, and in clinical executive positions.

Medicaid   In the United States, a joint federal and state program that provides healthcare coverage to more than 72 million Americans, including low-income families, parents, children, seniors, and individuals with disabilities. It is the single largest source of health coverage in the United States.

medical billing   (1) The transaction between provider and payer to receive reimbursement for services rendered; (2) the process of submitting and following up on claims in the US healthcare system.

medical device   A device or technology used to diagnose, prevent, monitor, or treat a disease, injury, or physiological process. It can be networked or stand-alone hardware, software, or applications. Health information and medical technology devices are regulated by the US Food and Drug Administration (FDA).

medical doctor (MD)   A medical practitioner, either a physician or surgeon with an advanced academic degree in medicine. After an internship and a residency assignment, in the United States, an MD must be tested and licensed by a certification board.

medical technician   A general category of healthcare employee who has received specialized training in administration and operation of various medical technologies such as medical devices and clinical systems. A medical technician has information protection responsibilities based on the particular equipment he or she uses and the PII and PHI collected, transferred, and stored.

Medicare   A program funded and administered by the federal government that provides health insurance coverage for individuals age 65 and over, or for citizens younger than 65 who are affected by long-term disabilities.

mitigation action   An action that involves prioritizing, evaluating, and implementing the appropriate risk-reducing controls recommended from the risk assessment process [NIST SP 800-30, ISO/IEC 27005].

monitoring   A component of detection security controls, an automated process for reviewing logs or actions, as well as monitoring the health and status of the system and its operations.

National Electrical Manufacturers Association (NEMA)   An association of nearly 325 electrical equipment and medical imaging manufacturers in the United States. Member companies manufacture safe, reliable, and efficient products used in the generation, transmission, distribution, control, and end use of electricity [https://www.nema.org].

National Health Service (NHS)   A government agency in the United Kingdom (UK) that is organized and resourced to provide universal health coverage. NHS is publicly funded via tax collection and is founded on the belief that all citizens have an entitlement to healthcare.

National Institutes of Standards and Technology (NIST)   A standard-setting agency that does not regulate industry but promotes innovation through measurement standards. The organization plays a critical role in helping industry and science create and implement these standards.

National Provider Identifier (NPI)   An identification standard for healthcare providers established by the US Health Insurance Portability and Accountability Act (HIPAA). The NPI is a unique identification number for healthcare organizations subject to HIPAA and used for administrative and financial transactions. It is permanently assigned to the provider regardless of location or job changes. The NPI is a 10-position, intelligence-free numeric identifier (a 10-digit number).

Nationwide Health Information Network (NHIN)   Within the United States, a proposed combination and interconnection of HIEs into an integrated network of national, state, regional, and local health information organizations.

notice of privacy practices   A HIPAA requirement that patients be informed of a covered entity's practices and procedures regarding use and disclosure of PHI. This is achieved by giving the patient, conspicuously posting, and making available the procedures the healthcare organization has in place to collect and use PHI. Under the EU DPA, data subjects should be given notice when their PHI is being collected.

notification   A regulated process for healthcare organizations and their third-party suppliers to announce adverse information incidents to help individuals manage potential unauthorized access and use of their PII and PHI. *See* breach notification.

nurse   The largest category of the healthcare workforce. The training and approach to patient care for nurses is comprehensive across many environments, specialties, and scopes of practice.

nurse practitioner   An advanced-level registered nurse who has completed additional academic training at a master's or doctoral degree level with advanced clinical training beyond that required of the generalist registered nurse (RN) role. Nurse practitioners have greater responsibilities than RNs and provide medical services similar to an MD.

nurses' aide   Assistants who work under a licensed nurse's supervision to provide basic patient care in a variety of healthcare settings, from a physician's office, to a hospital, to long-term care environments. A related occupation to hospital orderlies and attendants, nurses' aides perform services that include moving, repositioning, and lifting patients. Sometimes known as nursing assistant.

openness   Enables any member of the public who has legitimate interest to be provided information about the processing of healthcare data. Although this does not supply access to the data itself, it does mean that the organization should disclose how the data it maintains on behalf of others is kept secure, processed, or shared.

Organisation for Economic Co-operation and Development (OECD) principles
These categorize fair information practices for collecting, storing, and using PII. The organization aims to help individuals participate in the use of their own information. The principles assign responsibility for protecting information to the entities that collect and maintain it. The framework consists of the following principles: Collection limitation, Data quality, Purpose specification, Use limitation, Security safeguards, Openness, Individual participation, and Accountability.

overwriting   The process of replacing old data with new data. Data that has been overwritten is generally considered to be unrecoverable.

patient   A person who seeks assistance with matters of health (physical and mental), improvement of health status, or treatment of illness.

patient authorization   A detailed privacy-related document that gives covered entities permission to use PHI for specified purposes, which are generally purposes other than treatment, payment, or health care operations, or to disclose protected health information to a third party specified by the individual.

payer   Someone other than the patient who finances or reimburses the cost of healthcare. Commonly described as third-party payers or health insurers.

peer review   An assessment of processes, research, clinical records, and other medical work by qualified personnel with similar competency. This quality control method is a self-regulatory approach to maintaining standards and credibility within healthcare practices.

personal area network (PAN)   A small network consisting of a communications area near the individual, which may include a body area network (BAN), in which numerous devices are attached to convey information primarily over wireless channels. A PAN is sell-administered within a segment provided to it on the LAN of an organization or within an individual's home.

Personal Health Information Protection Act (PHIPA)   Ontario, Canada, legislation that is a component of the Health Information Protection Act that intends to protect the healthcare information of patients by healthcare organizations, called healthcare custodians in the regulation.

personal health record (PHR)   A record of personal health that is maintained by the patient as opposed to the provider organization. It is sometimes confused with an EHR or misidentified as part of a longitudinal EHR.

Personal Information Protection and Electronic Documents Act (PIPEDA)   A Canadian law relating to data privacy that applies to private sector organizations and regulates how they collect, use, and disclose personal information to conduct required business operations. PIPEDA includes provisions for paper as well as digital information protection.

personally identifiable information (PII)   Any information about an individual maintained by an agency, including any information that can be used to distinguish or trace an individual's identity, such as name, Social Security number, date and place of birth, mother's maiden name, or biometric records; and any other information that is linked or linkable to an individual, such as medical, educational, financial, and employment information [GAO Report 08-536].

pharmacist   A healthcare professional responsible for the proper and safe use and distribution of medications and who has advanced academic credentials with authorization to prepare and dispense medications prescribed by a qualified medical professional. Pharmacists are an integral part of the healthcare team in that they often provide meaningful education and counseling for patients who are receiving medication.

physical destruction   Options, such as shredding or incineration, of paper or digital data to destroy the physical characteristics of data storage.

physician   A healthcare professional whose role is to diagnose and treat injuries and illnesses for his or her patients. Surgeons are a specialized type of physician who performs operations.

physician assistant (PA)   Another general category of healthcare professional who has a license to practice medicine under the guidance of a physician.

point-of-service (POS) plan   A managed care plan that combines the most attractive elements of both HMOs and preferred provider organizations (PPOs). In exchange for a deductible and higher coinsurance payment on a one-time basis, an HMO enrollee can choose to use a service that falls outside of the HMO plan.

preferred provider organization (PPO)   A fee-for-service health plan with a number of providers who have aligned with the PPO. If the patient chooses a participating provider, the cost of medical care is discounted to the enrollee. If not, the service is covered at a lesser rate. A PPO offers more choice to the patient than other models, particularly an HMO. However, the out-of-pocket costs like deductibles and coinsurance payments to the patient are increased, generally. The costs are more when the patient exercises their prerogative and chooses a provider or service not included in the PPO plan.

privacy   Freedom from intrusion into the private life or affairs of an individual when that intrusion results from undue or illegal gathering and use of data about that individual [ISO/IEC 2382-8].

privacy shield   With the advent of GDPR, the replacement of Safe Harbor provisions. The European Union and the US Department of Commerce developed a way for US organizations to demonstrate adequate privacy protections to satisfy GDPR concerns and permit transnational PII and PHI data exchange.

processing authorization   Under the EU DPD, because of the vast levels of information use and sharing in healthcare, this authorization requires regulatory control and approval for transfer based on the nature of the information collection and transfer as well as prescribing appropriate safeguards.

proportionality   Addresses assurances that personal data that is collected and shared is limited only to that which is necessary and used for the intended and described purpose.

protected health information (PHI)   A subset of individually identifiable health information that includes demographic information collected from an individual by a health care provider, health plan, employer, or healthcare clearinghouse, and relates to the past, present, or future physical or mental health or condition of an individual; the provision of healthcare to an individual; or the past, present, or future payment for the provision of healthcare to an individual [45 CFR § 160.103 – Definitions].

provider   Any person or organization that is involved in or associated with the delivery of healthcare to a client, or is caring for a client's wellbeing [ISO/TS 27527].

pseudonymization   A particular type of anonymization that both removes the association with a data subject and adds an association between a particular set of characteristics relating to the data subject and one or more pseudonyms [ISO/TS 25237].

psychiatrist An MD who focuses on examining and treating mental illnesses and behavioral health issues with legal privileges to prescribe medication.

psychologist A PhD or PsyD who provides patient care with respect to behavior and mental processes. A psychologist provides counselling services and may conduct research within academic settings.

purpose A privacy principle included in most leading frameworks that asserts that data collected will be used for a specific reason and will be used only for reasons disclosed to the data subject or permissible under applicable law.

purpose specification (or limitation) A specification that is intended to protect data subjects by setting limits with regard to the collection and further processing of their data. It sets limits on how organizations are able to use PII or PHI data, while also offering some degree of flexibility for clinical and business requirements.

qualitative risk assessment An assessment process by which the components of the risk equations are valued at levels such as high, medium, and low. Subjective factors are used to measure and evaluate risk. Particularly useful when the assessment must be made in a short period of time or the assessors are familiar with the subjects of the assessment (such as systems, processes, vendors, or applications).

quantitative risk assessment An assessment process that includes the use of objective data such as financial impacts, revenue losses, historical frequency and probabilities, and risk scores associated with vulnerability management. Data can be difficult to obtain, so this approach is sometimes used in conjunction with qualitative methods.

quality A state of data that matches ideally to the concept of integrity as is applies to principles of security. Data should be relevant to the purpose for which it was collected, should be maintained to be accurate and complete, and should be updated to remain so.

registered nurse (RN) A nurse who has graduated from a nursing program at a college or university and has passed a licensing exam to obtain a nursing license.

reimbursement Repayment for expense incurred, the final step of the revenue cycle. As claims are processed and bills are submitted (and resubmitted), the desired outcome from the provider's perspective is to receive reimbursement for the cost of the provided healthcare.

remediation The method by which the organization responds to identified risks or weaknesses in controls. The process includes implementing changes to meet or exceed the requirements of a control or use of compensating controls to minimize risk.

residual risk A portion of the risk that remains after a risk assessment has been conducted and mitigation is implemented to the best extent possible. Note that some residual risk may be accepted, while other risks may be transferred or avoided.

retention The storage and maintenance of data by an organization. Policies are required to establish the length of time the records are useful; after this time, they are discarded. Regulatory requirements and the value of the information will determine how long an organization will keep the information.

risk The level of impact on the organization and information assets resulting from the operation of an information system given the potential impact of a threat and the likelihood of that threat occurring [NIST SP 800-47].

risk acceptance A conscious acceptance that a certain act may result in a negative consequence based on informed assessment and decision based on a process to identify the risk, best practices to address, and possible mitigation strategies implemented.

risk analysis The process of identification, recording, and determining action plans with regard to risk, both system and organizational in nature. It is a scientific approach to examining risks with probability and impact measures.

risk avoidance The decision not to perform an activity that potentially involves risk. An example would be not entering into a contract with a third party because of its previous history of data breaches.

risk communication A continuous process intended to improve collective and individual decision-making that includes providing awareness of the risk management process and the roles of each functional area, stating outcomes of risk assessments, and reporting on corrective action plans.

risk management lifecycle Applied to the healthcare organization and oversight of third-party relationships, includes activities identifying, assessing, and mitigating information risks.

risk planning A method of managing risk by developing a risk mitigation plan that prioritizes, implements, and maintains controls.

risk reduction Actions taken to lessen the severity of impacts or the likelihood of an incident from occurring. *See also* mitigation action.

risk transfer The process of shifting exposure to the organization by using other options to offset potential loss, such as purchasing cybersecurity insurance.

risk treatment Actions to be taken to address identified risks. Once risks have been identified and assessed, the organization must determine these actions, which are identified as risk treatments and include techniques to manage the risk. Techniques fall into one or more of four major categories: avoidance, transfer, mitigation, and acceptance.

role-based access A process implemented to match access to data or systems with the functional or structural role an individual provides within the organization. So, for example, a doctor who works in the emergency department will have the same access to data as another doctor in the emergency department, but the ER doc's access would not be the same as that of a doctor who works in the ophthalmology department.

rule-based access   A discretionary access approach that allows or restricts access based on parameters and properties not related to identity or function. For example, access could be based on IP address, geographic location, or time of day.

Safe Harbor   A provision within the HITECH Act that exempts HIPAA-covered entities and business associates from reporting and notifying external agencies and affected individuals when they have implemented specified technologies and methodologies so that the protected health information is not "unsecured." Encryption and de-identification are examples of specified technologies and methodologies that satisfy safe harbor exemption.

Safe Harbor Privacy Framework   A framework to provide an efficient and effective process for US organizations to demonstrate adherence to EU DPD privacy approaches. The US Department of Commerce in consultation with the European Commission developed this framework to accommodate the privacy programs of US firms and permit data transfer from EU organizations.

sanction policy   A human resources policy to apply disciplinary actions against members of the workforce who do not correctly handle protected health information.

sanitizing   Data and media disposal techniques that completely erase or securely cleanse all information from devices and storage platforms.

secure shredding   A physical data-destruction technique that destroys media such as a disc, tape, or hard drive by crushing, pulverizing, or processing through a shearer.

security   A process of assuring confidentiality, integrity, and availability of data, both in paper form and digital, via administrative, technical, and administrative controls.

security categorization   Means of determining the level of security required for a system based on the information (or data) type the system uses or maintains.

security controls   Measures that provide the capability to identify, protect, detect, respond, and recover from threats and attacks. These defenses or countermeasures are used to protect information, prevent physical asset destruction, and minimize risk.

segregation of duties   A sort of checks and balances system implemented to reduce the risk of accidental or deliberate misuse of information. It involves processes and controls that help create and maintain a separation of security roles and responsibilities within an organization to ensure that the integrity of security processes is not jeopardized, and to ensure that no single person has the ability to disrupt a critical computing process or security function.

service level agreement (SLA)   An obligating document that outlines the support or products the third party promises to provide and relevant measures against which the healthcare organization can assess fulfillment. One such support item and its measurement would be continuous network uptime.

single loss expectancy (SLE)   The value of the asset multiplied by the impact measurement as a one-time occurrence or single loss expectancy: (SLE) = asset value (AV) × exposure factor (EF).

social worker   A professional who concentrates on patients' quality of life and subjective well-being. Social workers administer to individuals, groups, and communities. Areas of practice include research, counseling, crisis intervention, and teaching.

staff augmentation   An outsourcing or contracting strategy that is used to increase a department staff temporarily. Additional personnel are integrated into a current workforce with similar day-to-day management and oversight.

stewardship   The responsibility for ownership and accountability in the managing or organizational data to ensure quality, accuracy, and availability.

supervisory authority   An independent body in each EU member state that oversees the data protection processes in its state. The position is an advisor to government and may take enforcement actions when there are infractions against privacy and data protection directives.

system recovery   Planning and processes that help ensure information systems are available in times of crisis and business disruption. Depends on adequate data backup processes to restore information assets as quickly as possible. *See also* disaster recovery.

Systematized Nomenclature of Medicine Clinical Terms (SNOMED CT)   A detailed terminology framework of concepts, descriptions, and relationships that works for developing inputs into healthcare systems and that resemble data flow diagrams or flowcharts. Used to describe extensive clinical terminology that is meant more as machine language to construct the EHR.

third party   A business external to the healthcare organization that provides supplies, services, and products. Third parties may also manage, maintain, or have access to sensitive information. In the United States, these entities are called business associates.

threat   A possible danger, an action, or a condition that presents a source of concern for the security of an organization, such as a phishing attack. A threat is any circumstance or event with the potential to adversely impact organizational operations and assets, individuals, and other organizations [NIST SP 800-12].

tort law   A civil action, as opposed to a criminal action, that establishes legal liability when injury or harm is caused by someone or an organization against another person or entity. Several categories of criminal acts can be affected by tort law: intentional, negligent, failure to fulfil a duty to act, and legal violation of law.

training   Part of security awareness as a security control, an approach to teach employees about proper information protection techniques, including incident reporting and password management.

trans-border concerns Jurisdictional considerations that affect data transferred and shared across national or state boundaries. Some regulatory guidance restricts or prohibits transfer of PII and PHI outside of the host country. Organizations that enter into third-party agreements with firms located in different regulatory jurisdictions will need to be aware of trans-border implications.

transparency When an individual's data is maintained by an organization, this process ensures that the individual is aware of how their data is maintained, processed, or shared.

unauthorized disclosure An impermissible use or prohibited access of PHI where the security or privacy of the information is potentially compromised.

use A general term for all actions that constitute handling information—collection, transfer, storage, analysis, and disposal are examples.

use limitation When disclosing PHI, the amount or content of data provided must be limited to what is required to satisfy the request and nothing more.

user-based access Access rights that are established based on an individual's attributes, specific to the person.

value stream mapping (VSM) A method, rooted in lean-management techniques made popular by Toyota decades ago, for analyzing the current state, reducing wastes, and designing an improved future state. The purpose of VSM is to increase efficiency by eliminating waste.

vendor An entity that sells, supplies, or provides a service or product. In healthcare, vendors do business with a provider organization. They may have many different customers, including those that are not healthcare organizations. Their service or product may or may not be healthcare related.

vulnerability A weakness in a computing environment based on ineffective security controls or a condition that puts an organization in danger of exploit by an information threat or natural disaster.

wide area network (WAN) An expansive, interconnected computer network that spans multiple cities and geographic areas across a telecommunication construction over public and private digital pathways.

wireless network Also called Wi-Fi, a generic term that refers to a wireless LAN that observes the IEEE 802.11 protocol to connect network nodes [NISTIR 7250].

INDEX

Single User License Terms and Conditions

Online access to the digital content included with this book is governed by the McGraw Hill License Agreement outlined next. By using this digital content you agree to the terms of that license.

Access   To register and activate your Total Seminars Training Hub account, simply follow these easy steps.

1. Go to this URL: **hub.totalsem.com/mheclaim**
2. To register and create a new Training Hub account, enter your email address, name, and password on the **Register** tab. No further information (such as credit card number) is required to create an account.
   If you already have a Total Seminars Training Hub account, enter your email address and password on the **Log in** tab.
3. Enter your Product Key: **3xqt-79gh-gfwn**
4. Click to accept the user license terms.
5. For new users, click the **Register and Claim** button to create your account. For existing users, click the **Log in and Claim** button.
   You will be taken to the Training Hub and have access to the content for this book.

Duration of License   Access to your online content through the Total Seminars Training Hub will expire one year from the date the publisher declares the book out of print.

Your purchase of this McGraw Hill product, including its access code, through a retail store is subject to the refund policy of that store.

The Content is a copyrighted work of McGraw Hill and McGraw Hill reserves all rights in and to the Content. The Work is © 2021 by McGraw Hill.

Restrictions on Transfer   The user is receiving only a limited right to use the Content for user's own internal and personal use, dependent on purchase and continued ownership of this book. The user may not reproduce, forward, modify, create derivative works based upon, transmit, distribute, disseminate, sell, publish, or sublicense the Content or in any way commingle the Content with other third-party content, without McGraw Hill's consent.

Limited Warranty   The McGraw Hill Content is provided on an "as is" basis. Neither McGraw Hill nor its licensors make any guarantees or warranties of any kind, either express or implied, including, but not limited to, implied warranties of merchantability or fitness for a particular purpose or use as to any McGraw Hill Content or the information therein or any warranties as to the accuracy, completeness, currentness, or results to be obtained from, accessing or using the McGraw Hill Content, or any material referenced in such Content or any information entered into licensee's product by users or other persons and/or any material available on or that can be accessed through the licensee's product (including via any hyperlink or otherwise) or as to non-infringement of third-party rights. Any warranties of any kind, whether express or implied, are disclaimed. Any material or data obtained through use of the McGraw Hill Content is at your own discretion and risk and user understands that it will be solely responsible for any resulting damage to its computer system or loss of data.

Neither McGraw Hill nor its licensors shall be liable to any subscriber or to any user or anyone else for any inaccuracy, delay, interruption in service, error or omission, regardless of cause, or for any damage resulting therefrom.

In no event will McGraw Hill or its licensors be liable for any indirect, special or consequential damages, including but not limited to, lost time, lost money, lost profits or good will, whether in contract, tort, strict liability or otherwise, and whether or not such damages are foreseen or unforeseen with respect to any use of the McGraw Hill Content.

www.ingramcontent.com/pod-product-compliance
Lightning Source LLC
Chambersburg PA
CBHW080126220326
41598CB00032B/4972